Understanding Research for Evidence-Based Practice

Understanding Research for Evidence-Based Practice

Fourth Edition

Cherie R. Rebar, PhD, RN, MBA, FNP, COI
Professor
Director, Division of Nursing
Chair, Prelicensure Nursing Programs
Kettering College
President, CONNECT: RN2ED
Dayton, Ohio

Carolyn J. Gersch, PhD-c, MSN, RN, CNE
Associate Professor
Associate Director, Division of Nursing
Chair, BSN-Completion Program
Kettering College
President, CONNECT: RN2ED
Dayton, Ohio

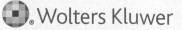

Philadelphia • Baltimore • New York • London
Buenos Aires • Hong Kong • Sydney • Tokyo

Acquisitions Editor: Chris Richardson
Product Development Manager: Meredith Brittain
Production Project Manager: Joan Sinclair
Design Coordinator: Joan Wendt
Manufacturing Coordinator: Karin Duffield
Prepress Vendor: S4Carlisle Publishing Services

4th edition

9 8 7 6 5 4 3 2 1

Printed in China

ISBN 978-1-4511-9107-3

Library of Congress Cataloging-in-Publication Data

Rebar, Cherie R., author.
  [Understanding nursing research]
  Understanding research for evidence-based practice / Cherie R. Rebar, Carolyn J. Gersch. — Fourth edition.
      p. ; cm.
  Preceded by Understanding nursing research : using research in evidence-based practice / Cherie R. Rebar . . . [et al.]. 3rd ed. c2011.
  Includes bibliographical references and index.
  ISBN 978-1-4511-9107-3
  I. Gersch, Carolyn J., author. II. Title.
  [DNLM: 1. Nursing Research—methods. 2. Evidence-Based Nursing—methods. 3. Qualitative Research. 4. Research Design—standards. 5. Research Report—standards. WY 20.5]
  RT81.5
  610.73072—dc23
                                                                                      2014008806

LWW.com

CCS0814

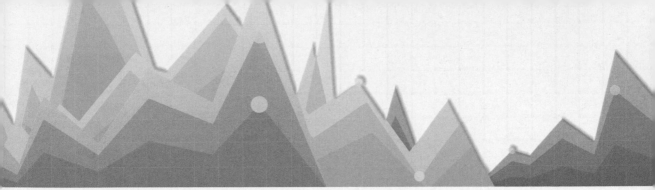

*This book is dedicated to the memory of
Carol L. Macnee and Susan McCabe.*

Reviewers

Barbara Baker, RN, MS(N), EdD, PHCNS-BC
Professor
College of Health Professions, Wilmington University
Georgetown, Delaware

Anne Bongiorno, PhD, APHN-BC, CNE
Associate Professor
SUNY Plattsburgh
Plattsburgh, New York

Jeanie Burt, MSN, MA, RN, CNE
Assistant Professor
Harding University
Searcy, Arkansas

Nathania Bush, DNP, APRN, BC
Associate Professor of Nursing
Morehead State University
Morehead, Kentucky

Karen Clark, EdD, RN
Dean of Nursing and Associate Professor
Indiana University East
Richmond, Indiana

Karan Dublin, MEd, RN
Professor
Tyler Junior College
Tyler, Texas

Sue Gabriel, EdD, MSN, MFS, RN, SANE-A, CFN, FACFEI, DABFN
Associate Professor
Bryan College of Health Science
Lincoln, Nebraska

Patricia Gagliano, PhD, RN
Professor of Nursing
Indian River State College
Fort Pierce, Florida

Elizabeth Gulledge, PhD, RN, CNE
Assistant Professor of Nursing/BSN Program Director
Jacksonville State University
Jacksonville, Alabama

Annette Gunderman, DEd, MSN, RN
Associate Professor of Nursing
Bloomsburg University
Bloomsburg, Pennsylvania

Susan Hendricks, EdD, MSN, CNE
Associate Dean for Undergraduate Programs
Indiana University
Indianapolis, Indiana

Kathy Holloway, MSN, DNP
Nursing Instructor
Franklin University
Shelby, Ohio

Cindy Hudson, DNSc, CNE, PHCNS-BC
Director of Round Rock Campus
Texas A&M Health Science Center
Round Rock, Texas

Teresa Isaacson, MSN
Undergraduate Nursing
Allen College
Waterloo, Iowa

Deborah Lawson, PhD
Adjunct Professor, Biology
Maryville University
St. Louis, Missouri

Arlene Lowenstein, PhD, RN
Professor and Director
Simmons College
Boston, Massachusetts

Ann Malecha, PhD, RN
Professor
Texas Woman's University
Houston, Texas

Rhonda Maneval, DEd, RN
Professor and Associate Chair
  of Nursing
Temple University
Philadelphia, Pennsylvania

Michelle McClave, MSN, RN
Associate Professor
Morehead State University
Morehead, Kentucky

Carole McKenzie, PhD, CNM, RN
Associate Professor
Texas A&M University
Commerce, Texas

Michael Perlow, DNS, RN
Professor of Nursing
Murray State University
Murray, Kentucky

Pammla Petrucka, PhD
Professor
University of Saskatchewan
Regina, Saskatchewan, Canada

Cheryl Pollard, PN, RN, BScN, MN, PhD
Assistant Professor
MacEwan University
Edmonton, Alberta, Canada

Deanna Reising, PhD
Associate Professor
Indiana University
Bloomington, Indiana

Amber Roache, DNP
Associate Professor of Nursing
King University
Knoxville, Tennessee

Rebecca Saxton, PhD, RN
Associate Professor
Research College of Nursing
Kansas City, Missouri

Theresa Schwindenhammer, MSN, RN
Assistant Professor
Methodist College
Peoria, Illinois

Kathy Sheppard, PhD, MA, MSN
Associate Dean and Professor
University of Mobile
Mobile, Alabama

Sharon Souter, RN, CNE, PhD
Dean and Professor
University of Mary Hardin-Baylor
Belton, Texas

Kathleen Sullivan, PhD, RN
Adjunct Professor
LaRoche College
Pittsburgh, Pennsylvania

Sharon Van Sell, BSN, MEd, MS, EdD
Professor
Texas Woman's University
Dallas, Texas

Laura Vasel, RN, MSN, CPNP, CNE
Assistant Professor/RN-BSN Coordinator
Bon Secours Memorial College of Nursing
Richmond, Virginia

**Anita Kay Williams-Prickett, PhD, RN,
  CDE**
Associate Professor
Jacksonville State University
Jacksonville, Alabama

Kathleen Williamson, PhD, RN
Assistant Professor
Widener University
Chester, Pennsylvania

For a list of the reviewers of the Test Generator accompanying this book, please visit http://thepoint.lww.com/Rebar4e.

Preface

We believe that learning should be fun and that learning happens best when students can relate new knowledge to something relevant to them. We also believe that when students are not expected to be researchers, they can enjoy learning how to read and use research as one important form of evidence on which to base practice. We love research, and we are fundamentally practitioners who find excitement and challenge in tackling new information to fill in the gaps in our knowledge about practice. We hope that some of our enthusiasm is communicated in these pages.

Understanding Research for Evidence-Based Practice differs from existing undergraduate research textbooks in a number of important ways. The first premise of this book is that students need to understand the language of research and the underlying concepts of the research process as it applies to evidence-based practice, but do not necessarily need to be prepared to conduct a research study. The second premise is that students and practicing healthcare professionals are motivated to read and apply research evidence only as it relates to their practice. Given these two premises, it is logical that many students and healthcare professionals read only the abstract and the conclusion sections of research reports. Those two sections usually contain less of the technical language of research and address most directly the clinical meaning of a research study, so they are viewed as both understandable and useful for practice. Following that reasoning, we organized this book around the sections of a research report, rather than the steps of the research process. It starts with what most practicing healthcare professionals are interested in—the conclusions—and then moves forward to the beginning of a research report. We believe that this will help the student recognize the relevance of each section of a typical research report in understanding and using research in evidence-based practice. If a student or a healthcare professional prefers to access information using the linear or forward approach to research, abstract through conclusion, they may do so by selecting the chapters in the order desired. In addition, five questions that a healthcare professional might ask when reading research are used to further organize the text, and throughout the chapters, the emphasis is on reading, understanding, and applying research in practice. In keeping with this, most chapters of the book begin with a clinical case that identifies what information the healthcare professional is seeking from research literature to answer a clinical question. One or two published research articles that directly relate to the clinical case are discussed throughout the chapter to provide specific examples of the concepts addressed; they are reprinted in full in Appendices A-1 through A-10.

It is a challenge to represent the breadth and depth of healthcare practice, research, and evidence-based practice in a single textbook. A real effort has been made to include clinical cases that reflect healthcare practice in a variety of settings, ranging from acute care to public health, and across a range of specialties. This text also differs from other undergraduate research texts in that we use the research articles as exemplars to discuss qualitative, quantitative, and mixed research methods. As healthcare science evolves, we recognize the need to use a variety of methods from both the positivist and the naturalist viewpoints to develop knowledge that reflects a holistic perspective. Qualitative, quantitative, and mixed methods are used to build knowledge in healthcare, and rather than artificially separating the discussion of these approaches, we contrast the approaches while identifying the broader conceptual base that is common.

Learners learn best by doing, so each chapter of this book ends with a specific learning activity that prepares students for the concepts addressed in the following chapter. To provide an opportunity for students to be active learners, an in-class questionnaire that can be used as a mini-research study is included in Appendix C. Appendix B is a fictional article that could have been based on the results from the in-class questionnaire. It intentionally contains flaws that are slightly more glaring than any likely to be found in a published, peer-reviewed research report. The fictional article is used throughout the text as an example, along with the authentic research reports.

The goal of this text is to enable students to read and comprehend published research, so that they can make professional decisions regarding the use of research reports in evidence-based practice. Associated with this goal is the hope that students will develop their interest and confidence in reading research, rather than avoiding it. Our text is designed to be user-friendly, taking a more casual tone than some research texts do, to minimize the intimidating nature of the language and concepts of research. For easy reference, each term in the glossary includes its chapter and page number in the text.

The sign of a successful textbook is that students decide to keep it to use in the future, rather than sell it after they complete their course. We hope ours will be one they keep. We believe that learning to understand and use published research can be fun, interesting, and useful for students, if they can see its direct relevance to their practice. The organization of this book is unconventional and the tone conversational, addressing the subject from the perspective of a reader and user of research, rather than from a creator of it. Students tell us this is a helpful perspective and one that they enjoy. As researchers, our greatest goal is to foster appreciation and enthusiasm for the process that we find so challenging and so clinically meaningful. We hope this text contributes to accomplish that goal. And we hope you have some fun!

TEACHING AND LEARNING PACKAGE

Instructor Resources

The following tools to assist you with teaching your course are available upon adoption of this text at http://thePoint.lww.com/Rebar4e:

- An **E-Book** allows access to the book's full text and images online.
- The **Test Generator** lets you generate new tests from a bank of NCLEX-style questions to help you assess your students' understanding of the course material.
- **PowerPoint Presentations** provide an easy way for you to integrate the textbook with your students' classroom experience, either via slide shows or handouts. Multiple-choice and True/False questions are integrated into the presentations to promote class participation and allow you to use i-clicker technology.
- **Case Studies** with answers can be used as a class activity or group assignment.
- **Assignments** with answers reinforce student learning.

- An **Image Bank** contains all the illustrations and tables from the book in formats suitable for printing and incorporating into PowerPoint presentations and Internet sites.
- **Strategies for Effective Teaching** offer creative approaches.
- **Learning Management System Cartridges.**
- Access to all student resources.

Student Resources

Students can also visit http://thePoint.lww.com/Rebar4e and access the following tools and resources using the codes printed in the front of their textbooks:

- **Interactive Critiquing Activities** enable students to read summaries of actual research examples and respond to a series of systematic questions, designed specifically for each study, to build students' confidence in critiquing articles. Responses can be printed or e-mailed directly to instructors for homework or testing.
- **Video Tutorials** explain difficult concepts.
- **Journal Articles** corresponding to book chapters offer access to current research available in Wolters Kluwer journals.
- Plus a **Spanish–English Audio Glossary** and **Nursing Professional Roles and Responsibilities.**

Carolyn J. Gersch
Cherie R. Rebar

Acknowledgments

We are forever grateful for the contributions to research and evidence-based practice that Carol L. Macnee and Susan McCabe provided to the first three editions of this text that have impacted practicing nurses, healthcare team members, and patients worldwide. May this and subsequent editions of *Understanding Research for Evidence-Based Practice* continue to honor their memory.

With gratitude and appreciation to our wonderful families, both at home and in the nursing profession, who have supported our endeavors, encouraged our creativity, and challenged us to lend our voices to the continuing evolution of evidence-based nursing.

Cherie R. Rebar & Carolyn J. Gersch

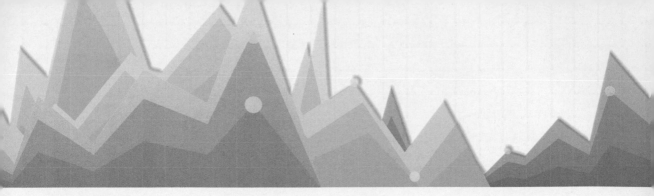

Contents

Reviewers vi
Preface viii
Acknowledgments xi

CHAPTER 1
Evidence-Based Healthcare: Using Research in Practice 1

Introduction 2
Role of Research in the Evolution of Healthcare Professions 3
History of Healthcare Research and EBP 4
Evidence-Based Bridge Theory 5
Evidence-Based Models 5
Questions for Patient Care 8
Where to Find Evidence for Practice 9
Developing Clinical Questions for Real-World Practice 12
Published Abstract: What Would you Conclude? 22
Systematic Reviews in EBP 23
Summary 25

CHAPTER 2
The Research Process: Components and Language of Research Reports 27

Introduction 28
The Language of Research 29
Components of Published Research Reports 30
The Research Process and the Nursing Process 40
Research Reports and the Research Process 46
Summary of the Research Process Contrasted to the Research Report 49
Critically Reading Research for Practice 50
Published Report—What did you Conclude? 51
Summary 53

CHAPTER 3
Discussions and Conclusions 55

The End of a Research Report—Discussions and Conclusions 57
Discussions 57
Conclusions 62
Common Errors in Research Reports 65
Critically Reading Discussion and Conclusion Sections of Reports 66
Published Reports—What would you Conclude? 67

CHAPTER 4
Descriptive Results 69

Differentiating Description from Inference 70
Understanding the Language of Results Sections 72
Connecting Results that Describe Conclusions 84
Common Errors in the Reports of Descriptive Results 84
Critically Reading Results Sections of Research Reports for use in Evidence-Based Healthcare Practice 85
Published Report—What would you Conclude? 86

CHAPTER 5
Inferential Results 89

The Purpose of Inferential Statistics 90
Probability and Significance 92
Parametric and Nonparametric Statistics 94
Bivariate and Multivariate Tests 95
Hypothesis Testing 102
In-Class Study Data 103
Connecting Inferential Statistical Results to Conclusions 103
Common Errors in Results Sections 105

Critically Reading the Results Section of a Report for use in Evidence-Based Nursing Practice—Revisited 106

Published Report—What would you Conclude? 107

CHAPTER 6
Samples 109

Samples versus Populations 110

Sampling in Qualitative Research 113

Sampling in Quantitative Research 116

Differences in Qualitative and Quantitative Sampling 123

Problems with the Sampling Process 124

Problems with Sampling Outcomes 126

Common Errors in Reports of Samples 128

Connecting Sampling to the Study Results and Conclusions 128

Critically Reading the Sample Section of Research Reports for use in Evidence-Based Nursing Practice 129

Published Reports—Would you Change your Practice? 131

CHAPTER 7
Ethics 133

Which Healthcare Team Member Actions are Research and Require Special Ethical Consideration? 134

Informed Consent 135

When Research is Exempt 143

Critically Reading Reports of Sampling and Recognizing Common Errors 144

Published Reports—What do they Say about Consent and the Sampling Process? 144

CHAPTER 8
Data Collection Methods 147

Revisiting Study Variables 149

Methods for Constructing the Meaning of Variables in Qualitative Research 152

Errors in Data Collection in Qualitative Research 154

Methods to Measure Variables in Quantitative Research 157

Errors in Data Collection in Quantitative Research 162

Common Errors in Written Reports of Data Collection Methods 168

Critically Reading Methods Sections of Research Reports 169

Connecting Data Collection Methods to Sampling, Results, and Discussion/Conclusion 170

Published Reports—Would you use these Studies in Clinical Practice? 171

CHAPTER 9
Research Designs: Planning the Study 173

Research Designs: Why are they Important? 175

Qualitative Research Designs 182

Quantitative Research Designs 186

How can One Get the Wrong Design for the Right Question? 192

Common Errors in Published Reports of Research Designs 194

Published Reports—Did Design Affect Your Conclusion? 195

Critically Reading the Description of the Study Design in a Research Report for use in Evidence-Based Nursing Practice 195

CHAPTER 10
Background and the Research Problem 199

Sources of Problems for Research 200

Background Section of Research Reports 202

Literature Review Sections of Research Reports 205

Linking the Literature Review to the Study Design 210

Published Reports—Has the Case Been Made for the Research Study? 211

Common Errors in Reports of the Background and Literature Review 212

Critically Reading Background and Literature Review Sections of a Research Report for Use in EBP 213

CHAPTER 11
The Research Process 217

The Research Process 218

Research Process Contrasted to the Research Report 227

Factors that Affect the Research Process 229

Generating Knowledge Through Research can be Fun! 230

Published Reports—What do you Conclude Now? 232

Conclusion 233

APPENDIX A Research Articles 235

Appendix A-1 Relationships Between Body Satisfaction and Psychological Functioning and Weight-Related Cognitions and Behaviors in Overweight Adolescents 237

Appendix A-2 Overweight or Obese Students' Perceptions of Caring in Urban Physical Education Programs 242

Appendix A-3 Leg Length Discrepancy in Cementless Total Hip Arthroplasty 255

Appendix A-4 Teaching Evidence-Based
Medicine Literature Searching Skills to Medical
Students During the Clinical Years: A Randomized
Controlled Trial 261

Appendix A-5 Predictors of Postconcussive
Symptoms 3 Months after Mild Traumatic
Brain Injury 271

Appendix A-6 The Affects of a Single Bout of
Exercise on Mood and Self-Esteem in Clinically
Diagnosed Mental Health Patients 286

Appendix A-7 The Use of Postoperative Restraints
in Children After Cleft Lip or Cleft Palate Repair:
A Preliminary Report 292

Appendix A-8 Investigating Risk Factors for
Psychological Morbidity Three Months after
Intensive Care: A Prospective Cohort Study 297

Appendix A-9 Quality-of-Life Outcomes between
Mastectomy Alone and Breast Reconstruction:
Comparison of Patient-Reported BREAST-Q and
Other Health-Related Quality-of-Life Measures 316

Appendix A-10 Why People Living with HIV/AIDS
Exclude Individuals from their Chosen Families 327

APPENDIX B Demographic Characteristics as
Predictors of Nursing Students' Choice of Type
of Clinical Practice 339

APPENDIX C Sample In-Class Data Collection
Tool 344

APPENDIX D In-Class Study Data for Practice Exercise
in Chapter 5 346

Glossary 347
Index 356

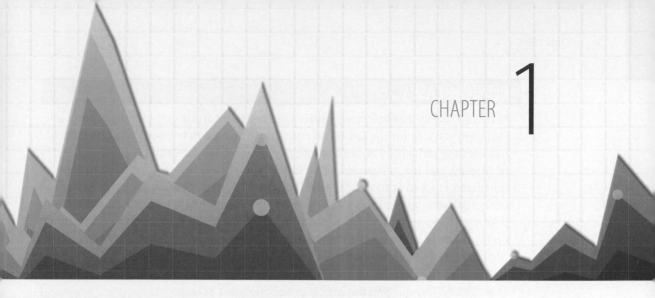

CHAPTER 1

Evidence-Based Healthcare: Using Research in Practice

LEARNING OBJECTIVE The student will relate research to the development of professional healthcare practice.

Introduction
Role of Research in the Evolution of Healthcare Professions
History of Healthcare Research and EBP
Evidence-Based Bridge Theory
Evidence-Based Models
Questions for Patient Care
Where to Find Evidence for Practice
Developing Clinical Questions for Real-World Practice

Determining the Best Available Evidence
Finding Answers Through Research

Published Abstract: What Would You Conclude?
Systematic Reviews in EBP

Evidence-Based Practice: Pros and Cons

Summary

KEY TERMS

Abstract
Bridge Theory
Electronic databases
Evidence-based models
Evidence-based practice (EBP)
Key words
Knowledge

Outcomes research
Peer reviewed
Printed indexes
Research literacy
Research process
Research utilization
Systematic review

CLINICAL CASE

M.D. is a 17-year-old adolescent who is a senior at a local public high school. She has had weight issues for the last 6 years and is considered to be medically obese. She has become concerned about the inability to lose weight, health problems related to obesity, and her self-esteem. She has discussed her concerns with the school nurse and is anxious to take action. The school nurse recognizes that M.D. needs both education and support in achieving her ideal weight. Using the key words *adolescent obesity*, *self-esteem*, and *health*, the RN completes a literature search and finds an article that appears to relate to M.D. and her weight. The article is titled "Relationships Between Body Satisfaction and Psychological Functioning and Weight-Related Cognitions and Behaviors in Overweight Adolescents" (Cromley et al., 2012). (You can find this article in Appendix A-1 of this text.)

INTRODUCTION

Understanding Research for Evidence-Based Practice discusses how you can use research in your practice. Its goal is to teach you, a practicing healthcare professional, to find answers to clinical questions you may have by using research. Another way to phrase this goal is that this book is about practice based on research evidence or evidence-based practice (EBP). To base your practice on research evidence, however, you must be able to understand the research language as well as the research process.

Because answering clinical questions is important for a practicing healthcare professional, this book begins at the end of the research process, with the conclusions, and moves forward through the process. While this may seem unusual, research study conclusions often lead to further questions. You may wonder, for example, why the author(s) reached these conclusions. That question may lead to the results section of the study, where specific numbers and measurements are described. You may also wonder to what types of patients these research results apply. That question may lead you to the description of the study sample. If you wonder why a certain patient was studied, or how the author(s) measured some aspect studied (e.g., pain), you must read and understand the methods section of the research study. Finally, the methods section may direct you to review what has been done before and what healthcare theory or theories may suggest about this clinical question. That information is in the beginning or background section of the research report.

Therefore, this book begins at the end and moves forward through a research report to understand both the research language and the process underlying it. The five general questions that are described in the paragraph below are used to organize the end-to-beginning approach. Each chapter discusses a different component of the research report and how that component can help to answer the five questions. These questions also can be used to organize your own reading and understanding of research so you can evaluate the appropriateness of applying the evidence (research findings) to practice (EBP). They are as follows:

- What is the answer to my practice question—what did the study conclude?
- Why did the author(s) reach these conclusions—what did they actually find?
- To what types of patients do these research conclusions apply—who was in the study?
- How were those people studied—why was the study performed that way?
- Why ask that question—what do we already know?

This book focuses on assisting you to read and understand research reports and to use them intelligently as evidence to guide your clinical practice. Therefore, each chapter begins with a clinical case that raises a clinical question that can be addressed by research. A published research report that is related to the clinical case is part of the required reading for the chapter, and each chapter focuses on what can be decided about practice based on an understanding of the article. To help bring the language and process of research to a practical level, you and your classmates also may participate in a small practice "study" that will be used in the text as a concrete example of different aspects of the research process.

When you finish reading this book, you will be prepared to read research critically and apply it intelligently to healthcare practice. Critically reading a research article means reading it with a questioning mind: knowing what information should be presented in a report, understanding what is reported, and asking yourself whether the research is good enough for you to accept and apply in your practice. You will not be prepared to be a researcher yourself, but you will understand some of the processes of research and how research can help you in your practice.

ROLE OF RESEARCH IN THE EVOLUTION OF HEALTHCARE PROFESSIONS

This text focuses on the healthcare professional's role in understanding and using research findings in **evidence-based practice (EBP)**, a process used by healthcare professionals to make clinical decisions and to answer clinical questions. It also has suggested some other ways that research may be part of the role of the healthcare professional. For example, healthcare professionals may be asked to use research findings as the basis for decisions about the development of clinical programs. They may be asked to participate in some step of the research process, particularly in acquiring informed consent and in collecting data. Equally important, as each healthcare profession recognizes the need for clinically relevant and informed research, healthcare professionals and healthcare groups may be asked to participate in all phases of a research study, from development and refinement of the purpose to interpretation of the results. For example, one of the hallmarks of hospitals that have the highest retention of nurses and quality of patient care—that is, hospitals that have received the American Nurses Credentialing Center (ANCC) Magnet Recognition Program status— is the inclusion of nursing research development and application in the clinical setting.

We begin this book by saying that it is not the goal of this text to give you the tools to implement research independently. Doctoral-level healthcare professionals are expected to be the experts in the research process. Those prepared at the master's level are expected to be sophisticated consumers of research, who are able to critically evaluate and actively participate in research. Nevertheless, baccalaureate-level healthcare professionals often are the foundation from which research is developed and are absolutely the focus for research utilization. **Research utilization** means the use of research in practice. Your understanding of the language and the process of research, coupled with your clinical experience, will allow you to be a contributor to a research team, should the opportunity arise. One hospital that perhaps best epitomizes the full extent of the potential role of research is housed on the grounds of the National Institutes of Health. Every patient there participates in at least one research study. Baccalaureate-level healthcare professionals there not only participate in research but also can develop their own cooperative research projects, with support from researchers with advanced preparation. Baccalaureate-level healthcare professionals can be members of Institutional Review Boards as well, bringing their knowledge of patients and patient care to assist in assuring that the rights of patients are protected.

Healthcare professions not only have a role in research that directly addresses questions generated within the profession, but it also addresses larger questions in healthcare. Healthcare has moved increasingly to interprofessional teams to address research problems. Healthcare professionals are also being sought increasingly to participate in research teams led by researchers from other disciplines. Healthcare professionals' unique understanding of health as it affects the whole person, family, and community is a perspective that often contributes important ideas to research studies. Professional healthcare providers are good at working with people. Thus, researchers from other disciplines often find that healthcare professionals can implement sampling plans effectively, with little subject loss.

Beyond generating and participating in research, healthcare professionals have an important role in formulating the national research agendas regarding health. The research supported and generated through various healthcare research organizations and housed at the National Institutes of Health has earned the respect of other, more established research disciplines. That development has contributed to ensuring health concerns particularly focused on healthcare have become part of national agendas for health-related research. Healthcare research has made great progress over the past century, and we can be proud not only of our heritage of research but also of our current and future contributions to meaningful research that improves the care of our patients.

HISTORY OF HEALTHCARE RESEARCH AND EBP

History helps us to understand the past and its continuing influence on the future. Healthcare research started slowly, but it has evolved at an ever-increasing and progressive rate.

Hippocrates played an essential role in understanding that illnesses and diseases had natural causes versus supernatural causes. He contended that physical factors such as food, water, and air impacted health of individuals. Hippocrates used logical reasoning and observation, the first methods of research in medicine. Forward a few centuries, and in the 20th and 21st centuries, medical research has vastly changed how diseases are diagnosed and treated due to the number of research studies conducted. Medical journals report research studies and their findings disseminating medical information to doctors and other healthcare professionals, such as the *Harvard Medical Journal*, *New England Journal of Medicine*, *British Medical Journal*, and the *Lancet Medical Journal*. These research findings are important to improving health outcomes.

In nursing, it is widely accepted that the history of nursing research begins with Florence Nightingale and her studies of environmental factors that affected the health of soldiers in the Crimean War. Throughout the 20th and into the 21st century, nursing research made significant strides in providing patient care, helping to improve patient outcomes. Many nursing research journals are used today to disseminate research findings such as *Nursing Research*, *Research in Nursing & Health*, *Advances in Nursing Science*, and *Western Journal of Nursing Research*.

Other healthcare professionals have similar research histories with research exploding in the 20th and 21st centuries. Research journals abound throughout healthcare professions to disseminate research findings to others. Journal clubs and professional healthcare organizations help to further disseminate and apply research findings to practice. National and international healthcare organizations have been created to advance research in healthcare and to be a repository for research-related information making it easier to find answers to clinical questions. Examples of these organizations include the National Institutes of Health, the National Institute for Medicine, National Institute of Nursing Research, and the National Institute of Mental Health. Examples of healthcare journals reporting research studies include *Respiratory Research*, *Occupational Therapy Journal of Research*, and *Nutrition Research*. Internet journals make research studies easier and faster to access such as the *Journal of Medical Internet Research* at http://www.jmir.org.

In the beginning of the 21st century, healthcare research continues to grow exponentially. The number of healthcare professionals preparing at the doctoral level, sources and opportunities for funding of research, and diversity of topics examined in healthcare research all have increased steadily. Since the 1990s, when qualitative approaches became recognized and respected as appropriate methods of scientific inquiry, healthcare has been implementing mixtures of quantitative and qualitative methods for study design and analysis that fit the unique research problems of the healthcare field.

Probably most important, as research has grown in each healthcare profession, the body of healthcare knowledge also has developed and we have expanded our horizons to consider **outcomes research**, international research, and traditional laboratory research. We have replicated and expanded on previous findings. Healthcare researchers have completed multiple studies all related to the same problems, allowing us to truly build knowledge and to find real answers to complex questions. As a result, we now have Centers for Research housed in various universities, where groups of healthcare providers with research expertise in specific areas (such as health-promoting behaviors) can work and build their research together to achieve a better-connected and deeper knowledge. Healthcare professionals also have recognized their limits as well as their strengths, moving increasingly toward the creation of and participation in interprofessional teams of researchers, capitalizing on the strengths inherent in the blending of many different disciplines.

EVIDENCE-BASED BRIDGE THEORY

There is a gap between available research findings (evidence-based information [EBI]) and clinical practice. How do we bridge the gap? The Gersch & Rebar Evidence-Based Bridge Theory explains how individual healthcare professionals can use EBI in clinical practice. This theory states that there is a gap that exists between available research (EBI) and the need for active application of this research (EBI) to enact positive growth and/or change within the individual's professional environment. As in Figure 1.1, the train symbolizes the EBI moving across the research-to-practice gap. Notice how the bridge provides a structure which EBI can be supported as it is applied in practice. Strategies and activities throughout the text assist in helping you to build your bridge.

Each healthcare professional individual exists in some state of need for research literacy to effectively and efficiently discern and utilize research in practice. Every individual has specific and various needs in developing research literacy and applying EBI to clinical practice. Where do you fall in this gap? You are taking the first steps by reading this book and participating in learning activities to help you become research literate. Most simply, **research literacy** means that you have an understanding of research terms and processes and are able to discern the validity of the research study's findings or EBI. EBI is only derived from valid research studies. The goal of this text and associated learning resources is to help you to become research literate and use EBI to answer clinical questions. When you are successful in developing and honing your research literacy skills and applying EBI to address clinical questions, you will have bridged the gap!

EVIDENCE-BASED MODELS

Evidence-based models offer a philosophical and practical approach in applying valid research findings to clinical practice in any healthcare field. The philosophical approach is common with evidence-based models and bases the approach in critical thinking processes to guide clinical practice. Healthcare professionals use strategies to apply EBI to EBP. These strategies are the practical approach to evidence-based models and are centered on identifying and answering clinical questions.

A national initiative for promoting evidence-based health information was developed in association with the Agency for Healthcare Research and Quality (AHRQ). Two goals of the initiative entail raising awareness of EBI's impact on patient outcomes and disseminating research findings from evidence-based centers for use in clinical decision making. Evidence-based centers and the AHRQ are repositories for research studies and tools to enhance

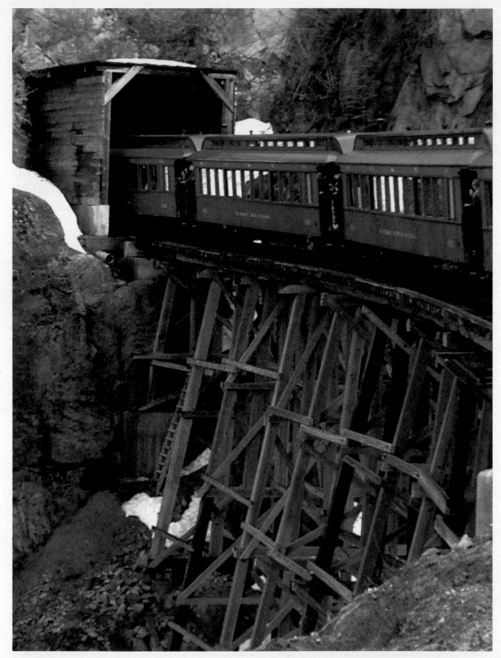

FIGURE 1.1   Gersch and Rebar Evidence-Based Bridge Theory: moving evidence-based information to practice.

patient outcomes (AHRQ, 2012). Evidence-based centers include Brown University: Center for Evidence-based Medicine, Johns Hopkins University, and Minnesota Evidence-based Practice Center (AHRQ, 2012). The Duke Evidence-based Practice Center is also funded by AHRQ and focuses on systematic reviews and meta-analyses to advance research and strategies to evaluate research findings (Duke University School of Medicine, 2013).

Several models for EBP have assisted in applying EPI to clinical practice including the Iowa model, the Ottawa model, and the Joanna Briggs Institute model (See Figs. 1.2 to 1.4). Models are frameworks that provide structures or guidelines for use. Each of these models contains specific steps in validating EBI and applying EBI to practice (EBP). EBP uses

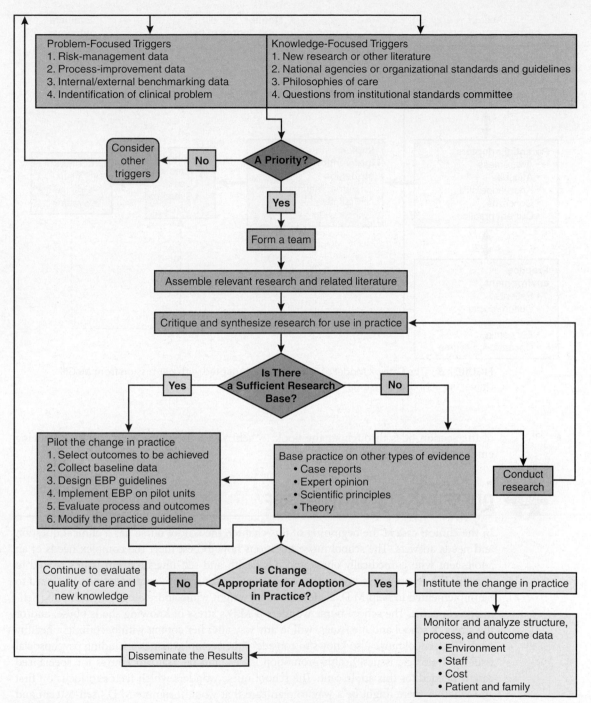

FIGURE 1.2   Iowa Model of Evidence-Based Practice to Promote Quality Care. (Redrawn with permission from Titler M, Kleiber C, Steelman V, et al. (2001). The Iowa Model of Evidence-Based Practice to Promote Quality Care. Critical Care Clinics of North America, 13(4), 497–509.)

decision-making skills that integrates clinical expertise, scientific evidence (EBI), and patient/community/population perspectives (American Speech-Language-Hearing Association, 2013). The six essential elements of an EBP model include assess, ask, acquire, appraise, apply, and evaluate (see Fig. 1.5 and Box 1.1). You will learn how to use each of the essential elements as we progress through the book. You will see these six elements listed with some

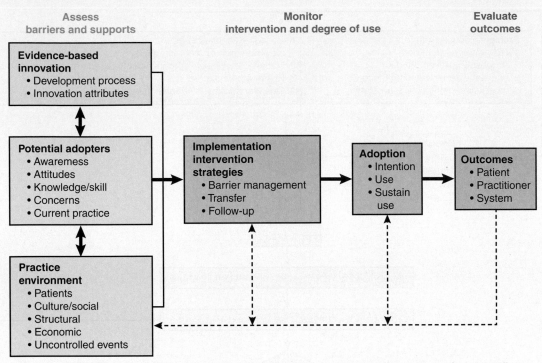

FIGURE 1.3 The Ottawa Model of Research Use. (Adapted with permission from McGill University School of Nursing.)

of the section titles throughout the book to help you understand which element is being emphasized in that section.

QUESTIONS FOR PATIENT CARE

In the clinical case at the beginning of this chapter, the school nurse has a clinical question and needs answers. The school nurse questions how to best meet the complex needs of an adolescent who is medically obese and has health and self-image/esteem issues related to obesity. The school nurse knows that educational and supportive interventions will need to be implemented to help M.D. achieve an ideal weight while addressing her health and self-image concerns. The school nurse wonders if M.D.'s stress of knowing she is obese, and/or the stress of school and life issues, will in any way alter her coping with becoming a healthy adult. The school nurse also knows to consider other complex issues, including psychosocial issues, physiologic issues, health-promotion issues, and referral procedures for specialized care if needed for this adolescent. The school nurse wonders which factor to focus on first and whether there might be a way to plan care that would promote M.D.'s self-esteem and also focus on several different issues at the same time, given the school nurse's busy workload.

This school nurse's question is just one example of the kinds of practice-related questions healthcare professionals face each day. Any healthcare student knows that not all healthcare professionals do everything the same way. Therefore, the questions arise, and you may already have had many questions yourself, such as which is the best way to flush a percutaneous endogastric (PEG) tube, teach incentive spirometry, or perform a radiological procedure? And then there are questions about the differences in patients. Why do male patients have a quicker postoperative recovery from coronary artery bypass grafts than do female patients? Why do some patients quit smoking when they are pregnant and

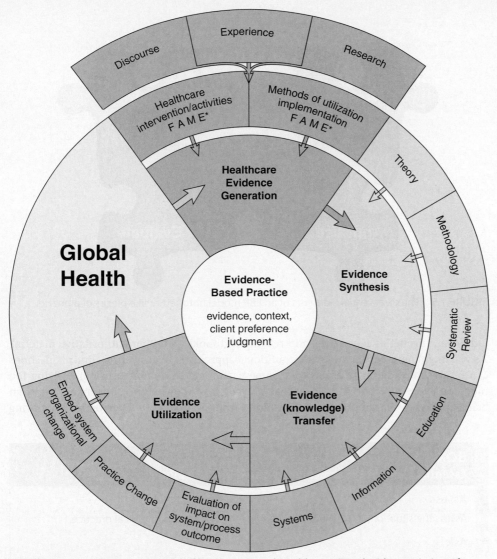

FIGURE 1.4 Joanna Briggs Model of Evidence-Based Healthcare. (Used with permission of the Joanna Briggs Institute.) F.A.M.E. Scale-Feasibility, Appropriateness, Meaningfulness or Effectiveness.

others do not? Why do some patients with AIDS keep recovering from infections, when others seem to weaken and die as soon as the first severe complications occur? Which is more helpful to patients with major depression—to urge them to get up and moving each day or to urge them to listen to themselves and follow their own natural schedules? Although healthcare knowledge has grown steadily and we know a great deal about providing optimal healthcare, there are still more questions than there are answers about how to promote health.

WHERE TO FIND EVIDENCE FOR PRACTICE

How do you, as a healthcare professional or student, find answers to clinical questions such as those listed in the previous section? Traditionally, four approaches have been taken, including consulting an authority or trusted individual, using intuition and subjective

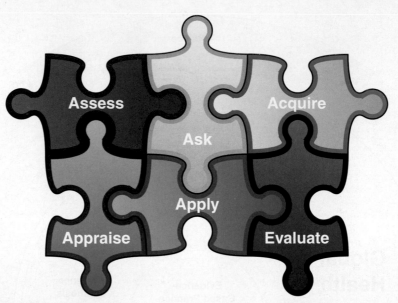

FIGURE 1.5   The six essential elements of an EBP model fit together like pieces of a puzzle.

judgment, turning to experience, and reading textbooks and other authoritative material. As you might guess, using these four traditional approaches to answering clinical questions can produce a wide range of answers, some useful and some not so useful. Relying too much on experience or on intuition may prevent new knowledge or understanding from being applied to clinical problems. Consulting with just one trusted person may not bring

---

BOX 1.1
Essential Elements of an Evidence-Based Practice Model

Assess

Assess the situation. Identifying an issue, concern, or question in clinical practice.

Ask

Ask a question. Using a questioning format, such as PICO, to ask a question relevant to a clinical situation.

Acquire

Find research applicable to the situation/question. Finding credible and current resources to find evidence from scientific research studies.

Appraise

Validate the research findings. Analyze, critique, and evaluate the research study for validity (truthfulness) and applicability.

Apply

Application of the EBI. Integrating clinical expertise, patient perspectives, and scientific knowledge (EBI) into a plan of action in the provision of care.

Evaluate

The last step in the process in evaluation. Evaluating or measuring patient outcomes as a result of your action is important in adding knowledge to the profession, providing support for policy changes, and incorporating EBI into clinical practice (EBP).

a range of thoughts and may result in a biased sense of perspective. Because of these concerns, a newer approach is being developed to standardize a healthcare professional's clinical decision-making process and to provide a framework for planning care that answers the kinds of clinical questions healthcare professionals may have. This approach is called EBP.

EBP is the term used to describe the process that healthcare professionals use to make clinical decisions and to answer clinical questions. Like traditional approaches, EBP also has four approaches to answer questions. But unlike the traditional approach in which you could choose to use an expert opinion or you could use a textbook, EBP uses ALL of the approaches ALL of the time for every clinical question. The approaches include

1. reviewing the best available evidence, most often the results of research;
2. using the healthcare professional's clinical expertise;
3. determining the values and cultural needs of the individual;
4. determining the preferences of the individual, family, and community.

To answer clinical questions using EBP strategies, the healthcare professional must know how to access the latest research, be able to correctly interpret the research findings, be able to apply the findings to the clinical problem using his or her clinical judgment and experience, and take into account the cultural and personal values and preferences of the patient (STTI, 2005). As more healthcare research is conducted, there is more and more evidence that practicing healthcare professionals can turn to in order to answer clinical questions. Using EBP allows a healthcare professional to determine the meaningfulness of the available evidence for the patient he or she is caring for and assists the healthcare professional to make decisions about diagnoses, procedures, treatments, and interventions on the basis of research evidence (EBI) that are justified as part of clinical practice.

EBP implies that one of the roles of a professional healthcare provider will be to frequently seek out the available evidence in order to plan and implement the best care possible. While the bulk of this book will focus on assisting you to know where to find research evidence and how to interpret it in order to have the research evidence influence your care, it is worth taking a minute to discuss when you should seek evidence. It is ideal to say that you will seek evidence for every patient care situation, but that may be unrealistic. Routine care is often based on protocols or procedures that apply evidence. But there will be moments in your clinical practice when you should actively and independently seek out evidence to inform your care.

Situations in which you should actively seek out research evidence on which to base your care include such times as when something in your clinical practice is out of the ordinary. It may be out of the ordinary because you are caring for a patient with a disease or health need you have not encountered before. An example of this would be if you were caring for an adolescent who has obesity-related physical and psychosocial complications, and although you had cared for adults with these health concerns, you had never cared for an adolescent. Or it may be a situation in which a patient has a characteristic that you have never encountered before, such as a cultural or religious one. An example of this would be if you were working with postrenal transplant patients and were caring for a Hasidic Jewish patient who has just emigrated from Russia. If you were unfamiliar with the patient care situation, this would be an ideal time to seek research-based evidence in order to improve care.

Another time that you should seek evidence is when the outcomes of the care you are delivering seem to differ in one or more patients without clear reasons. An example of this is a postsurgical patient whose rate of recovery is different from the typical patient the healthcare professional deals with in a specific healthcare setting. In this case, a search for research-based evidence may well provide increased knowledge, allowing the healthcare professional to provide the best care possible. Another time when a healthcare professional should seek out evidence is when there is a need to develop policy or plan standards for care. An example of this may be a healthcare professional who is a manager in an ambulatory care unit. The hospital has decided to initiate universal assessment for domestic violence for every patient, male and female, who presents for care. In deciding how to best initiate this change in routine care, the healthcare professional will find that a search of the available literature is very helpful.

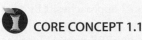 CORE CONCEPT 1.1

When to Seek Evidence

1. Something occurs out of the ordinary in your clinical practice.
2. Outcomes of care differ in one or more patients without clear reasons.
3. You need to develop a policy, procedure, or standards for care.

While there are four approaches used in EBP, it starts with the ability to locate and then interpret evidence, most often the results of research. This book focuses on how to review the best available evidence. The other pieces of EBP—using the healthcare professional's clinical expertise; determining the values and cultural needs of the individual; and determining the preferences of the individual, family, and community—also are very important and should always be considered (STTI, 2005).

DEVELOPING CLINICAL QUESTIONS FOR REAL-WORLD PRACTICE

We have been talking about EBP and the professional responsibilities of healthcare providers to identify and understand research-based evidence. We have used a clinical case as an example of the common nature of clinical questions that can be answered by examining research. But not every question can be answered by examining research evidence. Sometimes no researcher has studied anything similar to your question, or sometimes even though the health problem has been researched, the aspect of the clinical problem you are most interested in has not been studied. So it is important to be able to state your clinical question effectively and know when you can expect research-based evidence to be of help to you. An effective clinical question for EBP is one that has been asked before by someone else and, at least in part, has been explored by a researcher. In addition, a good clinical question has to focus on a healthcare issue that can be measured or described in some consistent manner. Finally, a good clinical question that may be answered by examining EBI has to provide information about what healthcare professionals want or need to do.

An example of an effective clinical question would be "What is the best patient teaching method for newly diagnosed adolescent diabetic patients treated in ambulatory care clinics?" This question is effective because it clearly focuses on what healthcare professionals need to do. Diabetes in adolescents is an area that has been researched, and it can be described or measured. We can use blood sugar levels to measure someone's diabetes. We can interview patients to describe how they learned to cope with their diabetes. A clinical question that is less effective would be "How can I help my young diabetic patient feel better?" While this question is healthcare related, it is less effective because it asks how a healthcare professional can make someone "feel better." Feeling better may mean different things to different people, and it is not easily measured. Another example would be the question from a respiratory therapist "Which insulin pump delivers the most consistent and accurate level of drug to adolescent diabetic patients?" While this is a specific and measurable question, it is less effective because it is not directly respiratory related. This type of question is most likely physician related or pharmacist related; it does not directly relate to respiratory actions.

❶ CORE CONCEPT 1.2 _____

An Effective Clinical Question

An effective clinical question for EBP includes a concern that someone has studied, focuses on a concern that can be measured or described, and is a concern that is relevant to your healthcare professional scope of practice. The question also addresses Who, Where, What, and When in terms of the clinical concern.

In addition to being related to a specific area of healthcare that has been researched and can be either described or measured, an effective clinical question includes a few other things. It identifies _Who_ you are interested in. In our example, the _Who_ are adolescent diabetic patients. An effective clinical question also identifies the _Where_. In our example, the healthcare professional identifies his or her interest in adolescent diabetic patients treated in ambulatory care clinics. In addition to _Who_ and _Where_, the effective question will identify the _What_ and the _When_. The _What_ is the health problem of interest or the desired outcome of care. In our example, the _What_ is patient teaching. The _When_ is often the least identified element of a clinical question, but an important one. The _When_ identifies where in the course of the clinical problem the question arises. In our example, we asked, "What is the best patient teaching method for newly diagnosed adolescent diabetic patients treated in ambulatory care clinics?" Our _When_ is "newly diagnosed." We are focusing our clinical question on patients who have just been diagnosed. As you can imagine, the patient teaching needs of individuals who have had diabetes for many years are different from those of patients who have just been diagnosed. We could have asked in our example, "What is the best patient teaching method for diabetic patients experiencing neuropathic pain treated in an ambulatory setting?" In this case, our _When_ focus is on a time in the course of diabetes that a person has begun to experience the complications of the chronic illness; therefore, the health needs of this person are different from what they were at the start of the illness. Using the _Who, What, When,_ and _Where_ approach to forming your clinical question will do a great deal to help you search for the best available evidence to answer your question. For first clinical question in this text, we will identify the _Who, What, When,_ and _Where_ in a table following the clinical vignette. Another method used in developing clinical questions is called PICO or PICOT. The PICO or PICOT method is similar to the Who, What, When, and Where method; yet, different in that the questions contains a comparison element (See Boxes 1.2 and 1.3).

Determining the Best Available Evidence

Practicing EBP implies that healthcare professionals use evidence to answer clinical questions. But what is evidence, and is all evidence equally useful for guiding a healthcare professional's decision making? Evidence should be thought of as information that provides a point of view or contributes to finding the solution to a clinical question. But all information is not always equally useful. Some information is from informal sources and is collected under less-than-rigorous conditions. Other information is obtained from very rigorous procedures, through formal methods. While both kinds of information may be useful, the more formally and rigorously the information is collected, the stronger it is considered as evidence on which to make evidence-based nursing (EBN) clinical decisions.

In considering what the best available evidence is, a healthcare professional needs to look at how the information that makes up the evidence was collected, how rigorous the method used to develop the evidence was, and what source was used to share the evidence. In this sense, evidence can be placed into two categories: research based and nonresearch based. Figure 1.6 shows examples of both. We will discuss nonresearch evidence first.

BOX 1.2
Designing Clinical Questions Using Who, What, When, and Where

The Four Ws

Who = who you are interested in studying; the population
What = the health problem of interest or the outcomes or care
When = the time of the health problem or outcomes of care occur
Where = the setting or situation

Example:

"What is the best patient teaching method for newly diagnosed adolescent diabetic patients treated in ambulatory care clinics?"

Who = adolescent diabetic patients
What = patient teaching method
When = newly diagnosed
Where = ambulatory care clinics

BOX 1.3
Designing Clinical Questions Using PICO or PICOT

PICO – PICOT

P = Population: Who you are interested in studying; the population
I = Intervention: the treatment or intervention of interest
C = Comparison: the intervention you are comparing "I" to in the question
O = Outcomes: the outcomes you are planning to measure
T = Time of data collection

Example:

What is the efficacy of individual versus group teaching methods for newly diagnosed adolescent diabetic patients on patient compliance with diabetic regimen?

P = adolescent diabetic patients
I = individual teaching method
C = group teaching method
O = patient compliance with diabetic regimen
T = new diagnosed through patient compliance measurement

Source: Riva, J. J., Malik, K. M. P., Burnie, S. J., Endicott, A. R., and Busse, J. W. (2012). What is your research question? An introduction to the PICOT format for clinicians. *The Journal of the Canadian Chiropractic Association, 56*(30), 167–171. PMCID: PMC3430448

Let us say that you have a clinical question regarding the transmission of the H1N1 flu virus. In order to plan how best to prevent the transmission of the flu, you could directly ask people who have had the flu recently how they think they got it. As you ask several people, you may notice some common answers that provide you with information (evidence). But it may not be the strongest evidence on which to base clinical interventions. You could consult a textbook. As a healthcare student, you will often use authorities, a type of non-research evidence, to answer your patient care questions. As a healthcare student, you will

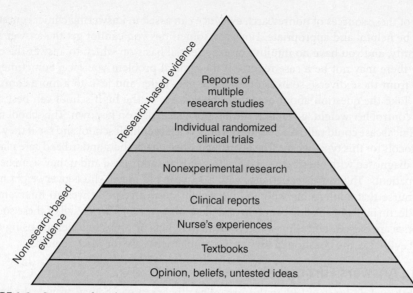

FIGURE 1.6   Sources of evidence.

regularly seek answers to questions from authoritative sources such as reference books, practice journals, other members of the healthcare team (such as patients, the pharmacist, chaplain, physician, and/or dietician). Notice that all these sources of evidence reflect the traditional approaches discussed earlier.

Another approach to answering clinical questions is to use your intuition or subjective judgment. This type of evidence is based on your own experience. Healthcare professional practices involve components of both science and art, and intuition or subjective judgment can be an important way of knowing what to do in clinical practice situations. Intuition can be a source of indirect evidence that is not explicit and articulated fully. Intuition can be thought of as a form of nonresearch evidence. It differs from common sense or arbitrary choice because it is knowledge—but knowledge that we cannot explicate in detail. Intuition may tell you that a particular day is not the day to push a depressed patient to get out of bed. Intuition may tell you that one patient with AIDS has given up and will not survive hospitalization, whereas another who is equally ill is determined to live. Such intuition will guide your care for each of these patients, perhaps leading to a focus on social support and spiritual care for the first patient and a focus on independence for the second patient. In this sense, intuition is evidence to consider in clinical decision making.

Other approaches to answering questions about your practice depend on your own experience as evidence. Experience may indicate that patients who had their indwelling urinary catheters changed every 72 hours had fewer urinary tract infections (UTIs) than did those who had theirs changed every 48 hours. Experience may also indicate that neonates who were treated using assist-control ventilators were discharged earlier than neonates treated with continuous positive airway pressure (CPAP). Personal experience with a health problem may also provide answers to clinical questions. You may know what worked for you or your family, so that is what you will offer or do for your patient.

Clinical reports are another source of nonresearch-based evidence for clinical decision making. This type of evidence is less personal, representing instead the formal experience of someone else. You may find a published article in a practice journal that discusses another healthcare professional's experience with a clinical issue. Or you may find an article that discusses the outcome of a particular approach to patient care. These case reports can provide a rich source of evidence, but the evidence is limited because it may pertain only to that one case and not reflect the unique needs of your patient or the factors that are present in your clinical question.

Each of these sources of nonresearch evidence can assist in answering clinical questions and can be helpful and appropriate. However, sometimes you cannot get the answer from an authority, and you have no intuitive or experiential basis on which to answer the question. Or there may not be a case report on the clinical problem you face. Sometimes the answers from these diverse sources of evidence may differ and lead to a more confusing picture. Take the question about how the school nurse at the high school can best assist M.D. to control her weight, given that she has not succeeded on her own. The school nurse in the clinical case could talk to a peer who works in a larger high school and see if they have any protocols for this type of care. The nurse could also check the standardized care plan for patients diagnosed with obesity to see if health needs are addressed and if they seem helpful to such patients. The nurse's experience with a 15-year-old niece who is overweight might tell the nurse that adolescents who are overweight do not respond well to interventions such as "lecturing," but sharing concerns and ideas may work. However, all of these sources of evidence are biased, reflecting subjectively held beliefs or opinions. Despite using these forms of evidence, the question of how to best implement care for M.D. remains.

Finding Answers Through Research

Research-based evidence or EBI, in the form of healthcare research, may provide the healthcare professional with an answer to a clinical question that avoids the subjective concerns or the informal nature of nonresearch evidence. Often it is exactly the types of questions that are not answered in textbooks, and that everyone has a different idea about or experience with, that are the questions studied in healthcare research. However, while very useful, reading and analyzing research is not necessarily the easiest way of gathering evidence for answering clinical questions.

Just as there are several sources of nonresearch-based evidence, there are several kinds of research-based evidence. Research-based evidence is considered to be stronger evidence on which to base decisions about healthcare. It is the result of carefully designed and implemented research that has been thoughtfully and precisely conducted to answer a specific question. The **research process**, as you will learn in this book, involves a set of systematic processes that formalize the development of evidence, which is why this type of evidence is stronger than nonresearch evidence.

The sources of research-based evidence are discussed in depth in later chapters. They include nonexperimental research and randomized clinical trials. The strongest forms of research-based evidence are reports that combine multiple research studies such as meta-synthesis, meta-analysis, and systematic reviews. We will discuss these further in this chapter as well as in later chapters.

In our clinical example, the school nurse asks the clinical question of how to best implement care for M.D. The school nurse can look to research to find answers. To look for answers in research, the school nurse must

1. identify research in the area of interest;
2. access the research report(s);
3. read and understand the research report(s);
4. decide whether the research finding is relevant and useful in answering the question;
5. decide whether to accept and use what is found as a result of the research.

Rather than completing all of these steps, it is easier to ask someone who is an expert or an authority, hoping that he or she has read the research. However, it is not uncommon for the answer to the question to be "I do not know" or for the answer to differ among sources. As a professional healthcare provider, you will be an authority from whom others will be seeking answers. This book will help you to gain the skills needed to use research intelligently in your practice, whether for answering direct clinical care questions on the basis of systematic reviews or individual research reports or for developing and evaluating quality of care standards. However, to read and understand research, you must first know more clearly what research is.

Identifying Applicable Research Reports

Finding research reports is the first step in using research in clinical practice. Identifying research articles has become easier with the widespread use of the Internet and the increasing numbers of journals that are published electronically. In the clinical case for this chapter, the school nurse used the high school's Internet to search for research articles about planning care for an adolescent who has obesity-related health issues. Not every article about a health condition is a research article. In fact, most information one can access through journals, texts, and the World Wide Web is not research based. So, what is healthcare research?

CORE CONCEPT 1.3

What Is Healthcare Research

Healthcare research is the systematic gathering of information to gain, expand, or validate knowledge about health and responses to health problems. EBP uses research-based evidence (EBI) to plan and implement quality care.

The definition of healthcare research includes two key components. First, for a written report or a Web site to be considered research based, it must describe the systematic gathering of information to answer some questions. Systematic means that a set of actions was planned and organized. The information-gathering actions may include interviews, observations, questionnaires, or laboratory tests, but they must have been guided by a plan and administered methodically or systematically.

Second, the information must have been gathered to answer a question that addresses a gap in our knowledge about healthcare. **Knowledge** is what is understood and recognized about a subject. Information can be gathered for many other purposes, including evaluation, reporting, or accounting for resources. Research seeks to gather information so that we can understand or learn something about which we do not yet have knowledge. Research begins with a question—an unknown—and develops new knowledge. In contrast, evaluation, reporting, and accounting usually describe or validate something that is already known or occurring.

What if an article, found by our school nurse working with M.D., describes, for example, the prevention and treatment of childhood obesity and mentions that adolescent obesity has increased? While this is of interest, it would not be considered a research report. Even if the article provided statistics or numbers about characteristics of adolescent obesity, it still would not be a report of research. A research report about the complications in children of all ages who are obese would formulate a question about those complications and then describe the process and results of a systematic effort to answer that question. Therefore, facts and numbers alone do not make a source of information a report of research. A research report provides a description of the systematic gathering of information to gain, expand, or validate knowledge.

Not only is it important to differentiate research reports from those that are not research, but also it is important to identify and find primary sources of research. A primary source is a report of the research written by the original author(s). Professional newsletters and journals often include summaries of research that have been presented at a conference or published elsewhere. Although these summaries are a quick source of information, they do not allow you to fully understand and evaluate the actual research because they are another individual's summary of that research. These summaries are helpful, however, for identifying research studies that may be potentially interesting and important in your practice. To use research findings intelligently, you must find and read the original research.

As you read more research, the difference between reports of research and other scholarly and informative work becomes clearer. In fact, many of the computer sources used to find research reports have an option that allows you to select only reports that are research, eliminating the need to even decide if an article is a research report. But it is important to understand that what you find when you read a research report is not just a description of facts, ideas, theories, or procedures but is also a question and a systematic effort to gain information to address that question.

Accessing Research Reports

Once you know what you are looking for, the next step in finding research reports is knowing where to look. As a healthcare student, you are probably already aware of numerous healthcare research reports. One of the obvious sources is a journal that includes the words associated with your particular healthcare profession such as "medical research" or "nursing research" in its title (i.e., *New England Journal of Medicine* or *Research in Nursing and Health* or *Nursing Research*). Most professional healthcare journals, even those whose primary purpose is not publishing research, often do include research articles, usually specifically labeled as research in the table of contents. However, simply picking up and scanning journals at the library or at a hospital is a somewhat hit-or-miss approach if you are interested in a specific clinical question. Three primary sources that allow you to search for research on a specific question or topic are (1) printed indexes, (2) the Internet, and (3) electronic databases. Table 1.1 lists examples of these three primary sources.

Printed Indexes. **Printed indexes** are written lists of professional articles that are organized and categorized by topic and author, and they cover articles written from 1956 to

TABLE 1.1	Sources to Search for Nursing Research about a Specific Clinical Topic		
TYPE OF SOURCE	LEVEL OF EVIDENCE FOR PRACTICE IMPLICATIONS	ADVANTAGES AND DISADVANTAGES	SPECIFIC EXAMPLES
Print			
Indexes: provide lists of articles that are organized by topic and author from a range of journals; include all types of articles, including research articles published as early as 1956	No evidence to support practice	Not available via computer/the Internet Studies that are older may not address research of clinical questions relevant to current healthcare, may provide "classic" information other sources may not. Tedious to use Can provide key words for use in searching for specific research articles	• Printed CINAHL (Cumulative Index to Nursing and Allied Health Literature), also known as Red books • Index Medicus • International Nursing Index
Card catalogs: list all materials held by the library, including books, audiovisuals, theses, and dissertations organized by topic and author	No evidence to support practice	Provides lists of sources available	
Abstract reviews: summaries of research studies and prepared bibliographies	Low level of evidence to support practice	Provides summaries of research and prepared bibliographies to assist in finding relevant research articles	• Dissertation Abstracts International • Psychological Abstracts • Sociological Abstracts

TABLE 1.1	Sources to Search for Nursing Research about a Specific Clinical Topic (*Continued*)		
Electronic World Wide Web (WWW)	No evidence to support practice	May not be reliable Can assist in finding relevant research articles Can assist in developing key words	Popular search engines include: • www.yahoo.com • www.go.com • www.altavista.com • www.dogpile.com • www.google.com
	Low to moderate level of evidence to support practice	Provides basic health information for consumers and healthcare professionals May or may not provide research articles Provides current information	Health/Medical search engines include: • www.health.com • www.healthfinders.gov • www.medscape.com • www.scirus.com
		Current and reliable sources in locating research articles and standards of practice based on research	Relevant healthcare-related Web sites include: • www.ana.org/American Association of Nursing • http://www.nih.gov/ and http://www.nih.gov/science/index.html/National Institutes of Health • www.cdc.gov/Centers for Disease Control and Prevention • www.dhhs.gov/Department of Health and Human Services • www.nursingsociety.org/ Sigma Theta Tau International Nursing Honor Society
Electronic databases: categorized lists of articles from a range of journals, organized by topic, author, and source	Level of evidence ranges from low to strongest for practice, depending on type of article (commentary, nonexperimental, or randomized clinical trials methodologies used)		• CINAHL—includes articles from 1982 to the present • MEDLINE (medical literature analysis and retrieval system) • PsycInfo (psychology information) • PubMed (database provided by the National Library of Medicine)
Systematic reviews	Strongest level of evidence for practice	Provides a review of multiple research articles May not be relevant for specific cases that have unusual or uncommon characteristics not addressed in articles	• Cochrane Reviews • Joanna Briggs Collection

today. They usually can only be found in formal academic libraries and are being used more infrequently since the development of computerized electronic databases. Printed indexes are, however, the only source that lists and categorizes research that was done before 1982. Because indexes are tedious to use, are not as available as other sources for finding research, and provide a catalog of studies that are older and thus not current, they should be considered a last resort for research. However, indexes can be helpful in providing ideas for key words to use in a computer search on a topic as well as indicating the kinds of research that have generally been done in your area of interest.

The Internet. Programs called *search engines* can be used to search the Internet; such as Google, Bing, and Yahoo. Because the Internet is a source of information from computers throughout the world, a tremendous and potentially overwhelming amount of information can be found on it. However, because almost anyone can put information on the Internet, the accuracy, completeness, and even honesty of information found there must be considered carefully.

When you use the Internet to look for research, it may help to use the word "research" in the search in addition to words that describe your question. Initially, you will probably get thousands of results, or "hits." These vary from connections to large databases, specific journals or newsletters, and organizations, to connections to individuals' Web pages. You then narrow the search to specific links that will give you research reports. Examples of sites that may provide links that could be helpful in answering clinical questions are those of the CDC (http://www.cdc.gov/) and the AHRQ (http://www.ahrq.gov/professionals/clinicians-providers/resources/nursing/). Links to large and well-established health-related organizations such as these can assure you high-quality information, and many of these sites provide selected research reports. Links to little-known organizations or sites, however, should be used cautiously because the information may be incorrect or incomplete.

When the RN in our clinical case used the Internet to search for ideas about helping M.D. resolve her health concerns, the search led to a link with a site that discussed resources associated with childhood obesity (http://www.aacap.org/cs/root/facts_for_families/obesity_in_children_and_teens). Another site provided the nurse with a practical overview of strategies for preventing and managing adolescent obesity-related complications (http://www.ncbi.nlm.nih.gov/pmc/articles/PMC3278864/) and provided ideas for planning care to help M.D.

Electronic Databases. Besides using search engines on the Internet, you can also use the Internet to make a connection with academic libraries through most university Web sites. Once you make that connection, you can usually access the large electronic databases available at these libraries. **Electronic databases**, the most commonly used source to find research reports, provide categorized lists and complete bibliographic citations of sources of information in a broad field of knowledge. Examples of computer databases include the Cumulative Index to Nursing and Allied Health Literature (CINAHL), which categorizes information that relates to the practice of nursing and allied health professions, and PubMed, which is a database provided by the National Library of Medicine that provides access to more than 11 million health-related and medicine-related citations. Electronic databases can be found in CD-ROM format as well as online. Most are organized similarly so that you can initiate a search for information using **key words**, terms that describe the information you are interested in getting. In the case of the clinical example, the nurse might have used key words such as "adolescent," "obesity," and "self-esteem." Sometimes the most difficult part of using an electronic database is determining which key words to use to narrow your search. Electronic databases also allow you to search for information written by a specific author, or for a specific article using its title. Searches can be limited by date of publication or type of information sought, such as research only. You can further refine the search to peer reviewed or scholarly articles or journals. **Peer reviewed** indicates that an article or journal has been evaluated by other professionals in the same field adding strength to the validity of the research findings. The results of an electronic search include a list of references with bibliographic citations and, usually, an abstract or summary of the article. Again, remember that not all articles found in a search will be research articles unless you have specified that you only want research articles. Although occasionally the title of an article alone may clearly tell you that it is relevant to the question you are asking, you may also need to read the abstract to decide whether it is relevant. Abstracts are discussed in detail later in this chapter.

After finding a citation for a possibly relevant research report, the next challenge may be to acquire a copy of it. Copies of research reports may be acquired in several ways. One way is to subscribe to those journals that usually print the types of research articles that are of interest to you. This allows the article you are interested in reading to be available at your home. A second way is to join one or more professional organizations that provide subscriptions to their journals as a membership benefit. For example, membership in Sigma Theta Tau International (2005) includes a subscription to *The Journal of Nursing Scholarship*, which includes many research reports. Another option for acquiring research reports is by obtaining them from your place of practice, as most healthcare organizations subscribe to several professional journals.

Because numerous journals are now published online as well as in print format, a third way to acquire a research report is to get it online. Although most online journals provide full-text articles only to subscribers, many academic libraries have subscriptions to both print and online journals. As a healthcare student, you may be able to get articles online. You also may be able to request an interlibrary loan of an article from a journal to which your library does not subscribe. If you do so, be sure to find out whether there is a charge for the article. Finally, you can acquire articles by visiting the closest academic library that subscribes to the journal that you need.

Reading and Understanding Research Abstracts

The school nurse in our clinical case will read the published online abstract to decide whether to take the time and trouble to acquire the entire text of the research article. However, reading and understanding the abstract to decide whether the report is potentially useful may be a challenge. Because the abstract for a research report is frequently available when a healthcare professional uses one of the different sources to find research, let us examine what usually is included in an abstract of a research report.

An **abstract** is a summary or condensed version of a research report. Although one meaning of *abstract* is "to summarize," another is "to take away." Because an abstract is a condensed summary, it does "take away" from the total picture or information about a research study and gives only limited information about the study itself. Therefore, the abstract should not be depended on for understanding a research study or making decisions about clinical care. However, if you are trying to decide whether to acquire the full report of a research study, the abstract can certainly be useful. Abstracts vary from journal to journal in format and length. They also vary depending on the type of research performed. Abstracts may be organized by headings, such as Background, Problem, or Results, or they may be written as a single paragraph. However they are organized, almost every abstract identifies the general problem or research question and the general approach taken to implement that research. Most abstracts also briefly describe the people included in the study (called the *subjects* or *participants*) and one or two of the most important findings. Abstracts vary in length from 100 to 500 or more words; those that are more limited in the number of words obviously provide less information. Even longer abstracts, however, provide only a "skeleton" of the key ideas from the research report.

Despite the abstracts' limitations, they still can be useful in determining whether the research study reported is one that you want to acquire and read. The abstract usually provides a clear idea about two important factors: (1) whether the research addressed the clinical question of interest and (2) whether it studied patients or situations that are similar to your clinical case, so that the research is relevant.

Often you can determine from reading an abstract whether the study addressed is the topic you are interested in exploring. For example, a search of the CINAHL database using the key words "adolescent" and "obesity" might return a citation for an article titled "Prediction of

Acceptance of Self in Obese Adolescents Using the Rosenberg Self Esteem Instrument"—a fictional title simply used as an example. This title suggests that the research might be relevant to caring for adolescents who are obese. The abstract for this article, however, might indicate that the purpose of the study was "to describe the relationship between how an adolescent accepts self and obesity." Because the school nurse in our clinical case is sure that the high school health clinic does not use this instrument for students, a review of the abstract would allow the school nurse to conclude that this article is not worth acquiring at this time. It is also possible that although the purpose of this study does not fit with the clinical question, the school nurse may choose to acquire this research report anyway because of its general clinical interest. Besides giving you information about the purpose of a study, most abstracts include information about who was included in the study. Regarding the question about obesity-related care, if an abstract tells you that the people (subjects) in the study were all boys who were involved with sports, you may decide that this study will probably not be helpful for your specific purpose. But if it said the people (subjects) in the study were all girls in high school, it might be very helpful. Be careful, because searching for research reports on a topic of interest can be a bit like eating peanuts—each one leads to yet another. It is easy to become distracted from the clinical question of interest by related studies. Because you may have limited time and resources, it is important to have as clear an idea as possible regarding the clinical question of interest before you begin searching and reading abstracts of research reports.

PUBLISHED ABSTRACT: WHAT WOULD YOU CONCLUDE?

To better understand the usefulness of reading and understanding research report abstracts, read the abstract of the article found by the school nurse in our clinical case: "Relationships Between Body Satisfaction and Psychological Functioning and Weight-Related Cognitions and Behaviors in Overweight Adolescents" (Cromley et al., 2012). You can find this article in Appendix A-1. Remember that the school nurse in the clinical case is trying to plan care to assist the adolescent patient who is medically obese. Consider the following questions as you read the abstract:

1. What do you understand or not understand in the abstract?
2. Do you believe that reading the entire report will be helpful in deciding what care would be necessary to assist M.D.? Why or why not?
3. Based on the abstract alone and what you know about the clinical question, can you make a decision about what would go into a plan of care for M.D.? Why or why not?

It is likely that you will not understand all the language in the abstract; do not be discouraged. The goal of this book is to help you learn to understand that language, and the next chapter directly addresses that topic. However, it is likely that you will understand some of the abstract, and reading even limited information about the research will add to your knowledge about adolescents and obesity. Some abstracts are organized by major headings (such as *Purpose*, *Methods*, or *Conclusions*) that can be helpful to your understanding, such as this example. The abstract addresses weight control may be impacted by body satisfaction. It states the researchers were looking for relationships between psychological well-being, weight control behaviors, eating, weight, and body satisfaction among 103 overweight high school students. It tells you that the study collected information about these adolescents from surveys that assessed these variables. The results indicated that higher body satisfaction was associated with higher self-esteem and lower chance of unhealthy weight control behaviors (Cromley et al., 2012). So even if you did not understand the entire abstract, you can make a decision about whether this research report is relevant to planning for the patient in our clinical case.

ⓘ CORE CONCEPT 1.4

How an Abstract Should Be Used

Abstracts from research reports are an important source of evidence and can be helpful in narrowing down or focusing on the appropriate research to acquire and read. They cannot, and should not, be depended on to provide a level of understanding of the research that would support clinical decision making.

Good, solid, practice-related decisions cannot, however, be based on information gleaned only from the abstract of a research report. Specifically, the research abstract does not give enough information for you to

1. understand all the results of the study;
2. identify who was in the study;
3. recognize how the results fit or do not fit with existing knowledge;
4. decide intelligently whether the study was performed in a way that makes the results realistic for clinical practice.

For example, the abstract from the Cromley et al. (2012) article does not tell you that the research participants were from the Minneapolis/St. Paul area and that they had to have a body mass index >85 percentile for their age and gender. The abstract also does not tell you how the subjects were assessed other than surveys. Because the school nurse in the clinical case is interested in how to implement care to assist the patient in the complex work of achieving ideal weight and health status, it is important to determine what assessment techniques were included in the study. The healthcare professional must read the entire research report to find the answer to these questions and to decide if the study's findings can be helpful in planning care for M.D.

SYSTEMATIC REVIEWS IN EBP

This book treats EBP in the broadest sense by including all types of research, as well as other sources of knowledge, as evidence. Currently, however, there is a particular emphasis in healthcare fields on a process of EBP that addresses clinical questions by searching the literature, evaluating evidence, and choosing an intervention. The product of this process is a **systematic review** of the research literature regarding a particular clinical question and is considered by many as one of the strongest forms of evidence for EBP. Thus, there is a *process* that is often referred to as implementing a systematic review as a basis for EBP, and there is a *product* that is also often referred to as a systematic review. Although it might be easier to refer to the process of implementing a systematic review as the process of EBP, doing so significantly limits the breadth of evidence that may be used in healthcare. Therefore, throughout this text whenever the term *systematic review* is used, the specific usage of the word will be made explicit to avoid confusion.

Like individual research reports, a systematic review includes an abstract and a statement of the problem. However, rather than developing a systematic plan to directly gather information from patients about that question, a systematic review gathers reports of research studies, which have already been completed, that address the problem. The review summarizes these studies, considering aspects of the research process (such as designs and samples) and then draws conclusions about what is known about the clinical question based on the entire group of studies. Here, as with abstracts of individual studies, a healthcare professional can review the abstract to decide whether the review is directly related to the question of interest. Again, even reviewing the abstract requires a basic understanding of the research language.

Dr. Archie Cochrane, a physician and epidemiologist, was the developer of the "Cochrane Reviews," an electronic database similar to CINAHL, which consists of systematic reviews in various healthcare fields (visit http://www.cochrane.org). If you search for topics in this database, you will find a short, focused systematic review, along with a list of relevant primary sources.

Another source for systematic reviews that is focused on the health professions is the Joanna Briggs Collaboration (visit http://www.joannabriggs.edu.au/). This collaboration is a coordinated effort by a group of centers from around the world to promote evidence-based healthcare, education, and training; conduct systematic reviews; develop Best Practice Information Sheets; implement EBP; and conduct evaluation cycles and primary research arising out of systematic reviews. There are currently more than 20 collaborating centers covering the disciplines of nursing, midwifery, physiotherapy, nutrition and dietetics, podiatry, occupational therapy, aged care, and medical radiation. Other databases are now incorporating systematic reviews as an option when searching for evidence-based literature.

The Cochrane Reviews, the Joanna Briggs Collaboration, and other databases all serve an important function in improving the use of research findings in practice because they pull together disparate studies into an easily accessible and organized form. This allows the healthcare professional to find multiple studies on the same clinical question already synthesized into a single review that ends with recommendations for practice. Clearly then, systematic reviews address the issues of access to research and, to some extent, applicability of research to practice.

EBP: Pros and Cons

Use of systematic reviews for EBP has limits as well as strengths. Just as a researcher implementing a traditional research study must make decisions about methods and sample, the author(s) of a systematic review must make decisions about what research to include. This raises the question of what constitutes the "best" evidence. Often, the standard set for appropriate studies included in a review that they be *empirical*, a term used for studies using quantitative approaches. Although there is no question that studies using a quantitative approach are important and useful for answering some questions in healthcare, many problems in healthcare do not lend themselves to the level of quantitative study. Therefore, an overdependence on systematic reviews of clinical research may limit both the types of problems that practitioners consider appropriate for research utilization and the dissemination of important knowledge acquired using other research methods.

Systematic reviews as a type of research have an important place in EBP. Reading and understanding systematic reviews should be conducted using the same five questions mentioned throughout this book and keeping the same openly questioning, critical mind. The difference in reading and understanding systematic reviews is that you must answer the five questions at two different levels, rather than just at one level. For example, when considering the question "How were those people studied—why was the study performed that way?" you must consider the methods for the different studies included in the review. However, you must also consider the rationale for use of a systematic review approach to this clinical question. Probably the toughest two-layered question will be "To what types of patients do these research conclusions apply—who was in the study?" To answer, you must consider the samples in the different studies in the review as well as the sample of "studies" that comprise the review. The second layer becomes "Why did the reviewer include those studies and not others?" Table 1.2 provides an overview of how one might apply the five questions to a systematic review.

TABLE 1.2	Five Research Questions Applied to Systematic Reviews
GUIDING QUESTIONS	**APPLICATION TO SYSTEMATIC REVIEWS**
Why ask that questions—what do we already know?	What do we already know that suggests the need for a systematic review?
How were those people studied—why was the study performed that way?	Why was a systematic review used? Why were the studies that were included in the review performed that way?
To what types of patients do these research conclusions apply—who was in the study?	What types of studies were included as evidence in the review? What types of samples were used in the studies reviewed?
Why did the author(s) reach that conclusion—what was found?	Why did the review reach its conclusions? What did the studies find?
What is the answer to the research questions—what did the study conclude?	What is the answer to the clinical question?

Systematic reviews are an important source of evidence for practice, but they are not the only evidence, and they are not even the only source of research evidence. As an intelligent reader and user of healthcare research, you must find how the use of evidence in the form of systematic reviews can be most useful to you in your clinical practice.

SUMMARY

In summary, we have examined the history of healthcare research and EBP and how that has led to today's professional healthcare practice. This chapter starts you on the way to understanding EBP and how to begin the process of validating EBI by critically reading, understanding, and intelligently using research in practice by (1) defining research, (2) describing sources of research reports, and (3) discussing how to use abstracts to select which research literature to read. You should now have a working sense of what is meant by EBP and how you might format a clinical question that could be answered through EBP strategies. The next chapter discusses the language of healthcare research as well as the components of published research reports and how they can guide your understanding and decisions about using the research in clinical practice.

OUT-OF-CLASS EXERCISE

Get Ready for the Next Chapter

To prepare for the next chapter and to give you a concrete example of the components of a research report, read the fictional research report titled "Demographic Characteristics as Predictors of Nursing Students' Choice of Type of Clinical Practice" in Appendix B. This report describes a fictional study similar to one in which you may participate during your first class period. As you read this report, make two lists: one containing important words or ideas that you understand in the report and one listing important words or ideas that you do not understand. Once you have read the report, you are ready to read the next chapter. Also, make sure you read the "Results" and "Discussion" sections of the article that our school nurse found in the clinical case (Cromley et al., 2012).

References

Agency for Healthcare Research and Quality. (2012). *About the national initiative for promoting evidence-based health information.* Retrieved from http://effectivehealthcare.ahrq.gov/index.cfm/who-is-involved-in-the-effective-health-care-program1/about-the-national-initiative-for-promoting-evidence-based-health-information

American Speech-Language-Hearing Association. (2013). *Evidence-based practice.* Retrieved from http://www.asha.org/members/ebp/

Cromely, T., Knatz, S., Rockwell, R. A., Neumark-Sztainer, D., Story, M., & Boutelle, K. (2012). Relationships between body satisfaction and psychological functioning and weight-related cognitions and behaviors in overweight adolescents. *Journal of Adolescent Health, 50*(2012), 651–653. doi:10.1016/j.jaohealth.2011.10.252

Duke University School of Medicine. (2013). Evidence-based practice. *Center for Clinical Health Policy Research.* Retrieved from http://clinpol.duhs.duke.edu/modules/chpr_rsch_prac/index.php?id=1

Riva, J. J., Malik, K. M. P., Burnie, S. J., Endicott, A. R., & Busse, J. W. (2012). What is your research question? An introduction to the PICOT format for clinicians. *Journal of the Canadian Chiropractic Association, 56*(30), 167–171. Retrieved from http://www.ncbi.nlm.nih.gov/pmc/articles/PMC3430448/

Sigma Theta Tau International. (2005). Evidence-based nursing position statement. *Honor Society of Nursing.* Retrieved from http://www.nursingsociety.org/aboutus/PositionPapers/Pages/EBN_positionpaper.aspx

Resources: Online

Agency for Healthcare Research and Quality—About Evidence-Based Practice Centers. http://effectivehealthcare.ahrq.gov/index.cfm/who-is-involved-in-the-effective-health-care-program1/about-evidence-based-practice-centers-epcs/

Agency for Healthcare Research and Quality—About the National Initiative for Promoting Evidence-based Health Information. http://effectivehealthcare.ahrq.gov/index.cfm/who-is-involved-in-the-effective-health-care-program1/about-the-national-initiative-for-promoting-evidence-based-health-information/

Agency for Healthcare Research and Quality—Nursing Research. http://www.ahrq.gov/professionals/clinicians-providers/resources/nursing/

Allied Health Research Institute. http://www.-cihr--irsc.-gc.-ca/-e/-

American Academy of Child and Adolescent Psychiatry. http://www.aacap.org/cs/root/facts_for_families/obesity_in_children_and_teens

American Nurses Association. http://www.nursingworld.org/EspeciallyForYou/Nurse-Researchers

Canadian Association for Nursing Research. http://www.canr.ca/index.php

Canadian Institutes of Health Research. http://www.cihr-irsc.gc.ca/e/193.html

Center for Clinical Health Policy Research. http://clinpol.duhs.duke.edu/modules/chpr_rsch_prac/index.php?id=1

Center for Disease Control and Prevention. http://www.cdc.gov/

Cochrane Collaboration. http://www.cochrane.org

Indiana State Department of Health—For Kids. http://www.in.gov/isdh/20064.htm

Joanna Briggs Institute. http://www.joannabriggs.edu.au/ and http://joannabriggs.org/jbi-approach.html#tabbed-nav=JBI-approach

Journal of Medical Internet Research. http://www.jmir.org

National Institute of Nursing Research. http://www.ninr.nih.gov/

The New England Journal of Medicine. http://www.nejm.org/

Sigma Theta Tau International: Honor Society of Nursing. http://www.nursingsociety.org/Pages/default.aspx

U.S. National Library of Medicine. http://www.nlm.nih.gov/

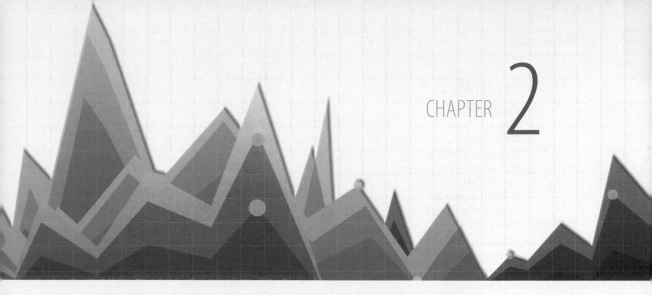

CHAPTER 2

The Research Process: Components and Language of Research Reports

---

LEARNING OBJECTIVE The student will differentiate the terminology in and the components of research reports.

Introduction

Paradigms for Research: What Do You Believe?

The Language of Research
Components of Published Research Reports

Conclusions
Results
Methods
Problem

The Research Process and the Nursing Process

Metasynthesis, Meta-Analyses, and Systematic Review Reports as Evidence for
   Healthcare Practice

Research Reports and the Research Process

Steps in the Research Process

Summary of the Research Process Contrasted to the Research Report

Critically Reading Research for Practice

Published Report—What Did You Conclude?
Summary

KEY TERMS

Conclusions	Problem
Data	Procedures
Data analysis	Process improvement
Descriptive results	*P* value
Hypothesis	Qualitative methods
Limitations	Quality improvement
Literature review	Quality improvement studies
Logistic regression	Quantitative methods
Mean	Results
Measures	Sample
Meta-analysis	Significance
Metasynthesis	Statistics
Methods	Systematic review
Mixed methods	Themes
Multivariate	Theory

CLINICAL CASE

The healthcare provider described in the case in Chapter 1 has found another article that addresses adolescent obesity, self-esteem, and health problems that may help provide answers to the clinical question. The article is titled "Overweight or Obese Students' Perceptions of Caring in Urban Physical Education Programs" by Li, Rukavina, and Foster (2013). It has been a long time since the healthcare provider has read research reports, and the healthcare provider is struggling with some of the language. But the healthcare provider is reminded of the overall similarity in the organization of research reports. The two articles found are available in Appendices A-1 and A-2. If you have not done so, read through them quickly to make the best use of the examples that are provided in this chapter. Do not worry about fully understanding the articles right now, but do keep a list of words or ideas that you do not understand.

INTRODUCTION

This chapter provides an overview of the major components or sections in most research reports as well as some of the unique research language that identifies these different sections. As you probably discovered when reading the articles in Appendices A-1 and A-2, not understanding certain terms in a research report is frustrating and creates barriers to your ability to use evidence-based information (EBI) intelligently in practice. You may even give up and decide not to use research because you can't understand all of the terms. Remember, using strategies to "bridge the gap" between research and clinical practice takes time and practice. This chapter discusses the meanings of some of the language of research and gives an overview of the research process. The remaining chapters will walk you through the individual sections of a research report and will elaborate on definitions of terms used in those sections. Viewing the entire report first will allow you to see the whole "picture" and will help you to understand where each section fits when we begin to review each specific part. Recognizing and understanding healthcare research language will make it easier for you to start reading and comprehending the research and to use it in your practice.

The language and style of research reports are unique and, therefore, can be difficult to read. They are generally written in a scientific writing style, the goals of which are to be clear, precise, and succinct. Like healthcare language, research language is formal, technical, and terse, with many ideas compounded into each sentence. This makes research reports reliable methods of communication for anyone immersed in the language of science, but it also makes them inscrutable to the novice who is just beginning to learn the language of research.

Learning to read research reports is similar to learning to read a patient's chart. The language of research is much like the language of healthcare—it, too, is packed with meaning in every sentence and uses unique terms that communicate clearly to anyone familiar with it. Just as you have mastered or are mastering the language of healthcare, you can master the basics of the language of research.

Paradigms for Research: What Do You Believe?

Have you ever found yourself thinking: What is research? Do I really believe in research? Is research overrated? What does research do for me, as a healthcare provider? I don't have time to look for research, is it easier to ask someone else or look in a book? If you have thought any of these thoughts, you are not alone.

Has your perception of the value of research in healthcare changed since reading Chapter 1? Chapter 1 defines research and its value to clinical practice in general. What about you as an individual healthcare provider? The first question is to ask yourself "How can research help me provide quality care?" In the past and still today, healthcare providers are using interventions that are scientifically weak. In other words, some healthcare actions are based in tradition; what they have learned in school, what more experienced healthcare providers have been doing for decades, and/or what they were taught by others. Currently, research is being used to provide healthcare providers evidence that can be translated to providing evidence-based care. This new knowledge assists healthcare providers in developing the most effective, safe, and competent care. Also, the fields of healthcare education are using research to assist healthcare providers in gaining the knowledge they need to enhance patient care. In the future, research has the potential to provide the healthcare professions with the knowledge needed to provide evidence-based care to any patient in any situation. Patients, whether individuals, families, groups, or communities, will benefit from EBP.

THE LANGUAGE OF RESEARCH

This chapter presents several terms that are unique to research. Each will be defined in this chapter, but do not be discouraged if you are not completely clear about all of them. They are also included and defined in the glossary, and we will revisit these terms as we discuss the different sections of a research report in more detail in the following chapters. The learning outcome for this chapter is that you differentiate the different sections or components of a research report and the language associated with each of those sections, not that you understand each of the terms in depth. Table 2.1 provides a summary of the sections of a research report and their associated language.

You were asked at the end of Chapter 1 to read the fictional article from Appendix B and compile a list of terms that you did and did not understand. Hopefully, this chapter will touch on some of the terms that were not clear to you and, perhaps, add to your understanding of those that you believed you already understood. Again, you can think of reading research as being similar to reading a patient's chart. The first time you read a patient's hospital chart, a great deal of the information in it may not have made sense to you, and you may not have even known which section to look in for different types of information. With time, however, you learned the unique language of the healthcare field and found

TABLE 2.1	The Sections of a Research Report and Associated Terms
RESEARCH REPORT SECTION	**ASSOCIATED TERMS**
Problem or Introduction: describes the gap in knowledge that will be addressed in the research study	• Literature review • Theory • Research question • Hypothesis
Methods: describes the process of implementing the research study	• Qualitative • Quantitative • Mixed methods • Measures • Sample • Procedures
Results: summarizes the specific information gathered in the research study	• Data • Data analysis • Themes • Descriptive results • Significance • Multivariate
Conclusions: describes the decisions or determinations that can be made about the research problem	• Limitations • Implications for practice

your way around a chart with ease. The same thing will happen with research reports. Just as you learned where to look for physicians' orders or diagnostic test results as well as the unique language used in those orders or results, you will learn where to look for specific information about a research study and to understand its unique research language. For example, you will learn where to look for information about procedures in a research study and some of the unique language used to describe those procedures so that you will have a good start at reading and better understanding research reports. As you read the different research reports used in this book, keep adding to your list of words or ideas that you do not understand, then periodically review it and cross out those words you believe you understand. You can use the list to guide your own reading and can share it with your fellow students and your faculty to assure clarification of the words to facilitate your own and fellow students' learning.

COMPONENTS OF PUBLISHED RESEARCH REPORTS

In addition to an abstract, almost every research report has at least four major sections:

- Introduction or Problem
- Methods
- Results
- Conclusions or Discussion

Table 2.1 describes each of these sections and lists some of their associated research terms. Because this book discusses research by beginning at the end or the conclusions of a research report and moving to the beginning of the report or introduction, we will look at each of the sections of a report, starting with the end.

Conclusions

The word *conclusions* is used in research reports much as it is generally used outside of the research setting. **Conclusions** identify what was found and complete a report by identifying an outcome. They specifically describe or discuss the researcher's final decisions or determinations regarding the research problem.

In healthcare research reports, conclusions usually include a description of implications for clinical practice. That is why practicing healthcare providers often start with the conclusions of a report. That section provides the "so what" by providing the meaning of the research for practice. What distinguishes conclusions in a research report from those in other reports is the expectation that they contain either new knowledge or confirmation of previous knowledge. This is a core concept. The goal of the research process is to generate knowledge that can be used in practice. This is another core concept. In the conclusions section of a research report, the findings or results of a study are directly translated into that new knowledge. So, you should expect that the conclusions go beyond simply saying what was found in a study; they present the implications or meaning of those findings for future practice. As such, the conclusions of research reports are powerful because they are the evidence for EBN. They are used as the basis for decisions about direct patient care, whether in program planning or in one-to-one direct patient care.

 CORE CONCEPT 2.1 _____

What distinguishes conclusions in a research report from those in other reports is the expectation that they contain either new knowledge or confirmation of previous knowledge.

 CORE CONCEPT 2.2 _____

The goal of the research process is to generate knowledge that can be used in practice.

Because of the power and importance attached to them, the statement or decisions described in the conclusions of a research report are carefully worded and should list any relevant cautions or limitations. This cautious presentation may, however, make the conclusions weak or not helpful to the healthcare provider who is looking for clear and direct answers to clinical questions.

For example, the school nurse in our clinical case is looking for specific advice about how to provide care for M.D. and finds the conclusions of the two reports (Appendices A-1 and A-2) described in sections labeled "Discussion and Implications" and "Discussions." From reading these sections, the school nurse learns that there is a relationship between lower body satisfaction and "less positive behavioral and emotional functioning" in overweight adolescents (Cromley et al., 2012). The school nurse also learned that enhancing body satisfaction in overweight adolescents can protect the teen against comorbidities related to obesity. In addition, the authors discuss strategies such as motivation and skills in weight-controlled behaviors to help adolescents who are overweight take control of their health. This is useful information for the school nurse, but it does not provide specifics about how to assist M.D. develop weight-controlled behaviors. Li et al. (2013) discuss caring perceptions in helping students from age 11 to 17 become engaged in physical education. The authors identify specific strategies in engaging adolescents who are obese or overweight including "empowering students with leadership opportunities and choices," "giving advice on living a healthy lifestyle," and "listening to students' voices" (Li et al., 2013). The authors of each article clearly express their conclusions cautiously by addressing specific limitations to the study and may do so for several reasons. Chapter 3 examines in more detail why conclusions are often constrained or hesitant.

The conclusions section of a research report usually has fewer unique research terms than does the rest of the report. This is probably another reason why the conclusions section is sometimes the first part read by healthcare providers. One term that regularly appears in the conclusions or discussion section is *limitations*. **Limitations** are the aspects of how the study was conducted that create uncertainty concerning the conclusion that can be derived from the study as well as the decisions that can be based on it. These limitations often address the information presented in the beginning sections of the report, such as the study's methods and sample.

Just as the cautious language used in the conclusions section can be frustrating when you are looking for practical answers to clinical questions, the limitations described may make you wonder whether you can use conclusions as evidence on which to practice. That is why the limitations are included in the conclusions: to remind the reader that there are constraints or limits to the knowledge being reported. Limitations do not mean that the results of a study are flawed or meaningless. They do, however, indicate the boundaries of or constraints to the knowledge generated by the research. To decide whether to use the knowledge described in a research report and how it will be used, you must understand not only the knowledge but also the limitations. This requires understanding of other aspects of the research process, such as sampling or methods that may place limits on the new knowledge.

Finally, the conclusions section of a research report usually contains recommendations for future research regarding the problem of interest. These recommendations often directly address the limitations that have been described and suggest additional studies that are needed to further build on the new knowledge generated and stretch the boundary of that knowledge. The research reports used in Chapter 1 and this chapter include a discussion on limitations of the study and suggestions for further research.

Results

The **results** section of a research report summarizes the specific findings from the study. Almost no research report can give all of the information that was gathered during a research study, so the results section contains a summary or condensed version of what the authors believe are the most important findings. *Data* is a word that is often used and has specific meaning in research. **Data** are the information collected in a study. Organizing and compiling data are called *data analysis*. **Data analysis** pulls elements or information together to present a clear picture of the information collected, but it does not interpret or describe the implications for practice of that picture of the information.

CORE CONCEPT 2.3

The difference between results and conclusions is that results are a summary of the actual findings or information collected in the research study, whereas conclusions summarize the potential meaning, decisions, or determinations that can be made based on the information collected.

Some of the unique language found in this section is a result of how the data were analyzed and what analysis methods were used to summarize the information collected. Results or findings may be reported in the form of numbers, words, or both. Which form is used depends on the type of information or data collected. If the study collected information about people's beliefs and experiences, the results section summarizes the words that were collected using terms such as *themes*, *categories*, and *concepts*. **Themes** are abstractions that reflect phrases, words, or ideas that appear repeatedly when a researcher analyzes what people have said about a particular experience, feeling, or situation. A theme summarizes and synthesizes discrete ideas or phrases to create a picture from the words collected in the research study. For example, in the fictional research report in Appendix B about nursing students' choices of type of clinical practice, the results section mentions "three distinct themes that represent the meaning of life experiences related to choice of field of nursing." The authors of this article do not list the answers given by 30 different nursing students; rather, they have looked for recurring ideas or words in those answers and have categorized them into themes or findings. In the perceptions of caring article, adolescents who were overweight or obese were interviewed about their experiences in feeling cared about or cared for from teachers and peers. Four themes were identified from the collected interview data and included "teachers' instructional adaptations, a positive, motivational climate, built interpersonal rapport, and supportive peers" (Li et al., 2013). These themes create a picture of meaning of situational experiences for the interviewed students.

In contrast, the data in the research study on body satisfaction and behaviors in overweight adolescents is primarily collected in the form of numbers, such as height, weight, and scores on the body mass index (BMI) and surveys including the Body Shape Satisfaction Scale and the Center for Epidemiological Studies Depression Scale for Children. Again, the authors do not list all the responses/results from the 103 different adolescents who completed assessment measures; rather, they summarize the numbers in different forms, such as means. The **mean** is an average for a set of numbers. The language that describes data analysis of information in numbers is called **statistics**, and the language of statistics is often one of the most intimidating languages to readers of research. We do not have to be statistical experts to develop a greater understanding of that language, and we will focus on the language of statistics in Chapters 4 and 5. However, a few key terms are worth highlighting here to help us get started.

Almost all research reports, even those that are mostly reporting results of interviews in the form of words, include descriptive results. **Descriptive results** summarize information without comparing it with other information. For example, descriptive results may state how many people were in a study, the average age of those studied, or the percentage who responded in a specific manner. In the perceptions of caring study, the authors place the descriptive results following the methods section and use numbers to describe the students. For example, the age of the participants had a range from 11 to 19 years of age with a mean of 14.86 and a standard deviation of 1.97. The mean is the average age of the participants (14.86 years of age). The standard deviation explains where the majority of the participants lie. A standard deviation of 1.97 indicates that 68% of all participants are within plus or minus 1.97 years of the mean (14.86). Means and standard deviations help readers create a picture of the participants in this article. We will be discussing the specifics of standard deviation in Chapter 4. In the body satisfaction and behaviors in overweight adolescents study, almost all of the results presented are descriptive. In Box 2.1, the

BOX 2.1
Descriptive Results Explanation on Eating-Related Behaviors and Cognitions

"Frequency of eating in secret and fear of losing control while eating (both in the past month) were measured by using items form the Eating Disorder Examination Questionnaire. Using the distribution median, these variables were dichotomized into ≥5 days versus ≤4 days. Importance of being thin was assessed with a 4-point Likert scale ranging from 'not at all important' to 'very important'" (Cromeley et al., 2012).

paragraph describing eating-related behaviors and cognitions from the article is repeated. Here, the authors describe how the variables were measured and how time was divided into two time divisions; greater than or equal to 5 days and less than or equal to 4 days. The authors provide this description to help readers understand what was measured. In contrast to more detailed research reports, the authors do not provide explanations of each of the descriptive values. The expectations are that the readers know how to read the descriptive data numbers. For new readers of research this expectation is overwhelming, however; understanding descriptive terms such as means and standard deviation provide a beginning for interpreting the results. Many healthcare programs require a statistics course as a prerequisite or corequisite to research and you can understand the "why" of this requirement. Thus far, we have talked about descriptive results, but the authors of the body satisfaction and behaviors in overweight adolescents study also provide some correlation statistics in the paragraph headed "Data analysis" and in Table 1 of the research report (Cromley et al., 2012). Here, the authors are doing more than just describing the findings because they are looking for connections between the variables in their study. Specifically, the authors are looking for a connection between the variables body satisfaction and weight loss or demographics. The computation of a correlation statistic to look for connections between variables requires consideration of two important statistical concepts: significance and p values.

Let us look at what *significance* means first. The second sentence in the data analysis section of the body satisfaction and behaviors in overweight states, "There were no significant differences between the 'high' (n = 50) and 'low' (n = 53) body satisfaction groups on demographics or weight loss (see Table 1)" (Cromley et al., 2012, pp. 652–653). **Significance** is a statistical term indicating a low likelihood that any differences or relationships found in a study happened by chance. In research, we often try to make decisions about clinical care for a large group of patients based on what we have found in a small group of patients. Statistical significance is important because we need to be sure that what was found in the small group of patients studied is not something that happened by chance rather than because of some factor we are studying. In the body satisfaction and behavior in overweight adolescents study, the authors do not provide any information on significance in the discussion other than stating there were no significant findings. This indicates the variables may be related by chance and not just the other variables studied. If the authors had found significance between the high body satisfaction and weight loss, then this indicates the findings did not occur by chance alone and we could expect that in another group of adolescents, we would find some relationship between high body satisfaction and weight loss. If a significant relationship was found, the author would provide a p value, which leads us to the second important statistical concept.

So if significance is indicated by p values, what is a p value? **P values** indicate what percentage of the time the results reported would have happened by chance alone. For example, a p value of .05 means that in only 5 out of 100 times would one expect to get the results by chance alone. If it is unlikely that the results happened by chance, then we can summarize the findings by saying that the results are statistically significant. In order to consider if the results of a study help to answer your clinical question, and in order to engage in EBP, you will need to look for these p values. For example, if a p value is given for the correlation between two variables as $P = <.01$, this would tell us the connection found between these two scores would happen by chance alone in $<1\%$ of samples. What that connection means and how it affects our clinical planning are not discussed until the conclusions section of the report. However, summarizing and reporting the finding of a connection that is not likely to happen by chance alone are important so that the reader knows why the researchers reached their conclusion.

Another term that is often found in the results section of a research report is *multivariate*. If you think about this term, it is easy to figure out that **multivariate** indicates that the study reports findings for three (multi) or more factors (variate) and includes the relationships among those different factors. The fictional article in Appendix B and the body satisfaction and behaviors in overweight adolescents report multivariate results because it looks at relationships and differences between more than two factors. For example, the fictional article does not use the word *multivariate*, but it does describe results of a statistical procedure called a *logistic regression*, which included the three factors of age, rating of health, and choice of field of nursing. Now that you know what the word means, you can count the number of factors analyzed and identify that this study is, indeed, multivariate. **Logistic regression** is a statistical procedure that allows us to look at relationships between more than two factors and test whether those relationships are likely to occur by chance. Statistical language such as this is discussed further in Chapters 4 and 5.

The information summarized in the results section of a report depends on who was studied, how the study was conducted, what the research question asked, and how the researcher(s) analyzed the information. To understand more completely what was implemented in a study and who was studied, we must look at the methods section of the research report.

Methods

The **methods** section of a research report describes the overall process of how the researchers went about implementing the research study, including who was included in the study, how information was collected, and what interventions, if any, were tested. Remember from Chapter 1 that one of the things that distinguish research from other ways of answering questions is its systematic collection of information. The methods section of a research report should describe those procedures used to collect information. Chapter 8 examines, in detail, the variety of research methods, along with the many names used for them. For now, remember that research methods can be broadly categorized under three major headings: qualitative, quantitative, and mixed methods. Because qualitative and quantitative methods are used both separately and together in healthcare research, the methods are discussed throughout this text. To assist you in understanding the differences between them and how the differences may affect your use of the research in practice, the following eight chapters will be organized so that general information relating to both approaches is described first, followed by specific information related to qualitative, quantitative, and then to mixed methods. The sections will be identified by use text colors for the first few chapters as noted above. Be sure to read carefully and take note of the different colors, as it is easy to get the three approaches confused. At this point, we will briefly differentiate qualitative, quantitative, and mixed methods.

Qualitative methods focus on understanding the complexity of humans within the context of their lives. Research that uses qualitative methods attempts to build a complete picture of a phenomenon of interest. Therefore, qualitative methods involve the collection of information as it is expressed by people within the normal context of their lives. Qualitative methods focus on subjective information and never attempt to predict or control the phenomenon of interest. The obese students' perceptions of caring study discussed in this chapter is a study using qualitative methods.

Quantitative methods focus on understanding and breaking down the phenomenon into parts to see how they do or do not connect. Therefore, quantitative methods involve collecting information that is specific and limited to the particular parts of events or phenomena being studied. Quantitative methods focus on objective information and can yield predictions and control. The body satisfaction and behaviors in overweight adolescents study used in Chapter 1 is a study using quantitative methods.

Mixed methods focuses on elements of both qualitative and quantitative methods by describing individuals' personal experiences, feelings, or perceptions and the measurable portions of the variables. In the past, mixed methods were deemed "less" scientific and useful. However, researchers are finding mixed methods valuable to the contribution of knowledge in particular to evaluation research. Evaluation research in healthcare studies healthcare programs and health-related phenomenon. For example, a mixed methods research for healthcare may be conducted on the rate of counting sponges/instruments used in a surgery and the surgical team members' view of the importance of counting sponges/instruments before, during, and after a surgical procedure. In this example, both

FIGURE 2.1 The differences between qualitative and quantitative methods.

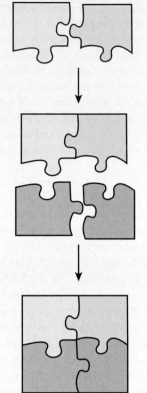

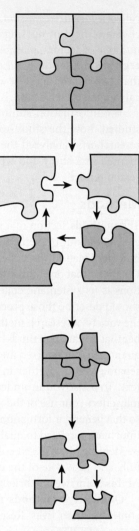

Qualitative knowledge building

Quantitative knowledge building

quantitative (rate of counting) and qualitative (individual's view) create a whole picture on the phenomenon of counting sponges, which impact patient outcomes.

Figure 2.1 illustrates the differences between knowledge building using qualitative versus quantitative methods: qualitative research assembles the pieces of a puzzle into a whole picture, whereas quantitative research selects pieces of a completed puzzle and breaks them down into their component parts. In mixed methods research, knowledge is built using both qualitative and quantitative methods so you can see how important mixed methods research can be to improving holistic patient outcomes.

Methods sections of research reports, whether they use qualitative, quantitative, or mixed methods, usually include information about three aspects of the research method: (1) the sample, (2) the data-collection procedures, and (3) the data analysis methods.

Sample

A **sample** is a smaller group, or subset of a group, of interest that is studied in a research. Using perceptions of caring study as an example, you will see that the researchers were interested in gaining knowledge to help a provider do a better job of caring for adolescents, but they only had the time and resources to study a group of 47 teenagers from one urban community.

Therefore, in planning care for M.D., the school nurse must consider whether the 47 adolescents from an urban community in the research report are similar to the adolescents in the school nurse's school. The effort to assure that the subgroup or sample and what happens to them is similar to the other patients or people being studied is emphasized in quantitative research methods. However, describing the sample, that is, who was studied, is important for understanding the results of a qualitative study as well as those of a quantitative study.

 ## CORE CONCEPT 2.4 _____

Most research attempts to gather information systematically about a subset, or smaller group of patients or people, to gain knowledge about other similar patients or people. Many of the methods in research are aimed at assuring that what happens in the subgroup or sample studied is as similar as possible to what would happen in other larger groups of patients or people.

The sampling subsection in the methods section of a research report describes how people were chosen, what was done to find them, and what, if any, limits or restrictions were placed on who or which research could be done in the study. It also usually describes how many patients or people declined to be in the study, withdrew from it, or were not included in it for specific reasons. For example, the fictional article states that the sample was one of convenience, meaning that no special efforts were made to get a particular type of student to participate. The students chose whether or not to participate in the study and did not provide identifying information on the questionnaire. Therefore, no restrictions were placed on who would participate; all the researcher did was approach a class of students and ask them to volunteer. This is an example of a simple sampling procedure.

In contrast, a research report using multiple studies to answer a clinical question such as a *metasynthesis* contains a more complex sampling method, involving the analysis of information about each individual study's report in order to identify the sample of reports that best met the criteria of the study. In this type of study, the investigators describe how studies were chosen and why studies were not chosen for the sample. Understanding samples and sampling is an important part of making intelligent decisions about the use of research in practice and is discussed in more detail in Chapters 6 and 7.

Procedures

In addition to information about samples, the methods section usually includes information about procedures used in the study. Healthcare providers are familiar with procedures within the context of healthcare. Research **procedures** are similar because they are the specific actions taken by researchers to gather information about the problem or phenomena being studied. Research procedures in qualitative, quantitative, and mixed methods studies differ because the purposes of the three approaches to research differ.

Because the systematic collection of information in a qualitative study involves looking as much as possible at the whole phenomenon being studied, procedures for qualitative studies are systematically planned activities—such as observations or open and unstructured interviews of people in their natural life situations—to see and hear as much as possible of the complexity of those situations. A qualitative researcher may videotape or audiotape interviews with individuals so that every word, expression, and pause can be carefully considered and studied. In addition, qualitative researchers keep detailed notes of their observations of the environment where the information is collected as well as the expressions and actions of those being studied. This is not a haphazard process but an organized, systematic, and intensive process to collect and then analyze the complexity of experiences.

In contrast, because the methods used in a quantitative study involve identifying specific aspects of a problem, the procedures involve actions to isolate and examine those particular aspects or pieces. The focus of a quantitative study is on clearly defining and examining that which is believed to be relevant to the problem being studied. Therefore, procedures may involve carefully defined repeated observations at set time intervals, such as taking a blood pressure reading immediately before and after a patient is suctioned. Another example may be a specific protocol for teaching each patient, in exactly the same manner, to use visualization to relax before surgery.

In summary, quantitative and qualitative methods lead to different approaches and procedures, whereas in mixed methods, both qualitative and quantitative approaches and procedures are used in a systematic and organized manner. Control and objectivity are hallmarks of quantitative methods, whereas naturally occurring conditions and subjectivity characterize qualitative methods.

Often, the procedures in a quantitative study involve taking measurements, sometimes directly, such as taking a blood pressure reading or measuring leg length during hip replacement surgery, but often indirectly, such as in a written questionnaire. **Measures** are the specific method(s) used to assign a number or numbers to an aspect or factor being studied. For example, in the article about body satisfaction and behaviors in overweight adolescents, the authors used a 10-item self-report to collect information about specific body features. They did not do extensive body testing on the adolescents; rather, they depended on the teenager's self-report of level of satisfaction of specific body features. The final numbers used in this study are the average or mean scores on this self-report of body satisfaction. Thus, the abstract concept of body satisfaction is converted into a number that can be analyzed.

Another example of the use of measures is found in the fictional article in Appendix B. The study examines factors that cannot be directly observed. The article has a section labeled "Measures," which describes a three-part written questionnaire. This questionnaire was used to assign numbers to aspects that were studied, such as perceived well-being or choice of field of study. So again, abstract concepts are converted into a number that can be analyzed using statistical procedures. Based on the previous discussion of qualitative and quantitative studies, it should make sense the body satisfaction and behaviors in overweight adolescents study used quantitative methods because the goal was to break down and describe aspects of overweight adolescents, whereas the perceptions of caring study used qualitative methods because the goal was to explore a phenomenon associated with overweight children. Both research reports carefully defined the factors to be studied and established a clear, easily reproduced approach to get information. Similarly, the fictional article not only describes measures used to translate the factors that were studied into numbers, indicating a quantitative approach, but also includes what the author calls a "qualitative question." By using the word *qualitative*, the author indicates that this part of the research attempted to look broadly or holistically at the students' experiences, without selecting specific pieces and asking focused questions. Therefore, the fictional article describes the mixed methods approach by using both qualitative and quantitative procedures in its methods section.

An important point to understand is that although this book describes and defines many of the terms used in the research process and found in research reports, the terms can have various meanings and can, at different times, be used broadly or more specifically. This can be frustrating or discouraging because the words or ideas are new, and you are just beginning to understand them. However, the more experience you gain from reading and learning about research, the easier understanding it will be. You will find the same situation with many of the words used in the healthcare field. For example, "normal" body temperature is defined as 98.8°F. Fever is clearly present when a patient has a temperature of 100.8°F or higher, but a temperature between 99.8°F and 100.8°F is not considered either febrile or "normal," and a patient can feel "feverish" with a "normal" temperature. With practice, healthcare providers learn to recognize these variations in the meaning of the words *fever* and *feverish*. Similarly, with practice, you will learn to recognize and be comfortable with the variations in meanings or use of research terms.

 CORE CONCEPT 2.5

Many of the terms used in research have a range of meanings rather than a single, discrete, locked-in meaning.

Data Analysis Plan

In addition to describing the sample and procedures used in a study, the methods section often includes a description of the data analysis. Remember that data are the information collected in a study, and data analysis is a description of what was done with that data to obtain a clearer picture of what the information tells us. Although the results section summarizes the outcome of data analysis, the methods section often describes in detail how the researchers worked with or analyzed the data. In the article, perceptions of caring, the authors describe some of the procedures they used to analyze data under heading titled "Data Coding and Analysis." In other reports, the authors may not have a specific heading for data analysis, so you may need to look for such headings as "Evaluation of Reports" and "Metasummary and Metasynthesis." The fictional article has a much shorter "Analysis" subsection, in which the author informs the reader that a specific computer program was used to analyze the data that were numbers and then describes the analysis procedures for the data that were words. Again, the approaches to analyze quantitative and qualitative data are different and are discussed further in Chapter 4.

Problem

So far, we have reviewed the conclusions, results, and methods sections of research reports: Conclusions discuss the outcomes, decisions, or potential meanings of the study; results summarize what was found; and methods describe how the study was implemented. This brings us to the beginning of a research report, a section often labeled "Problem" or "Introduction." Just as the word suggests, the **problem** section of a research report describes the gap in knowledge that is addressed by the research study. In this section, the researcher explains why the study was needed, why it was carried out in the manner that it was, and, often, what the researcher is specifically asking or predicting.

The introduction or problem section of a research report usually includes a background or **literature review** subsection, which is a focused summary of what has already been published regarding the question or problem. The literature review gives us a picture of what is already known or has already been studied in relation to the problem and identifies where the gaps in knowledge may be. It may report, for example, that studies have only been done with selected types of patients, such as with children but not with adults. Or, it may report that no one has ever tried to ask a particular question before: Perhaps studies have examined occurrence of one or two specific health problems in adolescents, but only a few have examined multiple physical and mental variables associated with obesity.

The literature review does not necessarily only include published *research* studies. It also may include published reports about issues related to practice or a description of a theory. A **theory** is a written description of how several factors may relate to and affect each other.

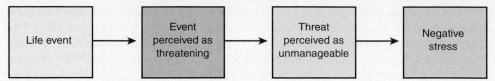

FIGURE 2.2 Proposed relationships among the four factors in Lazarus's theory of stress and coping (1993).

The factors described in a theory are usually abstract, that is, they are ideas or concepts—such as illness, stress, pain, or fatigue—that cannot be readily observed and immediately defined and recognized. For example, in nursing, theories such as Roy's theory of adaptation (1984), Neuman's system model (1982), and Watson's theory of human caring (1985) are examples of written descriptions of how the four major components of nursing (persons, health, environment, and nursing) may interrelate.

Lazarus's (1993) theory of stress and coping is another example of a theory that is somewhat simpler than many healthcare theories. It proposes relationships among four abstract factors: life events, perceptions of threat, perceptions of ability to manage a threat, and stress. The relationships proposed in the theory are if a life event occurs that is perceived as threatening, and there are no perceived approaches to manage or mitigate that threat, then stress results. Figure 2.2 illustrates the proposed relationships among these four factors.

When a research report discusses a theory in its introduction or problem section, the study usually tests or further explains the relationships proposed in that theory. Therefore, if a study report discussed Lazarus's theory of stress and coping (1993) in the introduction, we expect that the study will be based on, or will examine, some aspect of how life events and perceptions affect stress as described in that theory. If a research study is based on an existing theory, then the researcher often already has an idea of what relationships are expected to be found. These ideas are stated in the form of a **hypothesis**—a prediction regarding the relationships or effects of selected factors on other factors. Not every study will have a hypothesis. For a study to include a hypothesis, there must be some knowledge about a problem of interest so that we can propose or predict that certain relationships or effects will occur. If you remember from earlier in the chapter, qualitative research does not try to predict outcomes, and therefore, a hypothesis is seldom appropriate. The body satisfaction and behaviors in overweight adolescents study did not identify a theoretical framework (theory); however, the report does provide a purpose and a hypothesis for the study. This study also includes descriptions of several factors that may influence the problem of interest and suggests that the knowledge gap results from not knowing the effects or relationships among these factors.

THE RESEARCH PROCESS AND THE NURSING PROCESS

We started this book by stating that the goal was not to make you a researcher, but, rather, to give you the knowledge and tools needed to understand and use research intelligently. However, we do not want to continue this chapter with an emphasis on how complex and arduous the research process can be or the many potential barriers there can be to both implementing and publishing research. The research process is a wonderful and exciting challenge, like a giant interactive puzzle; as each piece is solved and fit into place, the rest of the pieces change and must be addressed in their new form based on what has already been completed. Fitting each piece into the puzzle can be extremely satisfying, and finishing small sections of the puzzle through completion of a research study can be rewarding.

Part of the reason the research process is fun is because it is a continuous learning experience for those involved. When one is trying to develop new knowledge, the challenges of planning and implementing a valid and meaningful study always require problem solving and creative solutions, so the opportunity to learn and create can be immense. More and more, we are recognizing that most research is best approached by using teams with members from different backgrounds and disciplines. This allows the knowledge brought to bear on a research problem to be wide ranging and to enhance the potential for a high-quality product.

It is the authors' hope that as you read and use research you will develop an interest in and excitement about the process of research as well as for the problems that it addresses. Although the baccalaureate-level healthcare provider is not expected to plan and implement research, there are several roles for healthcare providers in the research process, such as participation in planning a study or in subject recruitment and data collection.

As we discussed the research process, you may have noticed some similarities between it and healthcare processes, such as the nursing process. For one thing, both processes have been broken down into steps. In the broadest sense, the nursing and research processes are similar because they are used to solve problems. Both a research problem and a patient care problem (whether the patient is an individual, family, or community) can be viewed as a complicated puzzle, where often only some of the pieces are available at any time point.

Both types of problems are initially addressed through gathering information. In the nursing process, this gathering of information is referred to as assessment, and in the research process, it is referred to as describing and refining the knowledge gap or problem. However, in both cases, we are collecting information to guide us in understanding the problem and formulating a plan.

The second, third, and fourth steps of the nursing and research processes also initially may appear similar, although they differ in some major ways. Although the second step of the nursing process is planning and the second step of the research process is developing a detailed plan, the two processes differ because they have fundamentally different purposes. The purpose of the nursing process is to provide informed, scientifically based nursing care for human responses to potential or actual health problems. The purpose of the research process is to develop or validate knowledge. The goal of the nursing process is action to promote the established outcome of improved health. The goal of the research process is to acquire new knowledge, and the outcomes for that new knowledge cannot be known until the knowledge is established. Therefore, the second and third steps of the nursing process address planning and implementing care, whereas the second and third steps of the research process address planning and implementing acquisition of new information. As a result, the fourth steps of these two processes have different focuses because evaluation in the nursing process is concerned with outcomes, whereas data analysis and interpretation are concerned with understanding. Table 2.2 summarizes the similarities and differences

TABLE 2.2	Comparison of the Research Process and the Nursing Process	
	RESEARCH PROCESS	**NURSING PROCESS**
Similarities	• A process with steps • A form of problem solving • Complex "puzzle"	• A process with steps • A form of problem solving • Complex "puzzle"
Differences-based care	• Purpose is to develop knowledge • Plans and implements knowledge acquisition • Analysis and interpretation concerned with knowing	• Purpose is to provide scientifically • Plans and implements delivery of care • Evaluation concerned with outcomes

between the two processes. We discuss the roles of healthcare providers in research more in the next chapter.

Although there are some similarities and differences in the processes of nursing and research, it is essential that there be a strong relationship between the two. The research process should provide knowledge that is the basis for the nursing process. This is why this entire book focuses on understanding and intelligently using research in practice. In addition, the nursing process will often be the source of problems that need to be addressed using the research process. As we plan, implement, and evaluate patient care, we often find problems or face questions about the best ways to achieve our outcome of improved health. The nursing and research processes differ in purpose, but they are closely linked and together ensure the growth and development of nursing as a profession.

CORE CONCEPT 2.6

While different in purpose, the nursing process shares several steps and skills with the research process.

Metasynthesis, Meta-Analyses, and Systematic Review Reports as Evidence for Healthcare Practice

We have been discussing the sections and language in research reports in general; however, there are several unique types of reports we should recognize. These include reports of a single study, metasynthesis, meta-analysis, systematic reviews, and quality improvement.

Metasynthesis, meta-analysis, and systematic reviews can be used as evidence for healthcare practice. The two studies we have been using in Chapters 1 and 2 are reports of a single research study. These studies answer specific clinical questions in a specific situation that are often used in clinical practice. Another type of study that may be used as evidence for clinical practice is a **metasynthesis**, which is a report of a study of a group of single research studies using qualitative methods. A **meta-analysis** is a quantitative approach to knowledge development that applies statistics to numeric results from different studies that addressed the same research problem to look for combined results that would not happen by chance alone. Both of these methods examine a question or problem about which there have been a number of studies and actually take a sample of studies, rather than a sample of individuals. Metasynthesis and meta-analysis are similar to another special type of research report called a *systematic review*. As you recall from Chapter 1, a **systematic review** addresses a specific clinical question by summarizing multiple research studies, along with other evidence. Systematic reviews differ from metasynthesis and meta-analysis because they, by definition, will address a clinical question and they do not generally apply statistical procedures to the information collected from individual studies or develop a systematic metasummary of the content of each study.

The sections of reports of metasynthesis, meta-analyses, and systematic reviews resemble those of single studies but may differ in some important ways. Table 2.3 summarizes what you might expect to find in the different sections of reports of a systematic review, metasynthesis, and meta-analysis. All three begin with a section that identifies the problem of interest. In metasynthesis or meta-analysis, the problem identified may be anything that has been addressed in several individual research studies. In contrast, a systematic review addresses a specific patient care or clinical practice question because the intent of the review is to provide evidence for practice.

A systematic review has defined procedures, but they are not always described in the report under a heading titled "Methods." The procedures in a systematic review involve searching and identifying all published reports or primary studies that examine or are

TABLE 2.3 Components of Reports for Individual Research Studies, Metasynthesis, Meta-Analysis, Systematic Reviews, and Quality Improvement Reports

COMPONENTS OF REPORTS	TRADITIONAL RESEARCH STUDY	METASYNTHESIS	META-ANALYSIS	SYSTEMATIC REVIEW	QUALITY IMPROVEMENT STUDY
Problem or introduction	Review of the literature; theory; statement of a knowledge gap; predictions or hypotheses	Identification of a problem that has been addressed in only a few studies with limited findings	Identification of a problem that has been addressed in several studies with inconsistent results	Statement of a practice problem, including a broad overview of the relevant clinical questions related to the problem	Statement of a standard for patient care that is measurable and specific, usually including a summary of the research basis and clinical basis for the standard
Methods	Description of quantitative or qualitative procedures; sampling methods; data analysis methods	Description of the procedures used to find and select the individual research studies; description of the procedures used to analyze the individual studies	Description of the procedures used to find and select the individual research studies; description of procedures used to code and analyze results from the individual studies; usually includes a table of studies	Description of search strategies and criteria used for including a study in the review	Description of the procedures used to identify selected patient care situations and methods used to collect information about the care in those situations
Results	Description of findings; summary of themes or concepts or results of statistical procedures	Summary of findings, concepts, or themes across the sample of studies	Summary of results of statistical tests on groups of results from individual studies	Summary of research findings categorized and synthesized under clinically meaningful topics; usually includes a table of studies	Summary of the patient care practices that were identified
Discussion or conclusions	Summary of key findings; comparison of results to previous studies; speculation about the meaning of results in relation to theory; description of limitations; recommendations for additional research and final conclusions	Summary of key findings and identification of how these might differ from what is generally accepted understanding; identification of needs for additional research and of limitations in existing studies	Summary of key findings and identification of how these might differ from what is generally accepted understanding; identification of needs for additional research and of limitations in existing studies	Specific identification of practice implications derived from the synthesis of the literature; identification of needs for additional research	Summary of key findings; comparison of findings to established standards; speculation about reasons for differences found; recommendations for changes to remedy any deficits found

related to a particular clinical care problem. The researcher has to define the problem and determine which studies are and are not related to that problem. The researcher also describes the procedures used to search the literature after describing the problem, or perhaps at the end of the report, under a heading such as "Search Strategies."

In contrast, metasynthesis or meta-analysis reports usually have clearly identified methods sections in which the search strategies used, the inclusion and exclusion criteria used for the sample of studies, and the analysis methods applied to the sample of studies are all described. Remember that a metasynthesis or meta-analysis examines a sample of research studies rather than a sample of patients.

The results sections of metasynthesis or meta-analysis and systematic reviews differ because the metasynthesis reports specific integrated concepts extracted from the individual reports, while meta-analysis specifically describes the numeric values from findings of the different studies and the statistical tests used to test those numbers. A systematic review usually summarizes the available studies that address a clinical care question but does not yield new findings in either numerical or written form. A metasynthesis or meta-analysis may summarize the nature of the studies used, but the core of the findings will be new knowledge in either a numeric or conceptual form. Both systematic reviews and meta-analyses usually provide a table identifying the basic characteristics of the individual research studies that were included, which allows the reader to view the individual studies as needed.

Finally, metasynthesis, meta-analyses, and systematic reviews all have a conclusions section in which the potential meaning of the findings is described. As with single research reports, these types of reports may identify limits to what has been reported and usually recommend areas for future research. A systematic review always addresses implications for clinical practice.

Although systematic reviews are an important form of research that can be used in practice, quality improvement is a process that resembles, yet differs from, the research process. **Quality improvement** is a process of evaluation of healthcare services to see if they meet specified standards or outcomes of care and to identify how they can be improved. Quality improvement is often based on research, and the process and product resemble the research process. The questions in quality improvement are whether a certain set of actions is occurring and how desirable outcomes can be facilitated. This is a form of a descriptive research question. The standard or outcome itself is usually based on earlier research that indicates the set of actions or outcome that can and should be achieved. Standards of care change as research findings suggest better approaches to and potential outcomes of care.

In addition to asking a descriptive question about the presence or frequency of a set of actions or outcomes, **quality improvement studies** also often examine relationships among factors that may affect the outcome or actions of interest. Just as we want to know what factors may influence a clinical problem of interest, we want to know what factors influence the consistency of achievement of standards or outcomes.

In such ways, traditional research often serves as the basis for quality improvement standards. Moreover, many of the methods used in research directly apply to the process of evaluating quality. Finally, gaps in quality of care may indicate fresh areas requiring research as well as needs for changes in practice.

Although quality improvement studies are an important form of research that can be used in practice, process improvement is a process that resembles, yet differs from, the quality improvement and research process. **Process improvement** is a management system in which all participants involved strive to improve customer satisfaction. While meta-analysis, metasynthesis, and systematic reviews seek to find the best practices and development of standards of care to improve patient outcomes, process improvement methods seek to improve the process in which decisions/changes in care delivery are carried out. For example, a traditional research study may seek to answer whether customer satisfaction is improved when a professional translator is assigned to a patient versus the use of a family member for a patient who is Chinese, whereas a process improvement method seeks to improve an approach that increases customer satisfaction for all patients within an organization.

Therefore, process improvement is a management system, whereas quality improvement seeks to find practice-related answers. However, process improvement reports can resemble a quality improvement study by identifying problems using data, planning and implementing a change, and evaluating results. Quality improvement and process improvement systems use the same quality principles. Although we have explained differences between quality improvement studies and process improvement, the terms are often considered synonymous. Process improvement methods are based extensively in the business industry to remove process errors and increase efficiency within an organization leading to overall customer satisfaction. Healthcare organizations are successfully using these methods to increase patient satisfaction, efficiency, and effectiveness and decrease costs. In other words, these methods focus on meeting and/or exceeding customer requirements, needs, and expectations.

How does quality improvement play a role in healthcare services? According to the Health Care Improvement (HCI) project, quality improvement can be defined as "all activities that contribute to defining, designing, assessing, monitoring, and improving the quality of healthcare". The HCI project uses quality management principles to develop tools and methods to improve healthcare services. These principles focus on four areas: patient, systems and processes, measurement, and teamwork. The HCI project has improved healthcare services in many arenas. Another healthcare organization known as Agency for Healthcare Research and Quality (AHRQ) uses quality improvement research to improve healthcare services. The AHRQ (http://www.ahcpr.gov) focuses on healthcare outcomes, quality, cost, use, and access. The Joint Commission (TJC) (http://www.jointcommission.org) works to improve the quality of care and safety of patients within the United States. The TJC evaluates and uses accreditation to verify healthcare organizations and programs provide safe, quality care to individuals and communities. The TJC Center for Transforming Healthcare uses the Lean Six Sigma process improvement model to help healthcare entities reduce waste, decrease healthcare errors, and to improve quality of care (TJC Center for Transforming Healthcare, 2010). These organizations, along with The Institute for Healthcare Improvement, National Association for Healthcare Quality, The Institute for Safe Medication Practices, American Society for Quality, and Canadian Foundation for Healthcare Improvement are committed to using quality/process improvement principles to improve quality in healthcare services.

Healthcare organizations using process improvement methods rely on each employee at every level to strive for continuous improvement in healthcare services. The results could and do have drastically changed how healthcare providers practice. For example, data are collected on a surgical unit in a local hospital regarding the number of surgical wounds that have developed an infection. Healthcare providers identified possible causes of the infection and developed a procedure in caring for surgical wounds based on research indicating actions that decrease the risk of infection. Data were collected for several months after the procedure was initiated and the number of infected surgical wounds decreased. What do you think happened to the patient satisfaction scores after the procedure was followed?

There are several process improvement methods currently being used in healthcare organizations. Each method uses quantitative data to assess for process improvement opportunities. Total Quality Management (TQM) is a management system involving all organizational shareholders and requires a change in attitude that allows and encourages the participants to focus on quality and meeting customer's needs. The first priority in TQM is the customer. What can be done to improve customer satisfaction? What do customers want/need/expect? The Deming Cycle, also known as the PDCA model uses four steps in improving quality: plan, do, check, and act. In the planning step, a healthcare provider might identify an issue and plans for a change. The healthcare provider implements the plan/change on a small scale and then collects data to determine if the results were significant. If the change had significant results, the change may be broadened to include other areas. Results are then collected and the cycle continues. Continuous Quality Improvement (CQI) is another management system based in the belief that products, processes, and services can always be improved. CQI research focuses on customer satisfaction, scientific approach, and teamwork to develop strategies in improving the health and well-being of individuals.

A written report of a quality improvement study resembles a report of a traditional research study, but there are some differences between the two. The problem addressed in a quality improvement study usually concerns whether certain expected clinical care was completed, so the question involves discovering what is being done or what has happened, rather than trying to understand a phenomenon. As with traditional research, a quality improvement study usually examines only a subset of all the occasions when a specified type of care was given. Methods to collect data for a quality improvement study include questionnaires, direct observation, and chart reviews. The report of a quality improvement study describes how information was collected concerning the clinical care and a summary of what was found. This is similar to the methods and results sections of a research report. The conclusions of this type of report include recommendations for improving the quality of care based on what was found regarding the care currently given. The recommendations are similar to the conclusions that are drawn from a research study. See Table 2.3 for a summary of the sections of quality improvement reports compared with individual research reports, metasynthesis, meta-analyses, and systematic reviews.

The usefulness of a quality improvement study can be understood using the same five questions discussed throughout this book. Table 1.2 outlines how they might be applied. We can consider why the standard or outcome was established—what is the evidence for that standard? We can ask about the manner by which the study was implemented because various methods can be used to implement quality improvement, including chart review, observation, interviews, and questionnaires. Various approaches can be taken to the "sample" for a quality improvement study, including convenience, random selection, and purposive sampling. Similarly, data from a quality improvement study can be handled and analyzed in several ways, making the fourth question about what was actually found appropriate to consider. The last question of what the study concluded is obviously also relevant to quality improvement studies. Just as an accurate and meaningful research study can inform clinical practice, an accurate and meaningful quality assurance study can evaluate and strengthen practice. Findings from a quality improvement study that indicate standards are being met support continuation of existing practices. Findings indicating that standards are not being met should guide revision of existing practices to improve care. As with traditional research, findings from a quality improvement study may lead to the need for another study to further clarify issues that may relate to meeting standards or outcomes.

RESEARCH REPORTS AND THE RESEARCH PROCESS

So far, we have discussed the elements of a published research report. However, in doing so, we have had to at least touch on what a researcher does to conduct a research study. Although this book is not intended to teach you how to be a researcher, it is impossible to use research intelligently if you do not understand the basics of the research process. Just as you do not have to be a cardiac surgeon to understand what open heart surgery entails, you do not have to be a researcher to read and use research in EBP. Fortunately, the research report is written in a manner that closely mirrors the actual research process, so as we focus on understanding and intelligently using research, we can also learn the basics of the process. We will provide an overview of the steps in that process now, and then discuss the different steps further in the following chapters.

Steps in the Research Process

Figure 2.3 illustrates the five steps in the research process and the relationship between them and the sections of a research report. The first step is to define and describe a knowledge gap or problem. Frequently, this step begins with a clinical question or problem, such as the one raised by the school nurse in the clinical case who wants to find evidence to guide care of M.D. A researcher interested in this type of clinical question then performs a literature review to determine what is already known about the problem. Performing a literature review requires using databases, as discussed in Chapter 1, and the researcher should search for and read as many pertinent published articles on the topic as possible. As part of defining and describing the knowledge gap, the researcher also investigates whether anyone has ever implemented a study addressing the clinical question as well as how other people have studied or described aspects of the problem. Although this process may help the researcher to gain a clearer picture of how to construct a study to address the clinical question, it may also make the problem more complicated and confusing. Often, a researcher's question changes as he or she learns about what has already been studied or described. Therefore, the focus of the first step is to narrow and identify something specific for the study, and its culmination is a statement of a problem or purpose. The problem section of a research report partially reflects this step by providing a description of the relevant literature, possibly a theory, and one or more of the following: a research problem, question, or hypothesis. However, the neatly written problem or introduction section of a research report certainly

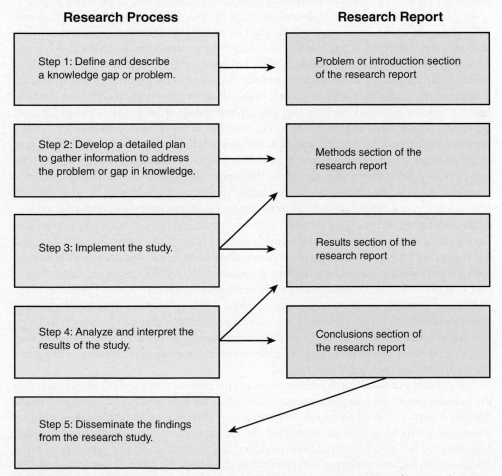

FIGURE 2.3 The relationship between the research process and the sections of a research report.

will not reflect all of the thinking, sorting, and comparing involved in the first step of the research process.

The second step is to develop a detailed plan for gathering information to address the identified knowledge gap. Planning the study depends on the problem or question being asked and the designs of qualitative, quantitative, and mixed methods, partly because of the type of questions asked and partly because of the researcher's beliefs about how best to gain meaningful knowledge.

Knowledge gaps that lend themselves to studies using qualitative methods are usually related to the experiences, beliefs, feelings, or perceptions of individuals, and often, little is known about the area in question. Because of this limited knowledge, qualitative methods provide a broad picture by describing the whole experience from the patient's viewpoint. In addition, a researcher may approach knowledge gaps by using qualitative methods because he or she believes that we can best learn and understand the phenomenon of interest by examining the phenomenon in its usual context. For example, in the perception of caring study, the researchers "explore" perceptions to help increase understanding about the experiences of students who are overweight or obese. In contrast, knowledge gaps that involve a concrete response or action, such as the relationships between body satisfaction, psychological functioning, weight-related cognitions and behaviors, lend themselves to a quantitative approach in which each factor that might contribute to understand a problem is identified, defined, and measured. A researcher who uses a quantitative approach believes that knowledge can best be generated by breaking down a phenomenon into its different pieces and objectively measuring and examining each piece and its relationship to the other pieces.

In this step, the specific methods used to study the problem are planned, including who will participate in the study, what will be done to collect information, and how that information will be analyzed. It requires understanding the various approaches used to systematically gather information, considering what has been done in the past and what kinds of problems have occurred, and planning carefully to maximize the knowledge that will be the product of the study. The methods section of the research report, like the problem section, summarizes the decisions made in this step by specifically describing the sample, procedures, and data analysis used in the study. For example, in the fictional article about nursing students' preferences for first clinical jobs, we are told that the study included junior-year undergraduate nursing students and that, in this program, traditional 4-year, RN-to-BSN and LPN-to-BSN students were included. The report also tells us that a written questionnaire was used to collect the data. The researcher in this study could have decided to study graduating seniors rather than juniors or to conduct in-depth interviews with selected students rather than using a questionnaire. The researcher had reasons for using juniors and having them complete a questionnaire, such as time constraints, student availability, and the researcher's view on meaningful ways to gather knowledge. What we read in the research report usually only reflects the final decisions of the second step of the research process, and the researcher will likely only provide a limited explanation of the methods used.

Because research is a process, a study may not occur as it was designed and planned; therefore, the methods section also may describe any changes made to the study plan as it was implemented. Neither the body satisfaction and behaviors of overweight adolescents or the perceptions of caring study indicate a deviation in the study plan, however; changes in the study plan are commonly experienced.

The third step in the research process is to implement the study by gathering and analyzing the information in the systematic manner planned in the second step. As mentioned in the discussion of procedures, this may involve numerous different actions, such as tape-recording interviews, performing carefully controlled clinical experiments, or mailing and compiling responses to a questionnaire. In addition to gathering the information, this step involves managing, organizing, and analyzing the information to address the problem being studied. The outcome of this step is reported in the results section of the research report, which is why that section describes the sample and summarizes the answers or outcomes for each measure. Those results may not directly answer the research question, but they do allow the reader to have a better understanding of what happened during the study. For example, the researchers in the perceptions of caring study collected data from a Southern urban city school district. The number of students was limited by the study's criteria of the participants having to be overweight or obese. Students were first identified by the researchers or physical education teachers within the district and then BMI was used to determine final selection into the study. It is likely that the researchers did not plan on only having such a small percentage of students who agreed to be in the study. We do not know if one type of student was more likely than another to participate as the researchers did not indicate if the ethnic/racial distribution between the community's population and the participants was similar. It is important to remember this when reviewing the conclusions because they may or may not apply equally to all patients.

The fourth step is the detailed analysis and interpretation of the results. In qualitative research methods, this step is woven closely with the third step, with analysis often guiding additional data collection. In quantitative methods, some preliminary analysis and summary of the data usually occur during the implementation step. However, additional analysis and careful interpretation of the meaning of the findings occur only after all the information from the study is gathered. The researchers will analyze the data, compare their findings to those from previous studies, and decide what they can conclude from the study. At this point, the researcher hopes to answer the question posed, confirm or not confirm the prediction made, or create a meaningful understanding of the phenomenon of interest. The actual findings from the study are summarized in the results section of the research report, whereas the implications, or potential meaning of those findings, are included in the conclusions section. As with all the other sections of a report, what is actually included does not reflect everything that the researchers did during this step. They will distill their analysis into a few paragraphs to provide the reader with a succinct summary of what they found and what it may mean for clinical care.

The fifth and final step of the research process is the sharing or dissemination of the findings. Gathering information to gain new knowledge is not a particularly useful activity if no one ever learns about the new knowledge, so an important obligation and commitment of the researcher is to share that research through publications, presentations, posters, and teaching. Research reports, such as the perceptions of caring and the body satisfaction and behaviors in overweight adolescents, are obviously a major method for disseminating research. However, these reports do not accomplish the goal of disseminating research if the people who need the knowledge cannot understand them. This brings us back to the importance of understanding and intelligently reading and using research in healthcare practice.

SUMMARY OF THE RESEARCH PROCESS CONTRASTED TO THE RESEARCH REPORT

The first step of the research process—describing and defining the knowledge gap or problem—is summarized in the background and literature review sections of a research report. These sections give us the context for a research problem and tell us about relevant theory and research regarding aspects of it. The information included in the research report is a synopsis of the much more extensive information that was gathered and synthesized during the first step. The research purpose and specific questions or hypotheses that conclude the first sections reflect the final refinement of the research problem into specific variables and a specific type of research question.

The second step of the research process is reflected in the methods section of a research report. This section tells us the study design, sampling plan, methods of measurement, and procedures. Again, all the previous research, practicalities, and experience that enter into the decisions about settings for a study, the sample, and the measurement are distilled into a few paragraphs describing the final decisions that were reached about the study plan.

The third step of the research process—implementing the study—is usually reflected in the results section of a research report because it is there that we learn who actually participated in the study. We also may see part of the implementation reflected in the methods section if what occurred during the implementation process changed the sampling or measurement approaches taken. In either case, the information included in a report rarely reflects all of the details of a study's implementation.

The fourth step of analysis and interpretation of the results of a study is reflected in both the results and conclusions sections of a research report. Of all the steps of the research process, probably this one is the most fully described in the report. However, even with this step, a great deal more goes into the process than is reflected in the results and conclusions sections of most reports.

Finally, the fifth step in the research process is the research report itself. However, developing and publishing a research study report also require more effort than may be obvious when looking at the final product. Publication depends on several factors. These include the fit between the purpose of the study and the emphasis of journals that publish research, the relevance and quality of the research study, and the ability of the researcher to express clearly and succinctly all the pertinent elements that are needed to fully understand and use the research. The first two factors primarily affect those who will use the research because they affect what research is available through journals and online. Some research journals publish all types of research in each issue; others develop themes for different issues, limiting the types of studies they will publish at any particular time. Other journals reflect specialties, such as obstetric nursing, and are only interested in research that is relevant to that specialty. Some journals do not want to publish research that is highly theoretical because they target readers who want practical and practice-focused information. To disseminate the study findings, a researcher first has to find journals that fit with the purpose of the completed study.

Some research are not published because problems with the quality of the research are identified during the review process that decreases the meaningfulness or validity of the study's results. This does not mean that the research was bad but simply that some flaw or aspect of the study creates enough doubt about the findings or meaning of the results to preclude its warranting publication.

Another factor that affects publication is the ability of the researcher to express in writing adequate information to describe accurately the entire research process. Many of the common errors in research reports that we will discuss throughout this book are errors of omission or lack of complete information. The research process requires much more thought and work than can be described in a research report. The challenge for a researcher, then, and for the reviewers and editors who contribute to the final publication is to describe clearly and completely all the aspects of the research process that were relevant to their particular study. The goal is to provide the readers with enough information to allow them to understand the study fully and to make intelligent decisions about the usefulness and meaning of the research for practice. One way this is accomplished is by using the language of research to limit the need to fully explain each study aspect. Yet, that very language of research may interfere with using research in practice because the practitioner may not be familiar with or understand the language.

 ## CRITICALLY READING RESEARCH FOR PRACTICE

In Chapter 1, you were introduced to five questions that will be used to organize this text. These questions also provide a broad framework for critically reading reports to evaluate their usefulness as evidence for your EBP practice. As a bachelor's-prepared healthcare provider, you are not expected to critique research reports in depth for their scientific soundness; however, it is important that you are able to critically evaluate research reports to decide whether they can serve as evidence related to your clinical practice question. Therefore, at the end of most of the chapters, we will include a section about common errors in research reports and list a set of questions to ask yourself that will allow you to critically evaluate research reports. Figure 2.4 presents six boxes containing the critical reading questions for the five broad questions that organize this text. Each of these sets of questions will be discussed in detail in the later chapters and are included here primarily to introduce you to them.

PUBLISHED REPORT—WHAT DID YOU CONCLUDE?

We have discussed briefly all of the sections in the published research studies about adolescents and obesity. The authors of those studies report directly that adolescents with obesity face health-related issues affecting their experiences both as an adolescent and as

---

How to Critically Read the Conclusions Section of a Research Report

Does the report answer the question
"What is the answer to my practice question—what did the study conclude?"

- Did the report include a conclusions section?
- Did the conclusions section assist me with my clinical problem?
- Did the conclusions assist in a general manner or provide specific information about my clinical problem?
- Did the conclusions section include limitations of the study?
- Did the limitations diminish my ability to use the conclusions in practice?
- Do the conclusions seem reasonable or warranted based on the results of the study?

⇓

How to Critically Read the Results Section of a Research Report

Does the report answer the question
"Why did the authors reach these conclusions—what did they actually find?"

- Did the report include a clearly identified results section?
- Were the results presented appropriately for the information collected?
- Were descriptive versus inferential results identifiable if this is a quantitative study?
- Were themes or structure and meaning identifiable if this is a qualitative study?
- Were the results presented in a clear and logical manner?
- Did the results include information about the final sample for the study?

⇓

How to Critically Read the Sample Section of a Research Report

Does the report answer the question
"To what types of patients do these research conclusions apply—who was in the study?"

- Did the report include a clearly identified section or paragraphs about sampling?
- Did the report give me enough information to understand how and why this sample was chosen?
- Is there enough information about the sample to tell me if the research is relevant for my clinical population?
- Was enough information given for me to understand how rights of human subjects were protected?
- Would my patient population have been placed at risk if they had participated in this study?
- Can I identify how information was collected about the sample? *(continued)*

FIGURE 2.4 Questions for critically reading research reports.

How to Critically Read the Methods Section of a Research Report

Does the report answer the question
"How were those people studied—why was the study performed that way?"

• Did the report include a clearly identified section describing methods used in this study?
• Do the methods make this a quantitative or a qualitative study?
• Do I understand what my patient population would be doing if they were in this study or a study using similar methods?
• Do the measures and procedures in this study address my clinical problem?
• Do I think that the measures used in this study would provide helpful and useful information when used with my patient population?
• Do I think what the researcher collected and the method of collection was the best way to address the clinical question?
• Do I think that the researcher(s) should have planned the study differently in order to answer my clinical question?

⇓

How to Critically Read the Description of Study Design in a Research Report

Does the report answer the question
"How were those people studied—why was the study performed that way?"

• Did the report include a clearly identified section describing the research design?
• Does the design make this a quantitative, qualitative, or mixed method study?
• Does the report address approaches taken to assure study rigor, internal validity, and/or external validity?
• Do I think that the researcher(s) should have designed the study differently in order to answer my clinical question?

⇓

How to Critically Read the Background Section of a Research Report

Does the report answer the question
"Why ask that question—what do we know?"

• Did the report include a clearly identified background and/or literature review section?
• Do I think the background discusses aspects of my clinical question?
• Does the literature help me understand why the research question is important to nursing?
• Is the majority of the literature cited current (less than 5 years old) or very important to understanding the research question?
• If a nursing or other theory was presented, does it connect to my clinical question?
• Is the specific research question/problem/hypothesis connected logically to the literature and/or theory presented in the background section?
• Is the specific research question/problem/hypothesis relevant or related to my clinical question?

FIGURE 2.4 *(continued)*

an adult. The studies also report that adolescents need support for their weight concerns. If you were the healthcare provider in the clinical case, would you now know how to develop a plan of care for M.D.? Why or why not?

One reason it may be difficult to decide how to develop a care plan for M.D. based on the research report is because the healthcare provider may still have questions about the research. What kinds of questions do you think the school nurse may have about how to proceed in the care of M.D.? One question might be whether you can believe the results of the study about perceptions of caring or whether the results are "strong" enough that you are willing to develop a plan of care around that evidence. A second question might be why the study did not address the issue of health-promoting behaviors in relation to weight. A third question might pertain to what adolescents perceive as important to promote their own health. You can probably think of other questions. With a further understanding of the research language and the research process, it is possible to answer most of the questions posed by reading the published report in more detail. In the next chapter, we look more closely at the conclusions of research reports and what they can tell us about patient care questions.

SUMMARY

In this chapter, we have examined all the components of a research report and at least have begun to become familiar with the unique language of research. Specifically, we have learned that conclusions are the last section of most research reports and that they identify what was found and complete a report by identifying an outcome. We now understand that the results section of a report contains a summary or condensed version of what the authors believe are the most important findings and that results may be presented as numbers or as words, depending on the data collected for the study. We understand that the methods section of a research report describes the overall process of how the researchers went about implementing the research study, including who was included in the study, how information was collected, and what interventions, if any, were tested. We learned that there are three approaches to research: (1) qualitative methods, which focus on understanding the complexity of humans within the context of their lives and attempt to build a whole or complete picture of a phenomenon of interest, (2) quantitative methods, which focus on understanding and breaking down the different parts of a phenomenon into its parts to see how they do or do not connect as well as involve collecting information that is specific and limited to the particular parts of events or phenomena being studied, and (3) mixed method, which uses both qualitative and quantitative approaches to find and identify parts and determine connections of a phenomenon of interest. Last, we discussed the problem section of a research report, which describes the gap in knowledge addressed by the research study. In this section, the researcher explains why the study was needed, why it was carried out in the manner that it was, and, often, what the researcher is specifically asking or predicting.

Besides examining all the components of a research report, we looked at how those sections relate to the actual steps of the research process, and we considered some special types of research reports such as a metasynthesis, meta-analysis, systematic review, and quality improvement reports. We are now ready to begin looking at each section of a research report in detail in order to assure that you can read and use research as evidence for your professional practice.

OUT-OF-CLASS EXERCISE

Differing Conclusions From the Class Study

The fictional article in Appendix B represents the kind of report that might be written based on a questionnaire that you may have completed in class. In that article, the author suggests that older students may be interested in nonacute settings because they have had more experiences with healthcare in several settings. In preparation for the next chapter, write a concluding paragraph that could be used to end the fictional article by taking the position that nursing programs must focus on recruiting older students so that more nurses can be obtained for general care and nursing home settings. Then, write a different paragraph taking the opposite position that age should not be considered when recruiting nursing students because it is not clear whether it contributes to choice of nursing practice after graduation. Base your arguments on the findings reported in the fictional article—not solely on your opinions or ideas. Once you complete this exercise, you are ready to read Chapter 3.

References

Cromley, T., Knatz, S., Rockwell, R. A., Neumark-Sztainer, D., Story, M., & Boutelle, K. (2012). Relationships between body satisfaction and psychological functioning and weight-related cognitions and behaviors in overweight adolescents. *Journal of Adolescent Health*, *50*(2012), 651–653. doi:10.1016/j.jaohealth.2011.10.252

Lazarus, R. S. (1993). Coping, theory and research: Past, present and future. *Psychosomatic Medicine*, *55*, 234–247.

Li, W., Rukavina, P. B., & Foster, C. (2013). Overweight or obese students' perceptions of caring in Urban Physical Education Programs. *Journal of Sport Behavior*, *36*(2), 189–208.

Neuman, B. (1982). *The Neuman system model: Application to nursing education and practice*. East Norwalk, CT: Appleton-Century-Crofts.

Roy, C. (1984). *Introduction to nursing: An adaptation model* (2nd ed.). Englewood Cliffs, NJ: Prentice-Hall.

Watson, J. (1985). *Human science and human caring: A theory of nursing*. Norwalk, CT: Appleton-Century-Crofts.

Resources: Online

Agency for Healthcare Research and Quality. http://www.ahcpr.gov

American Society for Quality—Home. http://www.asq.org

American Society for Quality—Six Sigma. http://asq.org/six-sigma/

Canadian Foundation for Healthcare Improvement. http://www.cfhi-fcass.ca/whatwedo/AppliedResearchandPolicyAnalysis/PrimaryHealthcare/ImprovingPrimaryHealthcare.aspx

Institute for Health Care Improvement Project. http://www.hciproject.org

Institute for Safe Medication Practices. http://www.ismp.org/

The Joint Commission. http://www.jointcommission.org

Joint Commission Center for Transforming Healthcare. http://www.centerfortransforminghealthcare.org/

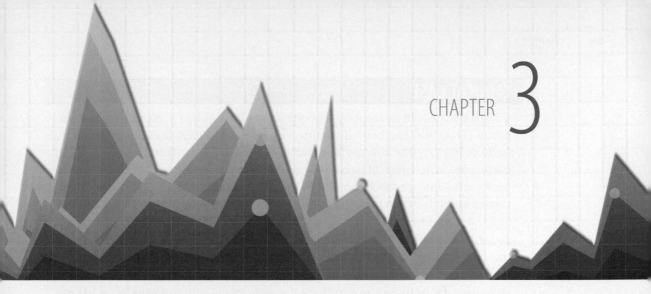

CHAPTER 3

Discussions and Conclusions

What Is the Answer to My Question—What Did the Study Conclude?

LEARNING OBJECTIVE The student will interpret the conclusions of research reports for their potential meaning for evidence-based practice (EBP).

The End of a Research Report—Discussions and Conclusions
Discussions

Summary
Comparison
Speculation
Implications for Practice

Conclusions

Can Conclusions Differ?
Do We Change Practice?

Common Errors in Research Reports
Critically Reading Discussion and Conclusion Sections of Reports
Published Reports—What Would You Conclude?

KEY TERMS

Conceptualization
Confirmation
Discussion
Generalization

Replication
Speculation
Study design

CLINICAL CASE

C.T. is a 63-year-old elementary schoolteacher who has had a left total hip arthroplasty (THA) and has been discharged home several days ago. She is currently undergoing physical therapy and home exercises. C.T. has been encouraged to participate in activities of daily living as much as possible; however, she is having back pain. During a follow-up visit at the orthopedic clinic, C.T. states she is concerned about her back pain. She mentions that she thinks that there is a difference in the length of her left leg and wonders if the cement used for her hip implant caused the problem. The orthopedic surgeon addresses C.T.'s concerns. Following the appointment, the orthopedic surgeon begins asking other orthopedic surgeons about leg length differences after THA surgery when cemented implants were used. From those conversations, the orthopedic surgeon wonders if the implant used (cementless vs. cemented) makes a difference in whether patients have more (or less) leg length differences. The orthopedic surgeon does a quick search in ProQuest using the keywords "total hip replacement," "cemented implants," and "leg length," which yields numerous hits. Several appear relevant, but one stuck out because the abstract addressed all three factors (key words) relative to the patient seen by the orthopedic surgeon, and the study was just completed. The article is titled "Leg Length Discrepancy in Cementless Total Hip Arthroplasty" (Peck, Malhotra, & Kim, 2011).

You can find this article in Appendix A-3. Reading the conclusion or discussion sections of this article will help you to understand the examples discussed in this chapter. In addition, Table 3.1 summarizes the clinical question and the key search words used by the orthopedic surgeon in the clinical case. We will include similar tables after clinical cases in later chapters to help you see how a good question for EBP is formed and how you could search for available evidence.

TABLE 3.1   Development of a Clinical Question from the Clinical Case

WHAT THA IMPLANT APPROACH (CEMENTED OR CEMENTLESS) CAN DECREASE POSTSURGICAL LEG LENGTH DIFFERENCES IN PATIENTS UNDERGOING THA SURGERY?

The *Who*	Patients having THA (replacements)
The *What*	Leg length differences
The *When*	During a THA surgical approach
The *Where*	Postsurgical
Key search terms useful in finding research-based evidence for this practice question	• Leg length • THA • Implant approach
PICO – PICOT	
P	Patients having THA (replacements)
I	Implant approach (cement or cementless)
C	Leg length equality
O	Postsurgery
T	N/A*

*Article does not address a specific length of time.

THE END OF A RESEARCH REPORT—DISCUSSIONS AND CONCLUSIONS

In this chapter, we address the first of the five questions that are used to organize this book: What is the answer to my practice question—what did the study conclude? As mentioned in Chapter 1, the major reason a practicing healthcare professional wants to read and understand research is to answer clinical questions; so the professional healthcare providers, such as the one in the clinical case, often go directly to the last section of a research report. That section is sometimes labeled "Discussion" or "Conclusions" or both, but its content usually includes both a discussion and conclusions, as described here.

When the healthcare provider who is interested in finding out whether the cemented hip implant impacts leg length discrepancies in patients who have undergone THA (replacement) reads the discussion section of the report on leg length discrepancies based on cemented or cementless implants study, the surgeon learns from the study that there are no significant differences in leg length discrepancies in patients who had cemented implants and those who had cementless implants. The surgeon continues reading the discussion and learns that other studies were done on leg length discrepancies between cemented and cementless implants. Peck et al. (2011) discuss a study by Leonard, Magill, Keily, and Khayyat that found a significant difference between cemented and cementless implants and leg length discrepancies. Leonard et al. found that cementless implants had a greater degree of leg lengthening than did cemented implants. The authors of the research report found by the orthopedic surgeon from our case study discuss the limitations of the research study in the discussion section of the research report. In the conclusion section of the study, the authors of the research report suggest that surgeons should be concerned with "preoperative templating both cemented and cementless procedures" to limit leg lengthening discrepancies (Peck et al., 2011), as both types of implants offer effective and safe treatment for degenerative hip disease. The surgeon's likely response to reading the discussion and conclusion sections of this report is "While I know that this study showed little leg length differences between cemented and cementless implants what do I do now?"

The discussion and conclusion sections of research reports initially may not be helpful in clinical questions for several reasons, including the following:

- The study may not address the question you are asking.
- The researchers may have had problems implementing the study, resulting in an unclear answer.
- The results of the study may have been unexpected or complex and increase, rather than decrease, possible answers to the question.

Later chapters address why research questions may not directly address clinical questions and the many problems that can occur when carrying out a research study. Although this chapter discusses briefly how unexpected results can affect clinical usefulness, understanding results and the results sections of research reports is discussed more completely in Chapter 4. This chapter focuses on a fourth reason why the conclusion of a report may not answer a clinical question: the healthcare provider having inappropriate or unclear expectations about what information can be found in the conclusion of a research report. Just what should we expect to find from the discussion and conclusion sections of research reports?

DISCUSSIONS

This book treats discussions and conclusions as two separate sections, but remember that you often find them combined in published reports. Table 3.2 summarizes the major components of most discussion and conclusion sections. The **discussion** section of a research

TABLE 3.2	General Components of the Discussion and Conclusion Sections of Research Reports
SECTION OF REPORT	MAJOR COMPONENTS OF THE SECTION
Discussion	• Summary of key findings • Comparison of results with those of previous studies • Description of whether findings confirm results of similar studies or predictions based on theory • Speculation about possible interpretations of results
Conclusion	• Description of the new knowledge that can be accepted on the basis of the study • A conceptualization of the meaning of the results or a generalization of the findings • A description of study limitations

report summarizes, compares, and speculates about the results of the study. Let us examine these pieces, starting with summarizing.

Summary

The first part of the discussion section in a research report usually includes a summary of the study's key results. This summary usually addresses the results that directly relate to the major research question posed by the researcher(s). It also includes the unexpected results and those that stood out as being particularly meaningful. However, this summary is usually brief because it follows a detailed description of the results. It is also likely, unless the study had few findings, that it will not include all of the results from the study. What the brief summary does include are the specific results from the study that the researcher believes are particularly important and meaningful.

For example, the discussion section on the leg length discrepancy study (Peck et al., 2011) discusses the impact of leg length discrepancies on "post-operative complications and patient dissatisfaction" and tells us that "studies confirm that a discrepancy in leg length has a direct adverse effect on clinical and functional outcome" (p. 184). The current study demonstrates that using either cemented or cementless implants for hip joint replacements can resolve functional problems associated with degenerative hip disease. The authors also discuss how surgeons can plan preoperative and intraoperative measuring methods to limit leg length discrepancies.

Comparison

After a brief summary of key or important results, the discussion section of a research report debates the possible meanings of the study results. Questions addressed in research studies are rarely simple or readily answered completely by only one study; therefore, the results provide information that can be explained or understood in several ways. Hence, the pros and cons of different explanations for the results may be described, forming a written debate. Further, the meaning of the findings must usually be interpreted within the context of existing knowledge, so the discussion section frequently compares the study's results with those of previous studies. The match or lack of match of results of a study to results from previous studies supports the different explanations offered regarding the results. Another important reason for comparing is to provide confirmation of previous findings. **Confirmation** is the verification of results from other studies. Rarely are we comfortable deciding that we are completely certain of the answer to a clinical question based on the findings of only one study. One goal of research is to build knowledge, with each research study adding a new piece to our understanding. However, as with the parts of any building that is going to be stable and strong, the pieces of knowledge must overlap and unite to make a cohesive whole. A study that is a duplication of an earlier study is called a

replication study, and its major purpose is confirmation. Usually, however, a research study differs from past studies in some ways by (for example) using a different patient group in the study or by using different procedures on the subjects. Whether a study is a replication or a variation of previous studies, the discussion section of the research report describes how the findings do or do not overlap with previous knowledge.

 CORE CONCEPT 3.1 _____

The summary of findings in the discussion section of a research report contains only selected results from the study. It does not give the reader a complete picture of the results, but does give information about some key or important results.

In addition to discussing how a study's results do or do not confirm those of previous studies, the authors may compare their findings with the predicted results that were based on existing theory. Theory might be considered to be the plans for the knowledge being built about a clinical question: like the blueprints of a building plan, a theory provides the description of how all the parts of a phenomenon should fit together. Not all research studies are based on a theory or test a prediction from a theory because not enough may be known about a clinical question. However, if the study tests a prediction or hypothesis that was based on a theory and the results show the pieces fitting together as the theory predicted, then the results are considered to confirm that theory. We discuss how theory directs and is built by research in Chapter 10.

The leg length discrepancy study that the surgeon found did not attempt to specifically test theory. Nor did the authors tell us whether the studies cited in the discussion section were based on theory. The discussion section of the article does cite previous studies in which to compare results. Some studies do demonstrate similar findings, helping to verify or confirm a study's results. However, the leg length discrepancy study resulted in a different finding than the other studies cited. This is why we usually need multiple studies to inform our EBP and to make clinical decisions. Results that differ from findings in previous studies require that the author(s) suggest reasons for those differences, which leads us to the third component of most discussion sections.

Speculation

In addition to comparison, the discussion section of a research report speculates about the reasons for the results of the study. **Speculation** is the process of reflecting on results and offering some explanation for them. The debate, or speculation, in a discussion generally considers several alternative explanations for the results and provides a rationale for the author's judgment about which is the best explanation.

 CORE CONCEPT 3.2 _____

The discussion section of a research report contains a debate on how the results of the study fit with existing knowledge and what those results may mean.

As Core Concept 2.3 from Chapter 2 stated, the results section provides the findings of the specific study, whereas the discussion and conclusion sections of a report interpret those findings in light of existing knowledge and theory. This interpretation is appropriately called a *discussion* because it is open to debate. It reflects not fact, but thoughtful, informed speculation. Although such speculation is thoughtful and informed and considers alternative possibilities, it is based on the author's knowledge and selection of previous research or theory. Another author might know or select a different theory or body of research to use in his or her discussion.

Why are the meanings of results from almost any study open to debate? The answer lies, in part, in the nature of research. We learned in Chapter 2 that research usually examines a question using a subgroup or sample of people. Although great pains are often taken to include diversity in the people, samples cannot possibly reflect all of the variation that exists in humans. What works with or happens to a few subjects is unlikely to always be exactly what happens with many patients or with everyone.

In fact, qualitative methods assume that experiences are subjectively unique and that although we can increase our understanding regarding a particular question, there may always be individual variations. Returning to our analogy of building knowledge piece by piece, the qualitative research perspective is that the picture of the phenomenon, which is the product in knowledge building, is constantly evolving because our world and our individual experiences are always changing.

Conceptualization is a process of creating a picture of an abstract idea; in the case of healthcare research, it is a picture of some aspect of health. Discussions and conclusions of qualitative studies conceptualize some phenomenon related to health as opposed to those of quantitative studies that objectify and isolate parts of the phenomenon. For example, a qualitative study might conceptualize patient satisfaction as a person's overall sense of the quality of the care that is received. A quantitative study may examine patient satisfaction as the total score on a survey of the patient's care experience. If theory is the blueprint or plan for a building, we can view a qualitative study as providing results that are an artist's rendition of how the building looks. Similarly, we can view quantitative results as a detailed parts list for constructing the building. The artist's rendition provides a clear sense of how a building might look or even feel and smell, whereas the parts list gives us a sense of how it looks when it is put together and how it might be used, but not of how we will actually experience the building. Figure 3.1 illustrates this concept.

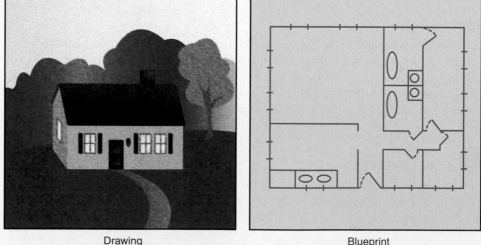

Drawing

Product of qualitative research is like
an artist's rendition.

Blueprint

Product of quantitative research is like a
blueprint, showing details and
how parts go together.

FIGURE 3.1 Products of qualitative versus quantitative research.

From a qualitative perspective, knowledge is built by creating a "picture album" filled with different "pictures" of a particular aspect of health. Each study result, or picture, gives a sense of the aspect of health at a unique moment in time. As we look at more and more pictures, we get a greater sense of the whole phenomenon. Each qualitative study provides a unique picture that adds to our overall understanding.

Quantitative methods do not assume that knowledge is always changing and evolving; they assume that there are answers to questions and that we can find those answers by reducing, objectifying, and quantifying the components of a phenomenon to understand the relationships among the components. For example, in the leg length discrepancy study (Peck et al., 2011), the researchers are using a quantitative research method to help understand how cemented and cementless hip implants relate to leg length. Quantitative methods assume that we get a greater sense of the whole phenomenon by breaking it down to smaller parts, and we get closer and closer to "knowing" the "real" answer to questions when we get the same results in different studies with different groups. The quantitative researcher expects that each study will add more details to the same detailed building plan.

By using both qualitative and quantitative approaches in one study, mixed methods research provides the best of both qualitative and quantitative qualities. Mixed methods research takes a picture of a unique moment in time and quantifies specific components of the phenomenon to study the relationships among the components. The mixed methods approach provides the researcher with better understanding of the building as a whole and more details about the building plan.

The goal of research is to generalize a study's results. **Generalization** is the ability to apply a particular study's findings to the broader population represented by the sample. Let's say, hypothetically, the authors of the leg length discrepancy study have found the cemented implants were better than the cementless implants in improving leg length equality for adults younger than 50 years of age and that this finding is supported by other research studies mentioned in the discussion section. If this study has valid and reliable findings (discussed in future chapters), this study's findings could then be generalized to other populations having THA. Qualitative, quantitative, and mixed methods research strives to develop knowledge that can be applied to a broader population. However, the term *generalization* is more commonly applied to quantitative research than to qualitative or mixed methods research. Nonetheless, a qualitative or mixed methods researcher will often do several procedures to make sure that the findings can also be applied to the population in the area of interest. The value of being able to generalize study findings is an important concept. If the study is conducted well, whether it is a qualitative, quantitative, or mixed method study, then a healthcare provider who reads the study can make better clinical decisions regarding the value of applying the research findings to work with similar populations.

Implications for Practice

The discussion in a research report often includes a debate on the meaning of the study results for clinical practice. For example, the leg length discrepancy article found that cemented or cementless implants did not make a significant difference in the amount of leg length discrepancy for patients undergoing THA. The authors suggest that preoperative measurements and planning and intraoperative measurements can reduce the amount of leg length discrepancy in either cemented or cementless implants. It is important to realize that choices are made concerning the best clinical interpretation of results, just as choices are made about how the results add to existing knowledge in general. This means that the discussion section needs to be read critically and with an awareness of the different meanings that could be assigned to the study findings.

The healthcare professional who reads the discussion section in the leg length discrepancy article is reading the author's interpretations of what is believed to be the key findings. The author clearly states that there is not a significant difference in leg length discrepancy between the use of cemented and cementless implants for hip replacements. The authors then compare key findings with previous studies. Be cautious when reading the comparisons as the authors have chosen which studies to include in comparing research findings. Some authors will provide a rationale as to why studies were chosen for comparison; for example, the same population was studied or the same therapeutic procedure was used, thus making the comparison easier to understand. The authors' speculation about the meaning of the results is most likely based on beliefs and past experiences as well as the results of previous research. The healthcare professional caring for C.T. has one possible answer to the clinical question about the use of cemented or cementless implants for other patients undergoing THA to limit leg length discrepancy. The healthcare professional must read previous sections of the report to decide whether the author's practice implications drawn from the results match the healthcare professional's beliefs and experiences. We return to the healthcare professional's dilemma later in this chapter.

CONCLUSIONS

The conclusions of a research report describe the knowledge that the researcher believes can be gained from the study, given its "fit" with other studies and theories. As stated in Chapter 2 in the discussion of sections of a research report, conclusions from a research study can be powerful because they are used to guide practice. Conclusions move beyond debate or speculation about the results to a statement of what is now "known" about a question or problem. As a result, they are generally worded carefully. Conclusions also may be statements about what we do not know, particularly if the study results do not fit with theory or replicate previous studies. Therefore, it is possible for a conclusion to state that we now know we cannot get the answer for our question using the methods or measures or sample that was used in the study being reported. More often, conclusions include recommendations for building knowledge about a clinical question or health aspect. In either case, the conclusion section almost always describes the limits that must be placed on the knowledge that has been gained from the study.

The leg length discrepancy study does not provide concrete answers to the orthopedic surgeon's questions. One reason for this is that when questions are complex, the research results are open to debate and interpretation. Another reason is that almost every study has limitations. A third reason is that researchers will often collect information via investigation, as opposed to constructing research questions to answer during the study. Remember from Chapter 2 that limitations are the aspects of a study that create uncertainty about the meaning or decisions that can be derived from it. You will note in the leg length discrepancy research report that limitations of the study are addressed in the discussions section. You will find research reports vary with regard to where limitations of the study are described. For example, some research reports have a specific "limitations" section separate from other sections. Wherever placed in the research report, limitations need to be discussed to help the reader appraise the findings before applying them to practice. Several aspects of a study may be viewed as limitations. We have already alluded to one factor that often limits a study: the sampling—who was included in the study. Although the leg length discrepancy study included a convenience sample from previous patient records (retrospective study) that included men and women between the ages of 30 and 88, and included data on leg length discrepancies, the study did not include data on race, health status, or other population characteristics. This aspect of the sample leaves us uncertain about the meaning of the results for patients with complex healthcare needs and patients who are of different racial backgrounds than those involved in the study. The study aims to produce findings that can be used in patients undergoing THA procedures. By using a convenience sample, the picture provided by the study results is limited to patients with degenerative hip disease.

As we will see in Chapters 6 and 7, many other sampling-related aspects can create limits to a research study.

A second factor that may be a limitation is the **study design**—the overall plan or organization of a study. Some study designs create more uncertainty than do others. For example, if the healthcare professional in the clinical case read a study that described nonoperative factors that may affect a patient's leg length, the healthcare professional would be uncertain about whether those factors were present before or after the operative intervention and thus whether they impacted the patient's postoperative leg length. However, the leg length discrepancy study uses a pretest and posttest design in which leg length measures were taken preoperatively, intraoperatively, and postoperatively; this design removes some of the uncertainty about the clinical use of results because we know the outcome change that occurred between the beginning and the end of the study. Many factors affect a researcher's decision about a study design, including the type of question being asked, the level of existing knowledge, and the availability of resources. Chapter 9 discusses research designs in more detail.

A third factor that may be a limitation involves the measures used in the study. Several problems can occur with study measures. For example, a study's measures may be inconsistent. If blood sugar is measured by using a glucometer that loses calibration halfway through the study, the resulting measures will be inconsistent. Sometimes paper-and-pencil questionnaires are unclear or confusing, causing people to be inconsistent in their understanding of, and therefore answers to, the questions. Another possible problem is that measures may be inaccurate or incomplete. Returning to the study using a glucometer for measuring blood sugars, if the glucometer had gone out of calibration before the study began, the resulting measures would be consistent but inaccurate throughout the study. That is, the measures would consistently be inaccurate. Accuracy and consistency of measures are referred to as *validity*, *rigor*, and *reliability* in research. The examples given in this paragraph are all reflective of quantitative research, although accuracy and consistency are also a problem in qualitative and mixed methods research. These ideas are the focus of Chapter 8 and will be explored in detail in that chapter.

Finding accurate measures of concepts in quantitative research is a problem in healthcare because it is difficult to find ways to quantify some concepts that are important to healthcare professionals such as anger, quality of life, pain, or self-confidence. If measures do not exist, the researcher will either have to make one or not include that factor in the study. Excluding an important factor limits the conclusions that can be drawn. For example, hypothetically, if a limitation was identified where the author did not assess leg length in the participants before the THA surgery, the researcher might assume that some of the leg length discrepancy findings are related to whether the implant was cemented or cementless. Without baseline measures taken before the THA surgery, the researcher's finding is just an assumption. This hypothetical lack of preoperative leg length measurement presents the possibility that findings of leg length discrepancies are actually the result of whether the implant was cemented or cementless when in fact both methods may limit discrepancies in leg length. Without a preassessment of leg length, how can the researcher make claims about which implant method improves leg length equality?

The methods used in a study are a fourth factor that may limit the conclusions. Not only does a measurement need to be consistent and accurate, but it must also be used consistently and accurately. An appropriately calibrated glucometer will still provide results that are inconclusive regarding a person's blood sugar if it is used at different times during the day and with different techniques to acquire blood samples. Similarly, a measure of a person's knowledge about HIV will not be conclusive if one group completed the measure immediately after a patient education program and the other group completed it 2 weeks after their education program. Therefore, the methods used to conduct a study also may lead to limitations in the conclusions.

The discussion and conclusions sections of a research report, then, include a summary of key results, a comparison of those results with findings from other studies or to existing theory, speculation and debate about the possible explanations for the results and how they fit with current knowledge, a description of study limitations, and, finally, some carefully worded decisions about new knowledge gained in the study. These sections include debate, speculation, and cautious language because research questions are complex, each study contributes only one new piece to the puzzle or one more picture to the phenomenon, and almost every study has some limitations.

Can Conclusions Differ?

At the end of Chapter 2, you were asked to write two concluding paragraphs for the fictional article in Appendix B, taking two different positions regarding who should be recruited for nursing programs, based on results reported in the article. Reviewing the results reported in that study, we find that age, type of program, and rating of health affected choice of nursing field. We assume that the goal is to focus recruitment of students on increasing the number of graduates who enter fields that are not considered acute, a goal with which you may not personally agree. One way to interpret the results is to focus on the finding that age was an important factor in choice of field and conclude that older students should be recruited. Therefore, the new knowledge gleaned from the study would be that recruiting older students will increase the numbers of new graduates entering nonacute nursing fields.

However, the finding that health rating was important could mean that the relevant factor is not age and experience, as the author suggests. Rather, the relevant factor may instead be level of health, with students who perceive themselves as less healthy selecting fields of practice that are generally considered less physically strenuous. If this is true, then age is not the relevant factor. Rather, schools of nursing must recruit students who want less physically strenuous positions. This second conclusion would probably be considered relatively implausible, but it illustrates that conclusions can differ depending on the interpretation of the results. Because the conclusions drawn from study results can differ as you read discussions and conclusions of research reports, you should carefully consider whether the interpretation provided makes sense to you in terms of your own knowledge and practice.

Do We Change Practice?

We have emphasized that the conclusions of research reports can be powerful because they are used to change practice. We have also pointed out some of the uncertainty that is reflected in most conclusions. Most importantly, we have said that the purpose for healthcare professionals to intelligently understand research is for them to apply and evaluate its use in practice. Recognizing the limitations of each research study and the complexity of building new knowledge does not imply that research cannot and should not be used in practice. However, it does mean that it is essential to have some understanding of more than just the study conclusions. We must understand why and how the limitations such as sampling, measures, methods, or design make the results uncertain, and we must look intelligently at the study findings to determine whether the author's interpretation is logical.

Each research study reflects only one piece or picture in the process of knowledge building, which is why healthcare professionals emphasize the use of systematic reviews. Systematic reviews include the results from many studies as evidence for practice. They compile the results of multiple studies regarding the same clinical question and organize the findings around key aspects related to practice. A systematic review also addresses differences in research studies, such as design, sample, and methods. The end of a systematic review is usually titled "Practice Implications" and summarizes the practice-related points that are most strongly supported by different research studies.

As with individual studies, however, systematic reviews are open to interpretation because the findings of particular studies can be given more or less attention. For example, the author of a systematic review may place less emphasis on negative findings about a procedure and interpret the positive findings to warrant a change in clinical practice. An author may also believe that any negative finding about a procedure questions its use and interprets any negative research to indicate that a procedure should not be adopted in practice. As in individual studies, the conclusions of systematic reviews include some hesitancy or caution and almost always include recommendations for further research. Systematic reviews as evidence for practice can be helpful, but the healthcare professional must still read the review carefully and intelligently to decide how the findings should be used in practice.

COMMON ERRORS IN RESEARCH REPORTS

To be read and used intelligently in practice, the research report must clearly and completely give the reader needed information. Many healthcare professionals assume that if they are not comfortable in their understanding of a research study, it is because they lack knowledge. While this may be the case, it is also possible that part of the problem is a lack of clarity in the research report. While we will summarize below the common ways in which a report can be unclear, we will also discuss common errors that may be found in research reports in later chapters. We do this to help you recognize that sometimes the problem lies not with your knowledge, but with the information provided to you. Appraising research reports allows you to make decisions about the report and associated findings.

As an example of errors in research reports, you may see a failure to include one or more major aspects of a discussion and conclusion. The authors should provide the information discussed in the discussion and conclusions sections. As a research reader, you should expect to find a summary of key findings, a comparison of the findings with previous research, and an interpretation of the meaning of the findings within the context of current knowledge. Also, you should find some discussion of the study limitations. The fictional article in Appendix B provides an example of a report that does not include important aspects because it neither compares its results with previous studies nor includes any discussion of study limitations.

A second common error is presenting a confusing summary of key findings or presenting new results. The summary should use language that is consistent with both the common use of terms and how the terms were used throughout the report. It should not include key findings that were not already described in more detail in the results section. Because we are starting at the end of a report, we might not know that information in the discussion was not addressed in the results, but we can quickly find this out if we read the results section. The summary of key findings is a brief, succinct summation. If a result is only provided at the end of a report in this manner, we will likely not have enough information about it to judge intelligently the usefulness of that finding for practice.

A third common error in research reports is overinterpreting the results. Like healthcare professionals in practice, researchers want answers to the questions they study. Therefore, it is tempting to overinterpret results by reading into them, generalizing them beyond what was actually found, or discounting the limitations. It is expected that a researcher will understate or be conservative when interpreting study results. However, occasionally, a report presents an interpretation that makes suggestions that are more than what can reasonably be concluded based on the results of the study. Similarly, occasionally, a research report draws conclusions that are not directly related to the question under study. It is important to read the conclusions of a study carefully and remember that conclusions are, in part, the speculation of the author. Part of being a healthcare professional who uses EBP effectively is to be a careful reader who thinks discriminately about the conclusions drawn from a study.

CRITICALLY READING DISCUSSION AND CONCLUSION SECTIONS OF REPORTS

In Chapter 1, you were introduced to five questions that will be used to organize this text. These questions also provide a broad framework for critically reading reports to evaluate their usefulness as evidence for your EBP. Remember, as a healthcare professional, you are not expected to critique research reports in depth for their scientific soundness. However, you are expected to be able to critically evaluate research reports to decide whether they can serve as evidence related to your clinical practice question. Therefore, Box 3.1 presents a set of six questions that you can use to help you in the process of critically reading the discussion and conclusion sections of a report.

BOX 3.1
How to Critically Read the Discussion and Conclusion Sections of a Report

Do the discussion and conclusion sections answer the question "Did the section provide an answer to my practice question—what did the study conclude?"

1. Did the report include a discussion and/or conclusion section?
2. Did the discussion/conclusion section assist me with my clinical problem?
3. Did the discussion/conclusion assist in a general manner or provide specific information about my clinical problem?
4. Did the discussion/conclusion section include limitations of the study?
5. Did the limitations diminish my ability to use the conclusions in practice?
6. Do the discussion/conclusions seem reasonable or warranted on the basis of the results of the study?

The first question to ask yourself is "Did the report include a discussion and/or conclusion section?" While this may seem like a simple question, some reports of research do not present much of a conclusion section, or it is not easy to find and may be buried toward the end of the article. The leg length discrepancy research report includes both a "conclusions" and "discussions" section. A second question to consider when critically reading the discussion and conclusion sections of a report is "Did the discussion/conclusion section assist me with my clinical problem?" To answer this, one needs to compare the *Who*, *Where*, *What*, and *When* contained in the discussion with that of your clinical question. The healthcare professional in our clinical case asks the question "What implant approach can decrease postoperative leg length differences in patients undergoing THA surgery?" If we look at the discussion section of the leg length discrepancy article, we find that it discusses implant approaches (cemented and cementless) and resulting leg length differences, making it a very good match to our orthopedic surgeon's clinical question. The orthopedic surgeon in our clinical case would learn how the implant approach could be used in trying to decrease leg length discrepancy in patients undergoing THA surgery.

The third question to ask yourself as you critically read the discussion and conclusion sections of a report is "Did the discussion/conclusion assist in a general manner or provide specific information about my clinical problem?" The answer is based on the healthcare professional's sense of how easily he or she can change their practice after reading the conclusions of the leg length discrepancy report. While the report assisted the healthcare provider in knowing that leg length discrepancies were commonly associated with THA surgery, the results were not totally supported by other studies mentioned in the discussion section of the report. A fourth question "Did the discussion/conclusion section include limitations of the study?" is answered by examining the discussion section of the report. The leg length discrepancy study described limitations within the discussion section of the article. The authors discuss limitations associated with the varied measurement methods used by five different orthopedic surgeons. The convenience sampling of the study is a limitation as well as the fact that the participants were patients from the same hospital. Limitations will be discussed in more detail in Chapters 6, 8, and 9. Studies may include patients that are not typical and may not closely resemble the patients our healthcare provider sees in the clinical case.

It is important to stop and think about statements such as the ones made by the researcher in the "Limitations" section, which leads us to the next question we need to ask ourselves when critically reading the discussion and conclusion sections of a report: "Did the limitations diminish my ability to use the conclusions in practice?" What do you think it means that the authors used a convenience sampling? How could it influence the interpretation of the findings that are presented? Does it increase, decrease, or not affect the healthcare provider's willingness to use these results in resolving the clinical question? This is the process of critically thinking about the evidence for EBP. As you answer these questions, it is important to remember that all studies will have limitations. It is an unavoidable aspect of studying living patients. The question to answer is whether or not the limitations are so limiting that the results cannot be generalized to your patients.

The final question to ask when critically reading the discussion and conclusion sections of a report is "Do discussion/conclusions seem reasonable or warranted based on the results of the study?" To answer this, you need to think about what the conclusions seem to say that a healthcare provider should do, and then see if the results section of the report supports this. To know whether this is a logical and clear conclusion, we will need to read the results section carefully. How this should be done is presented in Chapters 4 and 5. We will revisit this question after we learn more about critically reading the results section of research reports.

PUBLISHED REPORTS—WHAT WOULD YOU CONCLUDE?

The discussion and conclusion sections of the report found by the healthcare provider in the clinical case tell us several different things. They tell us that leg length discrepancies are common in patients undergoing THA surgeries and that cemented and cementless implant approaches are available. The discussion section tells us that other studies may have found different results and that using preoperative, intraoperative, and postoperative measures and planning is essential in reducing leg length discrepancies. This confirms the orthopedic surgeon's impression that there may be something that could be done to avoid leg length differences in patients undergoing THA. The conclusion section did not provide the healthcare provider with specific information about the findings, so the healthcare provider will need to read the results section to answer that question.

The conclusions from this report may contradict another report found by the orthopedic surgeon. This is often one of the most confusing and frustrating aspects of searching the literature for use in EBP. However, it is most often possible to fit the conclusions of apparently contradictory studies together in a meaningful way. For example, the orthopedic surgeon might decide from the leg length article that he or she must help other staff to preplan implant templating, use reliable measurements, and recognize and look for leg length discrepancies in all patients undergoing THA surgery. At the same time, another study may suggest that leg length differences in patients may be associated with underlying pathological conditions. With the results of the two studies combined, the orthopedic surgeon might plan to include additional assessments that may indicate the presence of an underlying condition before the THA is performed.

The discussion and conclusion section of a research report provides useful information for using research in practice, including a summary of key findings from the study, a comparison of the findings with previous research and theory, and an interpretation of the meaning of the findings. However, although the conclusions begin to answer the orthopedic surgeon's clinical question, he or she will probably want to know more about the assessments that were used in determining leg length discrepancies. This means that the orthopedic surgeon must read the preceding section of the research report—the methods section.

OUT-OF-CLASS EXERCISE

How Do We Organize a Large Amount of Information to Make Sense of It?

Chapters 4 and 5 discuss the results section of research reports. As we mentioned in Chapter 2, these sections often include some of the most complex and confusing language for those readers who are not advanced researchers. We look at some of the key terms in results sections that can readily be understood without having an advanced degree in statistics and discuss how to determine what you need to really understand and intelligently use nursing research in practice.

To prepare for Chapter 4, summarize some of the data from your in-class study exercise in a way that makes it easier to understand or that makes sense of it. When doing this, think about why your method of organization helps to make it easier to understand. If you did not have an in-class study, your faculty may provide you with some data to use for this out-of-class exercise. Once you have completed this exercise, you are ready to read Chapter 4.

Reference

Peck, C. N., Malhotra, K., & Kim, W. Y. (2011). Leg length discrepancy in cementless total hip arthroplasty. *Surgical Science*, *2*, e183–e187. doi:10.4236/ss.2011.24040

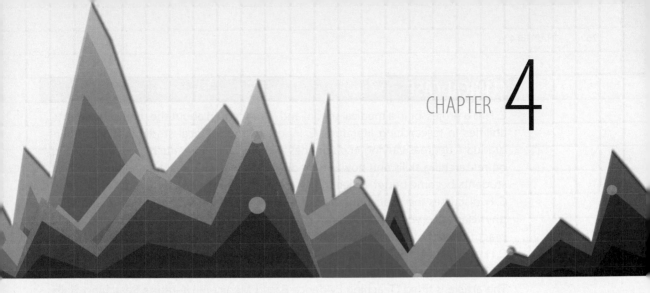

CHAPTER 4

Descriptive Results

Why Did the Authors Reach Their Conclusion—
What Did They Actually Find?

LEARNING OBJECTIVE The student will analyze the relationship between the descriptive results of research reports and the selected conclusion of the reports.

Differentiating Description From Inference
Understanding the Language of Results Sections

Language Describing Results From Qualitative Studies
Language Describing Results From Quantitative Studies

Connecting Results That Describe Conclusions
Common Errors in the Reports of Descriptive Results
Critically Reading Results Sections of Research Reports for Use in Evidence-Based Healthcare Practice
Published Report—What Would You Conclude?

KEY TERMS

Bivariate analysis	Frequency distribution	Normal curve
Categorization scheme	Independent variables	Predictor variables
Coding	Inferential statistics	Skew
Content analysis	Inference	Standard deviation
Data reduction	Mean	Theme
Data saturation	Measure of central	Univariate analysis
Demographic	tendency	Variable
Dependent variable	Median	Variance
Distribution	Mode	

CLINICAL CASE

C. H. is a professor in a medical school and is concerned about the medical students' abilities in researching literature. C. H. knows the medical students have under-graduate degrees varying in disciplines and wonders how much focus was placed on researching skills and how the medical school should react in helping medical students become better skilled at using literature in making decisions for practice. C. H. discusses the issue with other professors in the medical school and with local physicians. Everyone agrees literature searching skills are essential skills for medical practitioners, however; there is disagreement in how to help the medical students. C. H. conducts a literature search on Medline using the keywords "medical students" and "literature search" and finds a current article that may address the situation. The article is titled "Teaching Evidence-Based Medicine Literature Searching Skills to Medical Students During the Clinical Years: A Randomized Controlled Trial" by Ilic, Tepper, and Misso (2012).

You can find this article in Appendix A-4. Reading the results section on this article and the other articles in Appendix A and B will help you understand the examples discussed in this chapter. In addition, Table 4.1 summarizes the clinical question for this case study.

DIFFERENTIATING DESCRIPTION FROM INFERENCE

At the end of Chapter 3, we decided that to base clinical decisions on the conclusions of a research report, we need to have a better understanding of the study results. The results are the specific findings of a study that can provide an answer to the second question we are using to organize this book: Why did the authors reach their conclusion—what did they actually find? This chapter and Chapter 5 address this question.

The results sections of reports summarize findings with two broad goals: (1) to describe or explain the phenomenon of interest and (2) to predict aspects related to that phenomenon. Because qualitative studies approach knowledge development with an expectation of increasing understanding to inform practice, their results use data analysis methods to provide description and explanation. In contrast, quantitative studies may

TABLE 4.1 Development of Clinical Question From the Clinical Case	
WHAT STRATEGIES ASSIST MEDICAL STUDENTS IN PERFORMING EVIDENCE-BASED LITERATURE SEARCHING SKILLS DURING CLINICAL PRACTICE?	
The *Who*	Medical students
The *What*	Evidence-based literature searching skills
The *When*	During medical school clinical practice
The *Where*	Clinical practice locations
Key search to find research-based evidence for practice	• Medical students • Literature search
PICO – PICOT	
P	Medical student
I	Evidence-based literature searching strategy
C	No evidence-based literature searching strategy
O	Literature searching competencies
T	Third year of medical school for medical student

predict, as well as describe and explain, because the assumption behind them is that there is generalized objectivity. Quantitative data analysis aims not only to describe and explain but also allows us to infer what would happen with other similar groups based on what was found in the present study. **Inference** is the reasoning that goes into the process of drawing a conclusion based on evidence and is common in research work. It refers to the statistical procedures used in most quantitative studies, which therefore are called **inferential statistics**.

 CORE CONCEPT 4.1

1. Qualitative studies increase understanding of a phenomenon.
2. Quantitative studies describe and explain a phenomenon allowing us to infer what would happen to other similar groups.

It is important to differentiate between results that merely describe what the researcher found and results that are intended to allow inference because it directly affects what we can conclude from a study. The knowledge we gain from description can assist in the under-standing of a situation or phenomenon, and that understanding can help us in our clinical practice. Description does not allow us to predict the future or to understand what causes the phenomena that we have described.

To understand cause and effect and to make predictions, we must know not only what is present at a given point in time but also the order of factors or events and the timing of such events or factors. Why can't description allow us to predict? When we describe the presence of two or more factors, we know that they are present concurrently, but we do not know if one came before the other, if one caused the other, or if some other outside event caused both. Take the simple example of driving a car. If one were to describe the factors involved in driving, one would think of a car, a key, a driver, and a license. However, which factor must come first is not necessarily obvious from that description. Do we need a driver first to get a license? Or, do we need a car before we can have a driver? Description does not give us order and timing, so it does not allow us to predict.

 CORE CONCEPT 4.2

Results that allow us to predict include information about the order and timing of events or factors.

Only results that allow us to infer provide information that is useful to predict future responses or situations if the same set of circumstances applies. Results that allow us to pre-dict include information about the order of events or factors and the timing of those events or factors. Therefore, results that are intended to allow inference may be used in clinical practice to predict future health-related outcomes under similar circumstances. The article about literature searching skills found by C. H. in the clinical case for this chapter uses inferential statistics in the results section. These results indicate that there is not a signifi-cant difference in literature searching skills between a group of medical students who had a literature searching workshop and the group that did not have a workshop. These results could be used by C. H. and other professors in the medical school setting to predict that the medical students may not benefit from a one-time formal workshop and that other strate-gies to hone literature searching skills may be needed.

Not all inferential statistics lead to an understanding of causation, but all are used to infer that what was found in the specific results is also likely to be found in similar cases. Understanding some of the language that is used in the description of results and in inferential statistics is the first step in understanding what results mean for evidence-based practice (EBP). The article in Appendix B uses quantitative methods, which we will use in this chapter to gain a better understanding of the language in the results sections of research reports that reflect descriptive data analysis. We will look at the language of inferential statistics in Chapter 5 and will continue to use the fictional article and other articles found by the healthcare professionals in earlier chapters as examples in both chapters.

CORE CONCEPT 4.3

Research results that only describe or explain cannot be used to predict future outcomes or directly identify the cause of the findings.

UNDERSTANDING THE LANGUAGE OF RESULTS SECTIONS

To discuss the language in the results section of research reports, we must take a closer look at data and data analysis. As mentioned in Chapter 2, data are the information collected in a study. This information may take several forms—it may be numbers, words, or drawings, and it may be written, spoken, or observed. Once the information is collected, it has to be sorted and organized to be meaningful in answering the questions addressed in the research.

Most research reports' results sections begin by providing a summary of information about individual study variables. A variable is something that varies: It is not the same for everyone in every situation. Therefore, a **variable** is an aspect of the phenomenon of interest or research problem that differs among people or situations. Research aims to understand, explain, or predict those differences or variations. A variable may be some attribute of a person, such as age, health, or beliefs. It may be a test score, such as a score for anxiety level, or a physiologic parameter, such as body temperature. It may be an environmental aspect, such as community resources, family support, or employment rates. In all of these examples of variables, we know that there will be differences among people or situations.

Research attempts to gain new knowledge about variables that have been identified as important. In the research article for Chapter 1, the major variables studied included weight-control behaviors, eating-related behaviors and cognition, psychological functioning, body satisfaction, weight status, and demographics. Think about these for a moment. We can say that these are variables because we expect different people to have different levels of weight-control behaviors, eating-related behaviors and cognition, psychological functioning, body satisfaction, and weight status.

The goal of the body satisfaction and behaviors in overweight adolescents study was to understand and describe relationships among weight-control behaviors, eating-related behaviors and cognition, psychological functioning, and weight status and how they affected body satisfaction in teenagers. The researchers hoped to find key factors or connections that could guide them in the provision of care. The study variables found by C. H. in the clinical case for this chapter are identified in Table 4.2.

In Chapter 2, we said that multivariate analysis indicates there are more than two variables being discussed, and, in fact, most studies will probably include more than one variable. However, analysis of data at a given point that focuses on only one variable is called

TABLE 4.2	Identification of Specific Variables in the Teaching Evidence-Based Medicine Literature Searching Skills to Medical Students During the Clinical Years: A Randomized Controlled Trial

DEPENDENT VARIABLES	INDEPENDENT VARIABLES
Literature searching skills: • Writing a focused clinical question • Identifying information sources • Identifying an appropriate study type • Performing a literature search Confidence levels of literature searching skills—1 week after the workshop confidence levels of literature searching skills—6 months after the workshop	Formal workshop

univariate analysis. When you worked with the data from your in-class study, you were doing univariate analysis—that is, you were organizing data about individual variables.

Another word that you will often see in results sections is *bivariate*. **Bivariate analysis** refers to analysis with only two variables. Notice that the words themselves reveal their meanings: *uni* means "one," and *variate* means "to vary," so univariate is analysis of one variable; bivariate is analysis of two variables; and multivariate is analysis of more than two variables.

Both qualitative and quantitative studies have variables, but information about the variables for studies using these two approaches differs in how data are collected and how they are organized and reported in the results section of a report. The purpose of qualitative studies is to increase our understanding about some aspects of experiences. The results of those studies describe what was found, usually by organizing the data into concepts or themes and then by providing examples of the specific language used by participants to support and clarify the meaning of those concepts. The results describe findings about single variables, usually without using many numbers. Because quantitative studies use numbers to represent variables of interest and then often apply statistical tests to allow inference, we expect to see mostly numbers in the results section of a quantitative report.

CORE CONCEPT 4.4

Both qualitative and quantitative studies have variables, but information about variables for studies using these two approaches differs in how data are collected and how they are organized and reported in the results section of a report.

Language Describing Results From Qualitative Studies

In the Out-of-Class exercise in Chapter 3, you were asked to organize some numerical data so that it would be more informative. If the data had been words instead of numbers, the task of how to create some kind of order would not have been immediately obvious. For example, if you were given written paragraphs from a number of students and were asked to organize these data, you might break down the paragraphs into units that you could organize, such as individual sentences or groups of sentences that address the same idea. You could then organize the sentences according to shared ideas and determine how many different ideas occurred and how much agreement there was about the ideas. The goal of data analysis in a qualitative study is the same as that in a quantitative study: to organize the data and create some kind of an order so that meaning can be found.

BOX 4.1
Examples of Qualitative Data Collected in Response to the Question, "What Experiences in Your Life Have Led to Your Anticipated Choice for Field of Nursing Practice?"

"I have always loved movies where the nurses save the lives of people during a disaster. I guess, well, it seems like the best place to do that, you know, is, well, the emergency room."

"Nursing is all about caring for people. I mean, I don't know how I would have gotten through my son's illness without the nurses."

"The one thing I remember when I had my tonsils out was the nurse giving me ice cream. It made me feel safe."

"I come from a family of nurses who have all worked in hospitals, mostly the surgical or medical ICU."

"It was the nurse holding my hand when the doctor in the emergency room told me about my brother that made it possible for me to keep going."

"My roommate in college was a nursing student, and she always helped any of us who came to her, whether it was if we were sick or just feeling down."

"Every time I have had to go to the hospital with one of the kids, it was the nurses who really listened to me and made a difference."

"My aunt was a nurse. She always was so strong and sure of herself—I wanted to be just like her."

"The shows I've seen about the flying nurses—that is just such an exciting thing to do, I guess I figured I would never get bored."

"My best friend in high school was in a car accident and I was so scared to go see her. But the nurse, he just really helped me relax and not freak out seeing all the machines and things."

"There was no one like my Grandma Jane—she was the most caring person I ever knew; she nursed about everyone in the family until it was her turn to get sick and die."

Box 4.1 lists excerpts of data that might have been collected in response to "What experiences in your life have led to your anticipated choice for field of nursing practice?" the question identified in the fictional article as the measure used to collect subjective responses to help understand why students chose their fields of practice. Take a moment and read through those responses. Reading data in this form is even less helpful than reading a long list of individuals' ages. For the qualitative researcher, the organizing, ordering, and synthesizing of the data collected represent the heart of the research method. In fact, in most qualitative studies, data are analyzed throughout the process of implementing the study, and the results of this analysis are then used to guide additional data collection. This is in contrast to quantitative studies, in which the researcher usually does not analyze the data until all have been collected because changing the way data are collected, or changing which data are collected, undermines the results of the study.

Another difference between data analysis in qualitative studies and quantitative studies is that no absolute formulas are consistently applied to the data. Qualitative data analysis requires understanding, digesting, synthesizing, conceptualizing, and reconceptualizing descriptions of feelings, behaviors, experiences, and ideas. *Content analysis* is often the term used to describe this process of data analysis. **Content analysis** is the process of understanding, interpreting, and conceptualizing the meanings in qualitative data. To do this, the researcher starts by breaking down the data into units that are meaningful and then develops a categorization scheme. A **categorization scheme** is an orderly combination of categories carefully defined so that no overlap occurs. In qualitative analysis, the categorization scheme is developed based on the ideas found in the data; then pieces of data—units that reflect distinct ideas—are put into the categories. This process of breaking

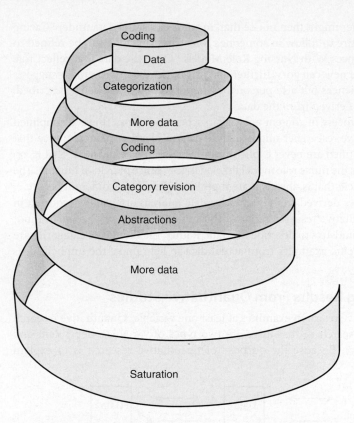

FIGURE 4.1 Spiraling process of qualitative data analysis.

(Spiral labels from top to bottom: Coding, Data, Categorization, More data, Coding, Category revision, Abstractions, More data, Saturation)

down and labeling large amounts of data to identify the category to which they belong is called **coding** or **data reduction**. When this coding or data reduction occurs, the researcher is also refining the categorization scheme and using the categories to guide further data collection.

One might say that there is a spiraling nature to the process of data analysis in qualitative studies, as illustrated in Figure 4.1. The process is not circular because it does not simply return to where it began but rather evolves to eventually identify key themes or concepts that reflect the meaning of the data. *Theme* is another term that is often found in the results section of a qualitative report. A **theme** is an idea or a concept that is implicit in and recurrent throughout the data. Themes are not the concrete, explicit words contained in the data; rather, they are the underlying ideas behind the words. Qualitative data analysis seeks to categorize and understand the data and the relationships among the categories to eventually conceptualize the data into themes. The spiral of qualitative data analysis occurs, in part, because as categories are developed through analysis, they are used to collect additional data, which is then coded and categorized. Eventually, data saturation occurs. **Data saturation** in qualitative research is the point at which all new information collected is redundant of information already collected. Data saturation occurs at a time when all new information fits into the newly established coding system so that the new information is saying the same thing as the data already collected. Therefore, no new information is being generated through continued data collection.

Look again at the data in Box 4.1, which have already been broken down into units, mostly sentences—and in a few cases, more than one sentence—that combine to express one idea. Content analysis to develop a categorization scheme might start by using a category for "Caring Experiences" and another for "Television and Movies." As the researcher examines the data and codes them into these two categories, you see that only two of the units fit under the "Television and Movies" category, whereas all the rest belong to "Caring

Experiences." The researcher might then notice that, in some cases, the data under "Caring Experiences" suggest a desire to follow in someone's footsteps. This idea can be refined to a category called "Experiences With Nursing Role Models." Once the data that reflect role models are moved into the new category, further analysis of the data that remain suggests that not only caring experiences but also personal caring experiences are being described. Thus, three themes can be derived from the data.

Figure 4.2 shows this process of content analysis in schematic form. This is a simplified example of how a qualitative researcher might analyze data to identify themes. Notice that the final three themes identified are never explicitly addressed in the actual data. That is, no piece of data says that it was the nurse role model that led to the choice of field of nursing. The themes identified are implicit; that is, the ideas are repeated differently by different people.

The themes or categories derived from qualitative data analysis are usually reported in the results sections of qualitative research reports. The author of this type of report cannot provide averages or other statistics to describe the data. Rather, the themes or categories are described, often using specific examples from actual data to help make the implicit ideas within the themes clearer.

Language Describing Results From Quantitative Studies

We have said that qualitative research examines at least one variable. Quantitative research differs from qualitative research in that there are two types of variables: dependent and independent (or predictor). Because the purpose of quantitative research is to explain

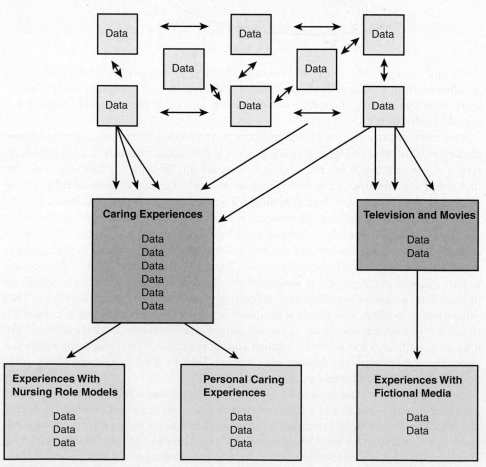

FIGURE 4.2 Schematic.

or predict a particular variable, we call that variable the **dependent variable**, which is determined by, or depends on, other variables in the study. It is the outcome variable of interest. In the fictional article about nursing students' preferences for practice, the outcome that the research is trying to explain or predict is choice of field of nursing practice, so it is the dependent variable.

Independent variables are those variables in a study that are used to explain or predict the outcome of interest, that is, the dependent variable. In the fictional article, the independent variables included age, perceived well-being, race, and marital status. These were factors that differed among students and that may explain or predict their choice of field, the dependent variable. Independent variables also are called **predictor variables** because they are used to predict the dependent variable.

Notice that Table 4.2 classifies the variables from literature searching skills to medical students study as dependent or independent. This study is quantitative and attempts to explain how a literature searching workshop affects literature searching competencies of medical students and confidence levels of medical students in searching literature. In some studies, you may notice that the variables may be identified as both a dependent variable and an independent variable. This is an example of a research term being "gray" rather than clearly "black and white." We discuss types of variables in quantitative research in more detail in Chapter 5.

In preparation for this chapter, you were asked to organize data from your in-class questionnaire to make it easy to understand. What did you do to make the information more understandable? Probably, your first thought was to create some kind of order in the data. The data given to you consisted of numbers. A logical way to create order is to list the numbers from smallest to largest (or vice versa). Doing so gives a sense of how alike or different people are in the values of the numbers, such as in age or marital status, by showing how many numbers are repeated or are close together and what the smallest and largest numbers are. The next thing you may have done was to determine the most common responses. This could be done by simply counting how many times each response was given, by calculating the percentage for each response out of the total responses, or by calculating an average of all the numbers.

Another approach to making sense out of a group of numbers includes using graphs, bar charts, or pie charts. This approach provides a visual representation of the data, which allows us to see the difference between the smallest and the largest numbers as well as the most common responses. Figure 4.3 is an example of a histogram (a type of bar chart) that could have been included in the fictional article on students' choices for clinical practice.

Hopefully, you found that organizing the data helped you to increase your understanding of what that information meant. Regardless of the approach taken, the product probably helped you to see two things: (1) how much diversity or difference occurred in the data and (2) the most common responses.

Variance, Standard Deviation, and Distribution

In the language of statistics, the diversity in data for a single variable is referred to as the variance, which reflects how the values for a variable are dispersed. The most common or frequent responses in a set of data are statistically described as the measures of central tendency. Each is discussed individually.

Variance is a statistic—a number—that can be used to show how much difference or variety exists in a group of numbers. Table 4.3 lists the ages of nursing students from three different classrooms. With short lists like this, you can look at the numbers and determine that there is more variety in the ages of students in classroom 2 than in classroom 1 or 3. But how do you objectively measure the variety or describe that variety in a way that can be consistently understood and interpreted by anyone? Obviously, just saying that classroom 2 has more variety in age than does classroom 1 or 3 is nonspecific—how much is "more?" You could also say that the ages range from 19 to 21 in classroom 1, compared with ages ranging

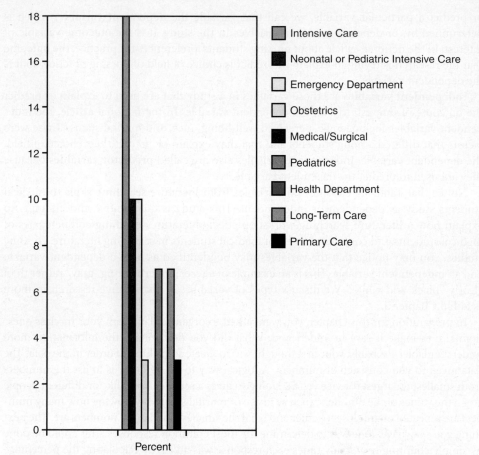

FIGURE 4.3 Histogram for the frequency distribution of students' choices of field of practice based on results in fictional article.

TABLE 4.3	Ages of Students in Three Different Classrooms With Variation and Central Tendency		
CLASSROOM 1*	**CLASSROOM 2***	**CLASSROOM 3***	
20	20	18	
21	24	20	
20	19	20	
20	21	24	
19	18	20	
21	23	20	
20	18	20	
20	19	18	
19	18	20	
20	20	20	
SD = .67	*SD* = 2.11	*SD* = 1.63	
M = 20	*M* = 20	*M* = 20	
Mode = 20	Mode = 18	Mode = 20	
Median = 20	Median = 19.5	Median = 20	

*Age in years.
SD, standard deviation; *M*, mean.

from 18 to 24 in classroom 2. This is certainly more specific and gives us a better sense of the differences, but the ages of students in classroom 3 also range from 18 to 24 years, yet there is more variety in ages in classroom 2 than in classroom 3. Therefore, there must be some way to represent the values in between the two numbers that give us the age range.

The variety in a group of numbers is explained statistically by computing a number appropriately called the **variance**, which is the sum of the squared differences between each value in the set of numbers and the mean (average) of those numbers, divided by how many numbers there were in the set minus 1. That can be understood by using the age of students in classroom 1 as an example. The variance is computed by subtracting the average of all 10 students' ages (20) from each student's age and squaring the difference, then adding those squared differences and dividing by 9. We square the differences between the mean to avoid negative and positive differences canceling each other. Therefore, the variance statistic is an average of the squared deviations from the mean. This is a mathematical definition, so you may still be wondering what it is you know when you see a value for a variance.

Whether or not you understand the formula for computing the variance, you can understand that variance tells you how much variety there is within a set of numbers. For example, the variance for the ages in classroom 1 is .44 ($s^2 = .44$), the variance for the ages in classroom 2 is 4.44 ($s^2 = 4.44$), and the variance in classroom 3 is 2.66 ($s^2 = 2.66$). These statistics reveal that there is more variety in age in classroom 3 than in classroom 1, but less variety in classroom 3 than in classroom 2. Although you can see the variety in the ages by looking at the short list of numbers in Table 4.3, if the list contained 100 numbers or 1,000 numbers, it would be much more difficult to get the variety without computing the variance. The variance gives us a specific statistic that represents differences or variety when reporting results for a single variable.

Thus far, we have discussed the variance for a single variable; however, more often the results section of a research report will use a statistic called the **standard deviation** instead of the variance. The standard deviation is simply the square root of the variance, so it also reflects variety among all the numbers. Remember that to compute the variance, we squared differences in values from the mean. This computational process results in the values for the variance being squared units of measurement, such as 4.44 squared years for the variance in classroom 2. The idea of "squared years," however, does not make much sense. If we take the square root of that variance, we get a standard deviation of 2.11 years (not squared years). The standard deviation is, in a sense, the average difference in ages from the overall average age. You can see by looking at the values for the ages in classroom 2 that it makes sense that the variety in ages can be accurately communicated by saying that there is an average of 2 years' difference from the overall average. This makes more sense than 4.44 squared years. In contrast, the standard deviation for the ages of students in classroom 1 is .67 years (or less than 1 year), and the standard deviation of the ages of the students in classroom 3 is 1.63 years. Standard deviation is usually abbreviated in research reports as *SD*, so a research report giving the standard deviation for classroom 3 would write "$SD = 1.63$." Although classrooms 2 and 3 both have a youngest and oldest student of 18 and 24 years, respectively, the average deviation from the overall average age is clearly greater in classroom 2.

Why do we care about variance and standard deviation? To understand the meaning of results for clinical practice, we must understand how much variety (variance) there is in the results. For example, if you were reading a research study that examined the effectiveness of an intervention to relieve pain, and the report tells you that the average rating of pain on a 10-point scale after the intervention was 2, that sounds good. Suppose that two different interventions each led to an average rating of 2, but the first had a standard deviation of 3.5, whereas the second had a standard deviation of .7. Although the first intervention led to the same average as the second intervention, the standard deviation tells us there was a great deal more variety in pain ratings with the first intervention. This means that some of the people who received the first intervention had higher scores or more pain as well as possibly lower scores or less pain. Although lower scores may be better, our goal in healthcare is to consistently improve pain, and higher scores in some of our patients definitely are not desirable. The second intervention led to much less variety in ratings of pain, which means that most of the subjects their pain close to a rating of 2 after the intervention. As a healthcare professional who understands standard deviations, you might decide that the second intervention is more consistent in relieving pain because it has a smaller standard deviation and choose to use that intervention rather than the first one.

A pain intervention study is an example in which we may not want variety because our clinical goal is to consistently decrease our patients' pain levels. In other cases, however, we may want variety to make the information useful clinically. For example, in the body satisfaction and behavior in overweight adolescents article, the authors reported the mean age of the teenagers in their sample was 15.2, with a standard deviation of 2.15 ($SD = 2.15$) (Cromley et al., 2011). This means that the average deviation around the age of 15.2 was 2.15 years, telling us that the individuals in the sample had a fairly narrow range of ages. Let's pretend the standard deviation for the study was 12.08 ($SD = 12.08$). This means that the average deviation around the age of 15.2 was 12.08 years, telling us that the individuals in the sample had a larger range of ages. So, the healthcare provider must decide if the range of ages of the adolescents in this study (or in the fictional results) will affect the usefulness of this study for evidence-based healthcare practice. What do you think?

Distribution is another term that is used in results sections to indicate the variety or differences found. In research, **distribution** refers to how the findings are dispersed. The variance and standard deviation for a set of numbers give us a clear sense of the spread of those numbers. However, it is not appropriate to compute the statistics of variance and standard deviation for variables that fit into discrete categories, such as type of job preference, rather than variables that are real numbers, such as age. For simplicity, often a researcher will assign numeric values to categories, such as 1 = professional employment, 2 = blue-collar employment. However, the actual numbers "1" and "2" are not a true measure of type of employment, and adding or subtracting the numbers will not tell us the "average" type of employment.

In cases where the variable is a category, we may find distribution described by using a table of percentages, histogram, or pie chart. For example, Table B.1 in Appendix B (the fictional article) shows us the frequency distribution of choices of field of nursing. A **frequency distribution** is the spread for how frequently each category occurs or is selected. We see from the table that 60% of students choose intensive care as their preferred field after graduation, and another 10% choose neonatal intensive care and emergency department fields. Figure 4.3 shows the same frequency distribution in a histogram format. Figure 4.4 shows what the frequency distribution would look like in histogram format if none of the students had selected the neonatal and emergency room fields and, instead, had selected the health department and long-term care fields. You can see that the distribution of choices would have looked different even with 60% still selecting intensive care. Just as the statistic for standard deviation can tell us about the distribution or variety in a numeric variable, a frequency table or histogram can tell us about distribution and variety in a categorical variable.

An important statistical concept that you may remember from your statistics courses is the **normal curve**. A normal curve is a type of distribution that is symmetric and bell shaped. Figure 4.5 shows two graphs with distribution curves; the one on the left is the familiar normal curve. Many of the variables in life that we are interested in understanding or using in research are distributed similarly to the normal curve. For example, height can range from small, in the case of a neonate, to tall, in the case of a few extraordinary individuals, but most people fall somewhere in the middle, with a relatively even balance on each side of the average height. The normal curve is a theoretical distribution. That means that if we could measure a variable, such as height, for every human on earth and plot all the heights, the result would be this perfectly symmetric bell-shaped curve. One thing that makes the normal curve unique is its symmetry; the normal curve can be folded in half at the center, which is the average, and the two sides will match. On the right side of

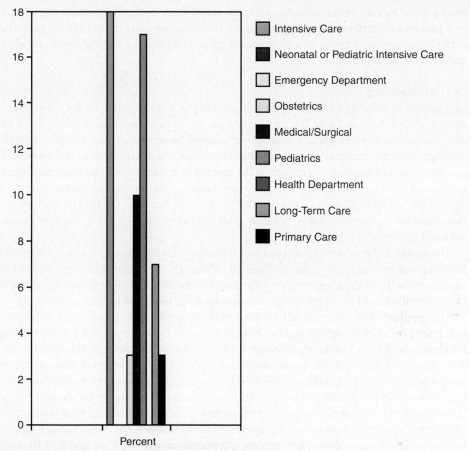

FIGURE 4.4 Example of histogram for distribution of field of study choices if health department and long-term care were endorsed more frequently.

Figure 4.5 is an example of a distribution that has a curved shape but is asymmetric. Much of inferential statistics is based on the assumption that the distribution of a variable would be normal or bell shaped if all the possible values for the variable were known. This assumption is based on experience with many variables of interest that are normally distributed. Therefore, when reading results, you will find references to a distribution of a variable being "approximately normal."

In summary, one of the important aspects of data that we expect to see described and summarized in the results section of reports is the diversity or variety in the data. This may

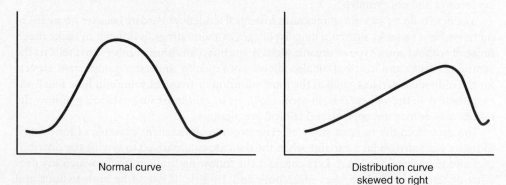

FIGURE 4.5 Examples of a normal curve and a curve that skews to the right.

be described by a univariate statistic called the *standard deviation* (or possibly the *variance*) or a frequency distribution, histogram, or pie chart. In any case, the variety for each study variable is important for us to understand because it affects the clinical decisions we can make based on the study.

Central Tendency

In addition to wanting to know about the diversity in a set of numbers for a variable, we almost always want to know the most common or average response or value for a variable. In quantitative research, a **measure of central tendency** shows common or typical numbers. Central tendency measures reflect the center of a distribution or the center of the spread. Three univariate statistics, called the mean, the mode, and the median, are the most commonly used measures of central tendency. Table 4.3 shows that the mean value for the ages of the students in each classroom is 20 years. The **mean** is simply the average of all the values for a variable—that is, the sum of all the values divided by the number of values summed and may be reported as $\bar{x}$.

The **mode** is the value that occurs most frequently: In classrooms 1 and 3, the mode is 20 years, but in classroom 2, the mode is 18. Although the mean of the ages in the three classrooms is the same, suggesting that the center of the distributions is the same, the center of the distribution of ages in the three classrooms differs when one looks at the mode.

The **median** is the value that falls in the middle of the distribution when the numbers are in numeric order. Although 20 years is the median age in classrooms 1 and 3, the median age for classroom 2 is 19.5 years (the average of $19 + 20$, the two most central values for age in that classroom). Although the mean, mode, and median are all measures of central tendency, comparing the three for a single variable also tells us something about the distribution. Looking at the mean (20 years), mode (18 years), and median (19.5 years) for students' ages in classroom 2, we see that although the average age was 20, more students were younger than age 20 than were older than age 20. The age distribution "leans" toward the younger ages. This leaning is described as **skew** when reporting research results. We have said that the mean, mode, and median are measures of "central" tendency, but if there is a skew in the distribution, these measures will have different values. This tells us that the middle of the distribution is not in the exact center of that distribution; it is off to the left or right of center. The second curve of Figure 4.5 has a skew to the right, which means that the middle of the distribution falls more to the higher range of the possible values. A normal curve does not have a skew. In fact, part of what defines a normal curve is that the mean, median, and mode are all equal.

Now, look at Figure 4.6, which shows curves drawn around the distribution of ages for the three classrooms we have been using as an example. Notice that the curve for classroom 1 is perfectly bell shaped and symmetric and that the mean, mode, and median are equal. The curve for classroom 2 is skewed to the left, is not symmetric, and the mean, mode, and median are not equal. The curve for classroom 3 looks similar to that for classroom 1, but it is narrower and not symmetric.

Again, why do we care about measures of central tendency? We care because a long list of numbers for a variable, such as a long list of ages or pain ratings, is difficult to make much sense of without some type of organization. A summary of those numbers that tells us the central tendency and distribution also allows us to quickly understand important aspects for the individual variable, such as the most common or frequent value and how much variety there is in the values. This, in turn, allows us to gain more understanding of how the results may or may not apply to real clinical practice.

The data from the in-class study exercise provide an excellent example of how much more we can learn about a variable when the data are summarized to give us the distribution and the central tendency. Let's consider the following study example, which involves a list of test scores from a class of 22 boys and 18 girls. It would be both tedious and frustrating to try to get a sense of their grades just by looking at the list of numbers.

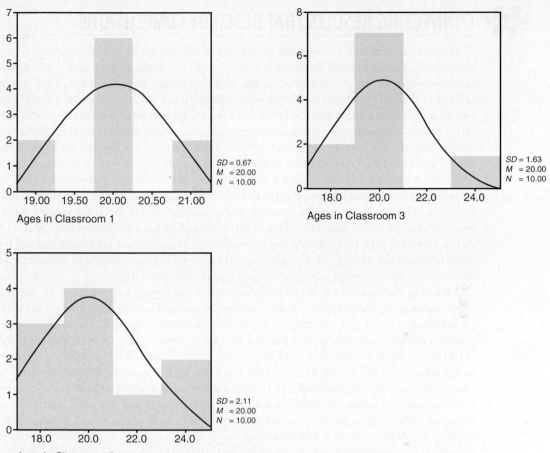

FIGURE 4.6 Frequency distribution histogram and curves for ages of students in three classrooms. *SD*, standard deviation; *M*, mean; *N*, number in sample.

However, when the author tells us that the range of scores is from 76 to 92 and that the mean and standard deviation for the test scores are 82 and 5.3, respectively, we have information that immediately tells us about the test grades in the study. A common way to report the mean and standard deviation results is to provide the mean with the standard deviation inside parentheses: 76–92 (5.3).

 CORE CONCEPT 4.5

Measures of central tendency and distribution are univariate statistics that summarize information about a variable.

The description of the variables in a study is always an important part of the results section of research reports. Description of data aims to summarize it in a way that makes it understandable and meaningful. Description of only one variable is called *univariate analysis*, and in quantitative research, that description almost always includes information that tells us about the distribution and central tendency for the variables. In reports of qualitative research, the entire results section is descriptive, taking units of data (words, pictures, and sentences) and developing categories and themes to describe that data.

CONNECTING RESULTS THAT DESCRIBE CONCLUSIONS

C. H. in our clinical case has read the results and discussion sections of the research report about medical students and literature searching skills. No **demographic** data—descriptive information about the characteristics of the people studied—were provided in the results section of the report. In this study, the only characteristics we know about the study participants is that they are in the third year of a medical school. Both quantitative and qualitative studies almost always include demographic data, although the reports of qualitative studies may not use statistics to describe those characteristics. The second sentence of the results section started with the overall finding of the study, "there was no statistical mean difference in evidence-based medicine literature searching skills between participants who attended the formal workshop and participants who did not" (Ilic et al., 2012). These results provide C. H. with an overview of the study and an understanding that there wasn't a difference between literature searching skills of those who attended a workshop and those who didn't. However, if C. H. read only this result, then C. H. would not know much about the other results of the study. C. H. needs to read the entire results sections as well as the conclusions section to fully understand the findings and results of the study.

Checking the descriptive results in Table A4.1 of the article (Appendix A-4), we find information about the student competency scores associated with literature searching skills including the overall and subcomponents of literature searching skills. The results section provides a supporting written summary of the results listed in the table. Tables A4.2 and A4.3 (Appendix A-4) have clear titles helping the reader to grasp what results are included in the tables. Specific results described are the basis for the new knowledge identified in the results and discussion sections. In the literature searching skills to medical student report, without the tables, we would not know the actual means or standard deviations of the results. The written description provides a quick summary of the results, and the tables provide details of the results. The reader can use both the table and written descriptions to understand the results of the study. These results then lead to inferences for clinical decision making and are reported in the conclusions section of the report. The discussion section of the literature searching skills to medical students study notes differences in results between this study and previous studies, leading the healthcare professional to seek more evidence.

 ## COMMON ERRORS IN THE REPORTS OF DESCRIPTIVE RESULTS

Two kinds of problems may be found when reading descriptive results in a research report: (1) incomplete information and (2) confusing information. We have emphasized the importance of understanding the distribution and central tendency in variables from quantitative studies to make clinical decisions. One problem that sometimes arises when reading the results is that this descriptive information cannot be found. The authors may fail to provide any univariate statistics about some of the variables in the study, or they may fail to provide all the information needed.

For example, a report may include only a measure of central tendency for an important variable without giving a range of values or the standard deviation. This absence of information about the variation in the variable makes it difficult to know how to interpret the findings related to that variable and can even lead to incorrect conclusions. The previous example of a study that examined two interventions to help pain whose results are a mean pain score of 2 for both interventions is a good example of this. Given the mean scores alone, one might conclude that the two interventions have exactly the same effect. This conclusion would be incorrect, however, because the standard deviations for the mean pain scores in this example (.7 and 3.5) are different.

Another example of a report with incomplete descriptive results is the fictional article. One of the variables that the author later indicates was important relative to the students' choices of field of practice was their health rating, but the only univariate information provided about the variable is that 20% of the subjects rated their health as fair or poor. We learn neither how the percentages broke down for ratings of "excellent health" or "good health" nor whether most of the 20% of subjects who rated their health at the lower end chose "fair" or "poor." This lack of information affects our ability to interpret the results that are reported later.

Aside from incomplete results, a second problem that may be found in the results section is a confusing presentation of the results. Descriptive results are often reported in tables, and sometimes those tables are not labeled or organized clearly. A table may use titles or identify variables that are inconsistent with the wording used in the text of the report. In fact, sometimes the text of a report fails to refer to the table at all. Another problem is that too much information may be put into the text, rather than used in a table. For example, the information provided in Table B.1 in Appendix B (the fictional article) would have been confusing and difficult to understand if the author had instead written a paragraph reporting those results as follows:

> Students chose several fields immediately after graduation, with 18 (60%) choosing intensive care, 3 (10%) choosing neonatal or pediatric intensive care, and 3 (10%) choosing emergency departments. One student (3%) chose obstetrics for field of study immediately after graduation, and no students chose either medical/surgical or health department. Two students (7% chose pediatrics, two students (7%) chose long-term care or nursing home care, and one student (3%) chose primary care.

Although this information could be sorted out by the reader, it is presented much more clearly in the table. A similar problem may occur in a qualitative report if the author does not give us clear descriptions of the categories or themes developed from the study. Look at the fictional article again and at the three themes identified that represented the meaning of experiences students identified as affecting their choice of practice. If the author had simply listed the themes as "personal life experience," "experiences with nursing role models," and "experiences with fictional media," it would be difficult to know how these types of experiences differ. The definitions and examples given in Table B.2 of Appendix B make it clear what those themes mean.

CRITICALLY READING RESULTS SECTIONS OF RESEARCH REPORTS FOR USE IN EVIDENCE-BASED HEALTHCARE PRACTICE

It should be clear from the examples just given that critically reading the descriptive results section of a research report is important. Box 4.2 presents a set of six questions that can be used when critically reading results sections. The first question, "Did the report include

---

BOX 4.2
How to Critically Read the Results Section of a Research Report

Do the Results Answer the Question, "Why Did the Authors Reach These Conclusions—What Did They Actually Find?"

1. Did the report include a clearly identified results section?
2. Were the results presented appropriately for the information collected?
3. Were descriptive versus inferential results identifiable if this is a quantitative study?
4. Were themes or structure and meaning identifiable if this is a qualitative study?
5. Were the results presented in a clear and logical manner?
6. Did the results include enough information about the final sample for the study?

a clearly identified results section?" may seem simplistic, but some reports do not present results in a specific section. The answer to the second question, "Were the results presented appropriately for the information collected?" refers to whether or not descriptions included information about distribution, central tendency, and variation that were appropriate for the study's variables. For example, was information about categories such as marital status presented as percentages, and were both the mean and the standard deviation included in information about variables such as age or scores on a measure? The third question is "Were descriptive versus inferential results identifiable if this is a quantitative study?" When we consider the results in the literature search skills to medical students article, we find that it includes descriptive and inferential results in both the written and tabular presentation of results.

If the study that you are reading used a qualitative method, a question to ask yourself in order to critically read the results section is "Were themes or structure and meaning identifiable if this is a qualitative study?" Not all reports of qualitative studies will be as clear. This leads us to the next question, "Were the results presented in a clear and logical manner?" For example, the perceptions of caring report from Chapter 2 organizes the results by using headings that represent the specific themes identified in the study. This is a logical and clear approach to present results. The last question to ask yourself as you read the results section of a report is "Did the results include enough information about the final sample for the study?" We have already discussed the importance of including demographic information in the report of results of a study, whether it is qualitative or quantitative. We also have identified that the authors of the literature searching skills to medical students did not include demographic information within the research report leaving some questions about the participants unanswered. We will revisit four of the six questions for critically reading results sections of research reports at the end of Chapter 5, after we finish learning a bit about inferential statistics.

PUBLISHED REPORT—WHAT WOULD YOU CONCLUDE?

Understanding what to expect in the reports of descriptive results makes it possible for you to know whether the research is something that might apply to your clinical practice. C. H. in our clinical case began the search with an interest in gaining a better understanding of what methods assist medical students in using literature searching skills in clinical practice. After reading the results and conclusions sections of the literature searching skills to medical students article, C. H. has a better understanding of how the literature searching skill development workshop may or may not impact literature searching skills of a future clinician. We will continue to look at the language of results sections of research reports in the next chapter.

OUT-OF-CLASS EXERCISE

Making Inferences About Well-Being and Marriage

Before proceeding to Chapter 5, look at the data collected from your in-class practice study, focusing on two variables: rating of well-being and marital status. Complete a univariate analysis of data for each of these variables to summarize distribution and central tendency. To do so, you will need to decide what is appropriate in terms of measure of central tendency (mean, median, or mode) and how to summarize distribution (range, standard deviation, and percentage). Then, determine what the data tell you in terms of answering the question, "Do married students have higher levels of well-being than unmarried students?" Based on the data obtained, answer the question and explain how you arrived at your answer. If you are not using an in-class study, a practice set of data about well-being and marital status is provided in Appendix D, which can be used for this exercise. Remember, this is an exercise to motivate you to think more about how results are presented in a research report and what they mean. You will then be ready to begin the next chapter.

References

Cromley, T., Knatz, S., Rockwell, R. A., Neumark-Sztainer, D., Story, M., & Boutelle, K. (2012). Relationships between body satisfaction and psychological functioning and weight-related cognitions and behaviors in overweight adolescents. *Journal of Adolescent Health*, *50*, 651–653. doi:10.1016/j.jaohealth.2011.10.252

Ilic, D., Tepper, K., & Misso, M. (2012). Teaching evidence-based medicine literature searching skills to medical students during the clinical years: a randomized controlled trial. *Journal of the Medical Library Association*, *100*(3), 190–196. doi:10.3163/1536-5050.100.3.009

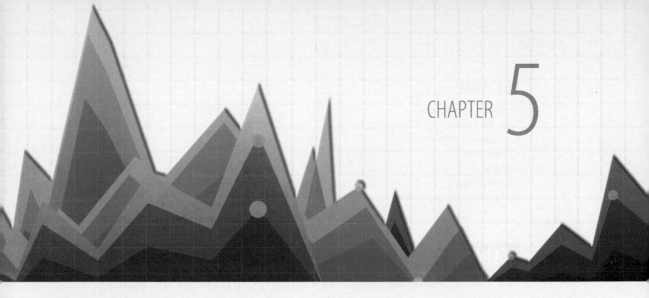

Inferential Results

Why Did the Authors Reach Their Conclusion—What Did They Actually Find?

> **LEARNING OBJECTIVE** The student will interpret inferential statistical results in relationship to their meaning for the conclusions of the study.

The Purpose of Inferential Statistics
Probability and Significance
Parametric and Nonparametric Statistics
Bivariate and Multivariate Tests

  Tests Looking for Differences Between Two Groups
  Tests Looking at Relationships Between Two Variables
  Tests Looking for Differences Among Three or More Groups
  Tests Looking at Relationships Among Three or More Variables
  Tests Looking at the Structure or Components of a Variable

Hypothesis Testing
In-Class Study Data
Connecting Inferential Statistical Results to Conclusions
Common Errors in Results Sections
Critically Reading the Results Section of a Report for Use in Evidence-Based Practice—Revisited
Published Report—What Would You Conclude?

KEY TERMS

Analysis of variance
Beta (β) value
Confidence intervals
Correlation
Covary
Factor analysis
Nonparametric statistics

Null hypothesis
Parametric statistics
Probability
Regression
Research hypothesis
t test

CLINICAL CASE

A team of healthcare professionals working in the Emergency Department have seen an increase in concerns about long-term effects of sports-related concussions. The healthcare team is wondering whether their current practices in identifying those patients who are more apt to have postconcussion syndrome (PCS) as a result of a concussion is still relevant and efficacious. After doing research, one member of the healthcare team brings an article to the next staff meeting to share findings. The article used a quantitative method to examine predictors of PCS following a minor traumatic brain injury (mTBI) (Ponsford, Cameron, Fiztgerald, Grant, & Mikocka-Walus, 2012). This article used several statistical terms, such as mean, standard deviation, and significance, in the results section, which the healthcare team must interpret to decide what the results mean for patients with suspected concussions and consider whether the evidence in the study can be used to guide healthcare practice in this situation. You can find this article in Appendix A-5. Reading the discussion sections of this article will help you to understand the examples discussed in this chapter.

THE PURPOSE OF INFERENTIAL STATISTICS

Chapter 4 discussed the meaning of the language used in research reports when descriptive results—those that describe or explain a variable or variables—are presented. This chapter continues the discussion of how to understand the results sections of research reports but focuses on inferential results—those intended to explain or predict a variable or variables. Note that the word *explain* is included in both of these definitions. This is because there is an overlap between simple description—a description that explains—and explanation that can be used for prediction. We are looking at a continuum of statistics that build from simple knowing, to understanding and explaining, and finally to predicting, as shown in Figure 5.1.

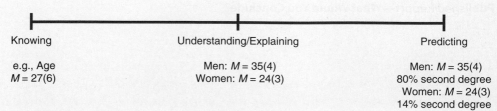

Knowing	Understanding/Explaining	Predicting
e.g., Age $M = 27(6)$	Men: $M = 35(4)$ Women: $M = 24(3)$	Men: $M = 35(4)$ 80% second degree Women: $M = 24(3)$ 14% second degree

FIGURE 5.1 A continuum for the purpose of data analysis.

SUBJECT NUMBER	AGE (IN YEARS)	GENDER	DEGREE STATUS
TABLE 5.1 Fictional Data for Ages, Gender, and Degree Status of a Nursing Student Class			
1	20	F	1st
2	23	F	1st
3	33	M	1st
4	21	F	1st
5	25	F	1st
6	40	M	2nd
7	32	F	2nd
8	20	F	1st
9	26	F	1st
10	25	F	1st
11	37	M	2nd
12	26	F	1st
13	23	F	1st
14	22	F	1st
15	24	F	2nd
16	30	M	2nd
17	35	M	2nd
18	21	F	1st
19	25	F	1st

Let us look at a simple example using the results about the ages, gender, and degree status of students in a nursing class shown in Table 5.1. The mean ($M = 27$) and standard deviation ($SD = 6$) for the age of the students is an example of simple description. Remember, the mean can also be represented as $\bar{x}$. Note in Figure 5.1 that the mean is followed by the standard deviation in parentheses. This is often the form used to report the mean and standard deviation in the results of a research report. This example of descriptive univariate statistics tells us that the students are relatively older and that there is a fair amount of variation in the ages, but we have no idea why the variation exists. To have some explanation of the variation, descriptive statistics might be used to give us information about the age of the men versus the age of the women in the class. In the example, the mean age for the male students is 35 ($SD = 4$), whereas the mean age of the female students is 24 ($SD = 3$). We now have a partial explanation of the variation in ages: There are both men and women in the class, and the men in the class are older than the women. The variation in age is explained to some extent, but we do not assume that we can use students' gender distribution to predict the age of students. However, if we discover that 80% of the male students are second-degree students, whereas only 14% of the females are second-degree students, this additional information can potentially be used for prediction. We can speculate that men may be more likely to pursue nursing as a second career and that the more second-degree students there are in a class, the older the students will be. To test whether we can use the number of second-degree students to predict the age of students in a classroom, we must use inferential statistics.

Why use inferential statistics instead of just descriptive statistics? At this point we do not know whether the differences and relationships among variables found in this classroom occurred by chance alone. We know that there are differences in this particular classroom, but we cannot know whether, in general, second-degree students are more likely to be men and older. Descriptive statistical results allow us to know and explain variables that we are interested in understanding, but we have to go a step further to use that explanation to predict or infer how those variables may occur in the future. This can be done through the use of inferential statistics, which are based on the concepts of probability and statistical significance. Therefore, to understand results that use inferential statistics, we must understand these terms.

PROBABILITY AND SIGNIFICANCE

As the healthcare team members in our clinical case start to read the section of the report titled "Results," they encounter the language of inferential statistics in the statement within the first paragraph of the section that states "There were no significant group differences in terms of gender, age, education, marital status, or employment status, or in history of previous mTBI" (Ponsford et al., 2012). In Chapter 2, we defined *significance* as a low likelihood that any relationship or difference found in a statistical test occurred by chance alone. Quantitative research often attempts to take what has been found in a specific situation, that is, one study, and infer that similar results would occur in other similar situations. The healthcare team in the clinical case not only is interested in what happened in the study by Ponsford et al. but also wants to predict that the same finding will occur in their practice setting if the information from the study is used to guide their EBP to improve patient outcomes.

In inferential statistics, we test for relationships, associations, and differences among variables that are statistically significant. We do this by creating distributions of test statistics that reflect variables having no connection between them, are unrelated, or are not different. In Chapter 4, we said that a distribution refers to how the findings are dispersed. A distribution of test statistics shows how the statistics from hundreds of samples would look if plotted on a graft. Then, we compute a test statistic for the results in our particular study and compare what we found in our sample or specific situation to what would be predicted to be found if there were not a relationship or difference in the variables. By convention, researchers say that if the test statistic falls into the range where we would expect 95% of all statistics to fall, given that there is no relationship or connection, then it is a nonsignificant statistic. Stated in the opposite way, if a test statistic falls *out of the range* of values that we would expect to occur 95% of the time, if there were no relationship among the variables, then we say it is a statistically significant value.

To illustrate this idea, we will use the statistic reported in the fictional article from Appendix B about the difference in ages of nursing students who choose acute settings versus nonacute settings. The article states that there was a significant difference in age and gives a test statistic of "$t = 2.1, p < .05$." The "t" value is a test statistic for differences in means between two groups, which we will discuss later in this chapter. In this case, the statistic was computed for the differences in the average ages of students who did and did not select an acute care setting for field of practice. Now look at Figure 5.2, which shows a distribution that is a normal curve, in this case a t distribution. Notice that for the t distribution, zero is at the center, and the possible values for the t test become larger at either end. A t distribution shows how the t tests for hundreds of different samples of two variables *that did not differ from each other in the "real" world* would be distributed. Now, returning to age as a variable of interest, if in the real world the ages of two groups are *not* different, then most of the time we would not get a big difference for the ages in any particular sample, and the t-test statistic would be a small number. However, occasionally, by chance alone, we get a large difference in age between groups in a sample (perhaps because a 12-year-old genius is in a particular sample).

Using the example from the fictional article, if students in the real world who did and did not pick acute settings were approximately the same age, then most of the time, if we took a sample of ages of students, choosing the two types of settings and computed a t test,

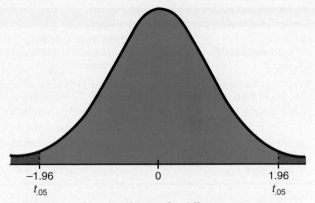

FIGURE 5.2 The *t* distribution for differences in two means in a sample when there is really no difference in the "real" world; green zone shows where 95% of values will fall, and two red zones show where 2.5% of the values will fall.

the value would be plotted on the distribution somewhere toward the middle, in the green zone. In fact, the green zone marks where a *t*-test value will fall 95% of the time if the two variables tested are not different. The red zones at either end of the normal curve are the areas where the *t* values will fall by chance alone 2.5% of the time if, in the real world, the two variables tested are not different. When we say that a test statistic is significant, we are saying that we will achieve that statistic only a small percentage of the time if there is no difference or connection between the variables.

When the healthcare team in the clinical case reads the section titled "Prediction of PCS at 3 Months for mTBI and Trauma Control Groups Separately," they found the study's results show the significant predictors for PCS at 3 months were "Hospital Anxiety and Depression Scale (HADS)" anxiety symptoms ($p = .01$) and higher age ($p = .04$). The healthcare team members know that what was found in this study probably did not happen by chance. How much "probably" means, or what the probability is that whatever was found happened by chance is reported by a *p* value. The *p* value represents the **probability** and is defined as the percentage of the time the result found would have happened by chance alone. In the predictors of postconcussive symptoms study, the authors indicate that the *p* value for the predictor of PCS, higher age was $p = .04$, which translates to 4%. This means that the statistic computed for the difference in scores from the first to the third month post injury would only happen 4 out of 100 times by chance alone. If the *p* value were .01, then the statistic would only occur by chance 1 out of 100 times (1%), and if the *p* value were .001, the statistic would only occur by chance 1 out of 1,000 times (1/10 of 1%). Statistical significance, no matter what test has been used, means that the results are unlikely to have happened by chance alone. Therefore, we infer from the finding of statistical significance that the difference, association, or relationship that we tested statistically is one that exists in the real world because we were unlikely to get our statistic by chance alone. Remember that inferential statistics are only used in quantitative methods because only in quantitative studies do we assume that the absolute truth can be found.

Statistical significance is also sometimes described in the results sections of research reports in the form of confidence intervals. **Confidence intervals** (CIs) state the range of actual values for the statistic we are computing (such as the difference in the mean ages of nursing students who do and do not choose acute care settings), in which 95 out of 100 values would fall. A CI for the differences in ages between nursing students choosing the two types of settings might be .8 to 6.2, and a research report might state that the differences in the means of ages for the two groups was 4.2, with a 95% CI (.8–6.2). This means that given the difference found in the study, 95 out of 100 times, the difference in ages between

TABLE 5.2	Comparison of *p* Values and Confidence Intervals	
	P VALUE	CONFIDENCE INTERVAL
Assumption	The relationship or difference tested is zero	The relationship or difference is that found in the data
Meaning	Gives the percentage of the time that we would get the test statistic by chance alone	Gives the range of values (biggest and smallest numbers) that would occur 95% of the time for the relationship or difference found
Interpretation	The smaller the value, the less likely that the test result occurred by chance alone	The smaller the range, without zero in it, the more confident we can be that the test statistic reflects the "real" world

the two groups of students will fall between .8 and 6.2 years. Note that this range does not include zero, so there is a low likelihood that there is zero or no difference. Another example occurs in the body satisfaction and behaviors in overweight adolescents article discussed in Chapter 1 (see Appendix A-1; Cromley et al., 2012). Table A1.2 provides the 95% CIs for the variables studied in relation to body satisfaction. CIs are almost always stated for the 95% range, whereas the probability of getting the result reported if there really were no difference or relationship is usually reported as one of three possible percentages: 5% ($p <.05$), 1% ($p <.01$), and .1% ($p <.001$). Table 5.2 summarizes the differences between p values and CIs.

 CORE CONCEPT 5.1

Inferential statistics are used to report whether the results found in the specific study are likely to have happened by chance alone. Statistical significance is not an absolute guarantee that the values are really different or related in the real world. Rather, statistical significance means that there is less than 5% chance that the amount of relationship or difference found happened by chance.

 CORE CONCEPT 5.2

Whether the report includes p values or CIs, the authors are telling you how likely it is that the results from the study were due to chance and, therefore, how likely it is that these results can be used to infer that there would be similar results in similar future situations.

PARAMETRIC AND NONPARAMETRIC STATISTICS

Before we begin to discuss some of the specific statistical tests that you are likely to find reported in the results sections, you must understand the difference between *parametric* and *nonparametric statistics*. These terms refer to the two broad classes of inferential statistical procedures that can be applied to numeric results from studies. **Parametric statistics** can be applied to numbers that meet two key criteria: (1) the numbers must generally be normally distributed—that is, the frequency distribution of the numbers is roughly bell shaped and (2) the numbers must be interval or ratio numbers, such as age or intelligence score—that is, the numbers must have an order, and there must be an equal distance between each value. **Nonparametric statistics** are used for numbers that do not have a bell-shaped distribution and are categoric or ordinal. Categoric or ordinal numbers represent variables for which there is no established equal distance between each category, such as numbers used to represent gender or rating of preference for car color. In the predictors of postconcussive symptoms, gender and litigation would be a nonparametric statistic, whereas age and education in years scores would be a parametric statistic.

Understanding that there is a difference between parametric and nonparametric statistics is important for two reasons. First, although it is the researcher's responsibility to decide which type of inferential statistics should be used, as an intelligent reader of research, you should understand that the decision is not always clear-cut. In fact, whole books are written about which types of statistics should or should not be used with selected data. Therefore, the author of a research report may include a sentence or two stating that either parametric or nonparametric statistics were used and the rationale for that decision. Second, types of statistical tests used in research differ depending on the kind of numbers in the results. Thus, more than one type of statistical procedure is needed to look for the same kind of relationship. For example, often research is looking for differences between two groups. If the variable that we expect to be different in the two groups has interval or ratio numeric values (and is distributed roughly normally or bell shaped), such as age, then the researcher can use a *t* test. But if the variable that we expect to be different for the two groups is a category, such as choice between red or green cars, then the researcher cannot use a *t* test and may use something called a Kruskal–Wallis one-way analysis of variance (ANOVA) test. The *t* test is a parametric statistical test, and the Kruskal–Wallis is a nonparametric test, but both help us to look for differences between groups. As we discuss some of the more common statistical tests that may be described in the results section of a research report, we will identify parametric and nonparametric statistics so that you will recognize and understand some of each class of statistical procedures.

CORE CONCEPT 5.3

Researchers use different types of statistics to test for the same kind of relationship, depending on the form of data collected. The research report may tell you why a particular type of statistical test was applied.

BIVARIATE AND MULTIVARIATE TESTS

The healthcare team members in our clinical case are not interested in becoming statisticians, but do want to know how and perhaps what predicts PCS for patients who have mTBIs. Table 5.3 summarizes some of the most common statistical tests used in nursing research by three general purposes for tests. In general, we use statistical tests to (1) look at differences between groups for one or more variables, (2) look at relationships among two or more variables, or (3) look at relationships of factors within a variable itself. Each of these general purposes addresses a different type of question. When we perform statistical tests to look at differences, we are asking some version of the question "Are groups unlike one another on a given variable or variables?" When we perform tests to look at relationships among variables, we might ask "Is there some natural connection between two or more variables?" For example, in the predictors of postconcussive symptoms study, the authors are looking for connections between gender, age, psychiatric history, physical health, post-traumatic amnesia, use of narcotic analgesics, and pain on PCS at 1 and 3 months post injury. Finally, when we look at relationships within a variable, this question might come to mind, "What are the natural components that make up a variable?" The statistical tests used when we are only looking at two variables or two groups are different from those we use with three or more variables or groups. We will first look at bivariate statistics—that is, statistical tests that are used with just two variables.

TABLE 5.3	Common Statistical Procedures Categorized by Type of Relationship Tested and Number of Variables Included	
TYPE OF RELATIONSHIP TESTED	TWO VARIABLES—BIVARIATE	THREE OR MORE VARIABLES—MULTIVARIATE
1. Differences—are groups unlike one another on a given variable or variables?		
Independent groups	• *t* test (parametric) • Sign test or median test (nonparametric) • Mann–Whitney *U* (nonparametric) • Wilcoxon rank test (nonparametric) • Fisher exact test (nonparametric)	• ANOVA (parametric) • ANCOVA, MANOVA, one-way ANOVA (parametric) • Kruskal–Wallis one-way ANOVA (nonparametric) • Chi-square for independent samples
Related groups usually overtime	• Paired *t* test (parametric) • McNemar change test (nonparametric)	• Repeated-measures ANOVA (parametric) • Friedman two-way ANOVA (nonparametric)
2. Relationships between variables—is there a natural connection between two or more variables?	• Pearson *r* (parametric) • Spearman rho (nonparametric) • Kendall tau (nonparametric) • Contingency coefficient (nonparametric)	• Multiple regression (parametric) • Canonical correlation (parametric) • Path analysis (parametric) • Structural equation modeling (parametric) • Discriminant analysis (parametric) • Logistic regression (nonparametric)
3. Relationships within a variable—is there a structure within a variable?		• Factor analysis (parametric) • Cluster analysis (nonparametric)

ANOVA, analysis of variance; ANCOVA, analysis of covariance; MANOVA, multiple analysis of variance.

Tests Looking for Differences Between Two Groups

In our discussion of significance and probability, we used an example from the fictional article from Appendix B in which the author wanted to explain or predict choice of field of practice. To do so, the author divided the students into two groups: those who chose an acute care setting and those who did not. The author then looked for variables that were significantly different between the groups, hoping that they might help to understand and predict which students would select nonacute practice settings. A *t* test was used to test for significant differences. A *t* test computes a statistic that reflects the differences in the means of a variable for two different groups or at two different times for one group. The two groups being tested might consist of anything of interest to nursing, such as men and women, single-parent families and two-parent families, those who quit smoking and those who did not, or hospitals with level-one trauma centers and hospitals without them. In all of these examples, one variable differentiates the two groups. Alternately, the "groups" might be the same unit at different points in time, such as families before and after a divorce, smokers before and after a smoking cessation program, or hospitals before and after a level-one trauma center is added. The variable tested can be anything that can be measured as a continuous number, such as age, family functioning, self-efficacy, or cost per patient visit.

The fictional article reports the results of two *t* tests. The two groups for both of these tests were the same: those who chose an acute setting and those who did not choose an acute setting. However, the tests looked for differences in two different variables. In the first test, the researcher tested to see whether age differed between the groups, and in the second test, the researcher tested to see whether health rating differed. In both cases, there was a statistically significant difference between the groups in the variables. The author also tells the reader that "there was no significant differences in number of years of postsecondary education and field of study." Because the test was not statistically significant, no test statistic is reported here, but the author believes it is important to tell you that the possibility of this difference was tested and was found not to be present. When using research in clinical practice, it is equally important to understand whether or not a difference or relationship is significant. Findings that there are no significant differences or relationships help us rule out factors that will affect our clinical care.

Other statistical tests that examine differences between two groups are mostly nonparametric and include the Fisher exact test, Mann–Whitney test, Wilcoxon signed rank test, McNemar test, and sign or median test (Table 5.3). It is not necessary to understand exactly how these tests are chosen and applied, but it is important to understand that whenever one of these tests is reported in the results section, it is being used to examine differences between two groups. If the p value that is reported with the test is <.05, then there was a difference between the groups that probably did not occur by chance alone. In the predictors of postconcussive symptoms report section "Analysis," the authors discuss the calculations of results between two groups using the Mann–Whitney test, Wilcoxin signed-ranks test, and the Friedman test "because the variables were not normally distributed" (Ponsford et al., 2012). This statement provides information about variable data and allows the reader to understand why these tests were chosen.

Tests Looking at Relationships Between Two Variables

In healthcare research, we often look for relationships or connections between two variables. When two variables are connected in some way, they are said to covary. Two variables **covary** when changes in one are connected to consistent changes in the other. For example, height and weight covary in healthy growing children. As the height of a child increases, the weight usually increases as well. Another example of covariance is found between the amount of practice of a procedure, such as urinary catheterization, and the number of errors. In this case, as the variable "amount of practice" increases, the variable "number of errors" consistently decreases. The statistical test used to examine how much two variables covary is called a **correlation**.

Two things are important to notice about a correlation statistic, also called a *correlation coefficient*. First, it is important to notice whether the number is negative or positive. In the example of the correlation between height and weight in children, the number for the correlation will be positive because the two variables move in the same direction—that is, they both increase. In the second example, the correlation between practice and errors will be negative because the two variables move in opposite directions. Figure 5.3 shows two graphs that can represent the two examples. Note that in the first graph, the points all fall along a line that moves diagonally from the bottom to the top. This shows that there is a positive connection or relationship between these two variables because as one goes up, the other goes up. In contrast, on the second graph, the points fall along a line that moves diagonally from the top and down toward the opposite end. This shows that there is a negative connection or relationship between the two variables because as one goes up, the other goes down.

Second, it is important to note the magnitude of the number for a correlation coefficient. Because of the way a correlation coefficient is calculated, it can only have a range of values from -1 to $+1$. A relationship between two variables that is "perfect"—as one goes up, the other goes up or down in exactly the same amount—will have a value of either -1 or $+1$. The lines drawn in the middle of the two graphs in Figure 5.3 show what perfect correlations look like. In real life, there is almost never a perfect correlation. Returning to the example of height and weight in children, we can observe that some children will become taller and not gain very much weight, and others will become only a little taller and gain more weight. Therefore, there will not be a consistent increase in weight each time there is an increase in height, as is shown in the scatter plot in Figure 5.3, where each spot represents one child,

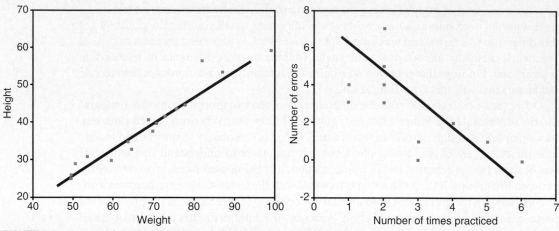

FIGURE 5.3   Scatter plots showing a positive relationship between height and weight in children and a negative relationship between practicing a procedure and number of errors.

and the spots do not all fall along a perfectly straight line. However, the bigger the value of the correlation coefficient, the more consistent and stronger the relationship is between the two variables.

To test whether or not two variables covary, a correlation statistic is computed and tested to see whether the computed value is likely to have occurred by chance. The predictors of postconcussive symptoms report includes several correlation statistics (as shown in Appendix A-5) providing an example of the use of a correlation coefficient. In the third paragraph, first sentence of the section titled "Predictors of Postconcussive Symptoms," the authors state "Examination of the intercorrelations of predictor variables revealed that initial Glasgow Coma Scale was significantly associated with posttraumatic amnesia duration" ($r = .572$, $p < .001$). The r is used to denote a Pearson correlation statistic (to be discussed later in the chapter); so you can see that this statistic shows covariation between the Glasgow Coma Scale and posttraumatic amnesia. From what we have just learned about correlation statistics, we know this means that the Glasgow Coma Scale and posttraumatic amnesia were connected to each other. We know that a *correlation* is a statistic looking at covariance or relationships between two variables.

If two variables covary, then they are connected to each other in some way. However, correlation does not tell us how the two variables are connected or whether one of the variables causes the change in the other. For example, if we had no other information besides the correlation statistic for height and weight of children, we would be left wondering whether weight causes growth in height, height causes increased weight, or both tend to increase because of some other factor we have not considered, such as age or nutrition. Therefore, correlations are inferential statistics that explain about relationships but cannot be used to predict because they do not tell us anything about which variable "causes" the other variable to change.

🕊 CORE CONCEPT 5.4

A correlation between two variables only tells us that they are connected in some way, not the cause of that connection.

For example, a study shows correlation statistics for each of the possible relationships between different pairs of variables. If we want to know whether there was a relationship between two variables, we would look at the statistical values. Taking the statistical value from the predictors of postconcussive symptoms article, $r = .572$, $p < .001$, this means 1 out of 1,000 chances would we get a statistic of .572 for the relationship between Glasgow Coma Scale scores and posttraumatic amnesia duration. Therefore, we decide that there is a relationship between Glasgow Coma Scale scores and posttraumatic amnesia duration and will expect to find such a relationship in other groups of patients who have had mTBIs. We also learn from this number that the connection or relationship between the variables are positive or negative. Finally, we know that the strength of the connection is on the moderate side because of where .572 falls between 0 (which indicates no connection at all) and 1 (which indicates a perfect connection).

Numerous types of correlation statistics can be computed between two variables, but the one you will probably find most frequently is the Pearson product–moment correlation, which uses the symbol "r" to represent the value of the bivariate relationship. Besides the Pearson product–moment correlation, other types of correlation statistics include the Spearman rho, the Kendall tau, and the phi. In all cases, the statistic gives the strength of the covariance between two variables. Remember a positive correlation occurs when both variables move in the same direction (if one goes up, the other does as well) and a negative correlation occurs when the variables move in opposite directions (one goes up and the other goes down).

For example, let us say you have two variables with the correlation value of $r = .50$, $p < .05$, because the size of the correlation coefficient reflects how strong the connection was between the two variables, we see that there was a moderate relationship between the variables. This would be in contrast to the correlation of variables with these values ($r = -.10$, $p < .01$). Although both of these connections are statistically significant, the strength of the relationships is different. What we understand from these statistics is that although in the first set of variables there is a moderately strong connection between them, in the second set of variables, the connection between the variables is not that strong.

Tests Looking for Differences Among Three or More Groups

Frequently, healthcare research addresses questions about more than just two groups. For example, we might be interested in comparing patients who smoke, patients who have never smoked, and patients who have quit smoking for their rates of respiratory complications after cardiac surgery. We can perform three different t tests to examine differences in complication rates between smokers and those who have never smoked, then between smokers and former smokers, and then between those who have never smoked and former smokers. Keeping up with these comparisons makes one's head whirl, and, obviously, the number of comparisons required would become more complicated with more groups we have. In addition, each time we get a result that is statistically significant, a small chance remains that we are wrong in our decision that the result did not happen by chance. These chances of being wrong add up when we do multiple statistical tests to answer just one question, making our chance of an error in our decision much larger when we do three or more tests on the same set of variables. The alternative is to use a different type of statistical test called ANOVA.

Analysis of variance tests for differences in the means for three or more groups. Although it is not necessary that you do the calculations for ANOVA, it may be helpful to know what the test does, which is reflected in its name. The ANOVA compares how much members of a group differ or vary among one another with how much the members of the group differ or vary from the members of other groups. In other words, the test analyzes variance, comparing the variance *within* a group with the variance *between* groups. For example, an ANOVA test of respiratory complications in three groups of patients categorized by smoking status calculates how much variation there is in respiratory complications within the patient group that smokes, the patient group that never smoked, and the patient group that formerly smoked. It then calculates the amount of variation in respiratory rate between the smoking patients, the patients who never smoked, and the former smokers. Finally, the test compares the variation inside the groups with the variation between the groups to see their differences or similarities. The test statistic in ANOVA is usually an "F ratio" value, and, like other statistical tests, the final test statistic is then compared with a set of statistics one would get if there were no differences between the groups. The F ratio compares the variation between groups with that within groups, and the larger the F ratio, the more variation between groups. However, the value of F ratios differs depending on the number of groups compared and the number of people studied, so it is not possible to make general statements about the meaning of the F ratio, except within the context of significance testing. If the F ratio value for a particular study falls into the area of statistics that has less than a 5% chance of occurring by chance, then we decide there is a statistically significant difference between the groups. In the example of respiratory complications, if the F ratio were significant, we would be able to decide that smoking and smoking history affect the rate of those complications.

Neither the fictional article nor the predictors of postconcussive symptoms article used ANOVA because neither study needed to compare the means of three or more groups. Other versions of the ANOVA allow the addition of more variables and various interconnections among variables into the ANOVA. Some of the most common are analysis of covariance (ANCOVA), multiple analysis of variance (MANOVA), and one-way ANOVA. For each of these, the basic purpose of the test is to compare means of an independent variable among three or more groups. Some of the most common nonparametric statistical tests that also test for differences among three or more groups are the Kruskal–Wallis and the chi-square test (Table 5.3).

In addition to comparing three or more groups, we often want to look for differences within groups during three or more points in time. Continuing with the example of patients who smoke and their respiratory complication rates, suppose that instead of comparing them with patients who never smoked, we compared smoking patients' respiratory complication rates before and after pulmonary toilet care over a 3-day period. In this case, we are not comparing different groups, but the same group over time. The statistical test used in this type of situation is a repeated-measures ANOVA. Like other ANOVA tests, it calculates differences in variance within the group at each time point but compares those variances with the variances between the time points. Commonly used nonparametric tests for differences within groups at three or more points in time include Friedman tests and the Cochran Q. Note the predictors in postconcussive symptoms article by Ponsford et al. (2012) used the Friedman test because of the three different times data were measured (at the acute stage, at 1 week, and at 3 months).

Tests Looking at Relationships Among Three or More Variables

Just as we are often interested in differences among three or more groups, we are also interested in how a group of more than two variables covaries. For example, in the predictors of postconcussive symptoms article (Appendix A-5) (Ponsford et al., 2012), the authors are interested in how a set of variables, such as the patients' age, gender, and educational level, all covary in relation to occurrence of PCS. If each of these variables is connected to PCS occurrences but is also connected to each other somewhat, how much does each variable independently contribute to the variation occurring in the occurrence of PCS? Our goal is to understand what factors or variables connect to occurrences of PCS and in what direction and to what extent so that we can use our knowledge of those connections to increase the potential that we can impact a patient's occurrence of PCS. If individuals' values reflecting PCS occurrence were a big pie, each of the factors studied might be a piece of that pie, although those pieces will overlap somewhat. We are interested in seeing not just how much each factor by itself connects, but how the factors overlap so that we know which of the many factors might be the most useful to focus on when planning evidence-based care to improve patient outcomes. The statistical procedure that we use to look at connections among three or more variables is called *regression*. **Regression** measures how much two or more independent variables explain the variation in a dependent variable. The regression procedure allows us to predict future values for the dependent variable based on values of the independent variables.

A regression analysis gives the information needed to know how much different factors independently contribute or connect to a dependent variable. Authors can use a table format to report the results of regression analysis in order to examine how much of an effect each of the factors that they had identified contributed to, let us say in this case, patient satisfaction. Suppose the table has two columns with results labeled "*b*" and "R 95% CI." Under the column labeled "*b*," the statistical value for relative contribution of each of the factors is listed. A **beta (β) value** tells us the relative contribution or connection of an independent variable to the dependent variable. The *R* refers to how much of the variation in scores the factor studied explains. The 95% CI refers to what we would expect the *b* value to be 95% of the time, given the results that we found in the study. In summary, what you should understand is that each variable in a regression analysis is tested to determine whether it is independently connected with the dependent variable. If it is connected, a test of how much or to what extent it is connected is provided. A healthcare provider must read the results section of an article to see what factors predict patient satisfaction. From this, the healthcare provider may see that the patients and patients' families have different contributing factors for patient satisfaction and must take this into consideration when trying to improve patient satisfaction of patients and patients' families. In addition to regression analysis, numerous statistical procedures examine relationships among three or more variables. The names of some of the most common types of procedures used in healthcare research are listed in Table 5.3 and include canonical correlation, path analysis, structural equation modeling, and discriminate analysis.

Tests Looking at the Structure or Components of a Variable

We have discussed bivariate statistical tests that look for differences between two variables and tests that look at relationships between two variables. We also have discussed multivariate tests that look at differences or relationships among three or more variables, and we have identified several parametric and nonparametric statistical tests for each purpose. The last general purpose for statistical procedures is to look at the structure or components within a variable of interest. These types of statistical tests are used when the variable of interest is complex and not easily measured using a single item or question. The researcher may collect information about the complex variable using several different questions or measures and then want to determine the connections among the questions or measures. For example, a nurse researcher might be interested in studying patient satisfaction associated with care. Several aspects of care may influence satisfaction, such as availability, communication with providers, cost, and whether expectations for care are met. The researcher might develop 60 statements for a survey, each of which affects some aspect of satisfaction. Responses to the survey may be scores on a scale to indicate the respondents' level of agreement with each of the statements. Scores to all 60 statements can be added together to produce a single score for satisfaction, but this does not help us to understand the important components of satisfaction that make up that score. Statistical procedures, called **factor analysis**, can be used to look for discrete groups of statements that are more closely connected to each other than to the other statements. Factors are the components or discrete groups of measures or statements that covary closely. In our example, the researcher might find that statements about paying bills, insurance, and difficulty getting referrals all covary more closely than statements about communication. These statements might be said to reflect a factor that could be called *barriers to satisfaction*. Factor analysis will identify groups of measures of a single variable that are connected closely enough that the connections are not likely to happen by chance. In clinical practice, a study that uses a factor analysis procedure has the potential to provide knowledge about some of the components or parts that comprise a health-related concept, such as fear, pain, or denial. The nonparametric statistical test that may be used to look at structure within a variable is called *cluster analysis*.

To summarize, several specific statistical procedures are used to test for differences and relationships. The types of tests differ depending on the type of data and whether two, or more than two, variables are to be tested. When any of these tests are applied to specific data, they produce a test statistic that will be symbolized in a unique manner, such as a "t" statistic, "F" statistic, or "r" statistic. The specific statistic from the study is compared with a distribution of statistics that would have occurred in similar data by chance alone if there were really no relationship or difference. If the statistic from the study falls into the range of values that occur <5% of the time, it is likely that there was a relationship or difference, and the result is statistically significant. Often, the level of statistical significance is specifically stated in the form of a p value or CI.

HYPOTHESIS TESTING

In Chapter 2, we defined *hypotheses* as predictions regarding the relationships or effects of selected factors on other factors. Inferential statistics are used to test whether the predictions in hypotheses are "accurate," so hypotheses direct which statistical procedures are used with the data. The results for two types of hypotheses may be described in a research report. The first type, a **research hypothesis**, is a prediction of the relationships or differences that will be found for selected variables in a study. You may find reports of research that authors have not used hypotheses. However, in the predictors of postconcussive symptoms article, the authors used a research hypothesis, "injury-related factors, including presence and severity of a mTBI, would have the strongest influence on outcome measured in terms of postconcussive symptoms at 1 week postinjury and that ongoing problems at 3 months postinjury would be predicted by a combination of mTBI presence and severity; psychological factors including anxiety, depression, pain and post-traumatic stress syndrome; and other life stressors" (Ponsford et al., 2012, 305). This hypothesis predicts that as mTBI severity, anxiety, depression, pain, posttraumatic stress syndrome, and life stresses increase, postconcussive symptoms will increase. This is a clear prediction that not only will there be a relationship, but it will also be positive. In some studies in which we are not given predictions in the form of hypotheses, the authors may use research objectives instead, and we will discuss these further in Chapter 10.

The second type of hypothesis that may be tested and reported about in the results section of a research report is a statistical hypothesis that is often called the *null hypothesis*. A **null hypothesis** always predicts that there will be no relationship or difference in selected variables. Remember that, in general, researchers want to be cautious about jumping to conclusions based on the results of a particular study. This is why researchers agree that statistical test results are acceptable only when they would occur by chance <5% of the time. Otherwise, even if we find a difference or relationship in the data, we decide that it was just a chance happening, and we cannot prove that there was a "real" relationship. The null hypothesis reflects this same thinking by stating our prediction about relationships or differences in the negative, predicting no relationship or difference. The researcher must then find enough evidence to reject that prediction, a statistically significant test result being the evidence that is required.

In summary, a research hypothesis is stated in the positive and predicts the nature and strength of a relationship or difference among variables. It is the researcher's hope that the results of a study support the prediction. A statistical hypothesis is stated in the negative, and it is the researcher's desire for statistical tests to be significant so that the null hypothesis can be rejected. Not all quantitative research studies use hypotheses, but if there are one or more hypotheses, they are usually identified in the section of the report that describes the research problem. Chapter 10 discusses hypotheses in more detail.

IN-CLASS STUDY DATA

To illustrate the use of inferential statistics, let us look at the data that were collected in your in-class study. If you are not using an in-class study, you can refer to a sample set of data in Appendix D that could have been collected in a nursing class. Suppose that before these data were collected, you had observed that your fellow students who were married were generally healthier than those who were not married. You wonder whether this is true and realize that the data from your in-class study could be used to test this idea because a question about marital status and a question about overall health is included. This means there are two variables of interest: (1) marital status and (2) rating of health. The question of interest concerns differences between two groups and might be stated as "Is there a difference in health rating between married and unmarried nursing students?"

To use the in-class data to answer this question, you must first divide the health ratings into two groups: the health ratings of students who indicated that they were married and those who indicated that they were single, divorced, or widowed. Once this is done, it is easy to get an average health rating for the two groups and to see whether they are different. If they are exactly the same, or close, you probably do not have to look any further for a tentative answer to your question based on these data. If there is a difference, the next question is whether the difference is in the direction you predicted and whether it is big enough that you can believe that it did not happen by chance alone. Looking at the average health ratings will tell you whether single students seemed to have higher or lower health ratings. However, you cannot judge whether the findings prove or disprove your hypothesis because the ratings may have been simply chance findings. This is the place where inferential statistics come in because if this information is entered into a statistical computer program, you can run a *t* test to calculate differences in the means for rating of health of married and unmarried students.

If you are using an in-class study, predict whether some difference found in your class data will be significant before your professor runs an independent *t* test to determine the *t* value for your in-class data. For the fictional data in Appendix D, the computer calculates that the mean health rating for single students is 3.1 and the mean rating of health for married students is 2.3. These ratings look different and are opposite to what was predicted before data were collected. When we do a *t* test, we get a *t* value of 2.7 ($p = .011$), so there is a significant difference in health ratings between single and married students. However, from these data, we can conclude that the evidence does not support the hypothesis that married students are healthier; instead, it supports the opposite idea. In this fictional study, single nursing students had significantly higher ratings of their health than did married nursing students. That it was a statistically significant difference tells us that we can be sure that the difference did not happen by chance alone.

CONNECTING INFERENTIAL STATISTICAL RESULTS TO CONCLUSIONS

There are several important connections between results and conclusions of reports that have used inferential statistics. If inferential statistics were used, we know that the goal of the researcher is to predict that the findings of the study apply to similar situations or groups in the future. Therefore, we expect to find in the discussion and conclusions statement both how the results can be applied to similar situations or groups in the future and what aspects of the study may limit our ability to draw conclusions about future situations or groups. In the fictional article, for example, the author summarizes the findings and then concludes that "Nursing programs that are particularly concerned about shortages in nonacute settings may be able to expand this workforce by focusing their recruitment efforts on older students and by further developing or expanding RN to BSN and LPN to BSN programs." The author is saying that in the future, age and type of program of study are likely to be connected with choice of field of study, just as they were in the article. Although the author fails to give any statement of the limitations of the conclusion, the size of the sample—one class of 30 nursing students—might be a reason to consider limiting it.

If the results of a report included hypothesis testing, we should also expect a statement in the conclusions of the report about whether the hypotheses were rejected or accepted. Most importantly, the meaningfulness of statistically significant results should be discussed in the discussion and conclusions section. Throughout this chapter, we have talked about statistical significance; however, the presence of statistical significance does not necessarily indicate that the results are meaningful for clinical practice. Conversely, lack of statistical significance does not necessarily mean that there is no clinical significance in the results. The presence of statistical significance depends on several factors, one of which is the number of cases in the study. This is logical, given that we are trying to use probability to help us to infer connections or differences in the real world. If the study only includes a few cases or subjects, then the chances of a "weird" or unusual case affecting the average result is pretty high. The test distribution for a study with only a few cases results in a large "green" zone and a small "red" zone because there is a good chance that a single odd case will change the actual test statistic (Fig. 5.2).

 CORE CONCEPT 5.5

The size of the sample, or number of cases, in a study affects the likelihood that a statistical significance will be found.

A study that has a large number of cases has a high likelihood of finding statistically significant findings, simply because whatever is found is not going to be affected easily by the chance that an odd case fell into the sample. However, the difference or connection that is found may not be large enough to have meaning for clinical practice. The author of the fictional article, for example, does not give the average ages of students who selected acute and nonacute settings. It is possible that the difference in age was only 1 or 2 years. A difference of this size may be statistically significant but may also be too small to have any meaning when one is trying to recruit individuals to nursing.

A clinical example of the difference between statistically significant and clinically meaningful findings might be a study of ratings of pain, such as the one discussed in Chapter 4. Suppose that this fictional study has 500 subjects and that after one group receives an intervention, the mean ratings of pain are 2.5 (1.3) for patients getting the intervention and 2 (1.5) for patients not getting the intervention. In Chapter 4, we used an example where the standard deviations were different, although the means were the same. In this example, the means are different, whereas the standard deviations are similar. The researcher might report that there was a statistically significant difference in pain ratings between the group that did and did not get the intervention. This means that the difference in ratings was not likely to happen by chance. However, if you look at the difference, it is not large and may not, in fact, be clinically meaningful. You must decide whether a difference of only one-half of a point is large enough to warrant implementation of the intervention, even though you may believe that this difference is unlikely to have occurred by chance. Thus, statistical significance does not necessarily imply clinical significance.

We would expect, therefore, that the conclusions of a research study that used inferential statistics would address whether the statistically significant findings were also meaningful findings. We also would expect that the conclusions would address whether findings that were *not* statistically significant might still warrant further consideration because they appear to be clinically meaningful.

CORE CONCEPT 5.6

Statistical significance does not directly equate with clinical meaningfulness.

COMMON ERRORS IN RESULTS SECTIONS

As with the reports of descriptive results, two kinds of problems may be found when reading inferential statistic results in a research report: (1) incomplete information and (2) confusing information. Incomplete information occurs when the results section of reports gives us the statistical test results, including the p value or CI, but does not give us the descriptive results needed to interpret the statistically significant result. For example, suppose that the author of the fictional article from Appendix B had told us that there was a significant difference in health rating ($t = 2.1$, $p < .05$) among students who chose acute versus nonacute fields of practice. The test statistic alone does not tell us which group had the higher health rating, so it is impossible to interpret the meaning of this statistically significant difference.

Another example of incomplete information might be a research report that includes a statement that there was a statistically significant finding but does not provide the test statistic. Because some of the statistics tell us a great deal, the lack of the statistic can limit our understanding of the results. If, for example, the authors of the predictors of postconcussive symptoms study in Appendix A-5 had told us only that there was a significant relationship between Glasgow Coma Scale and posttraumatic amnesia without providing statistical information, we would have no idea about the direction of that relationship or its strength. It would be conceivable that those who had high Glasgow Coma Scale results (normal) had had more posttraumatic amnesia, which would be a negative relationship with the value for "r" being negative. However, the authors did provide us with the correlation coefficient of r (.572); we would know that this tells us that there was a positive relationship and that it was moderate in strength.

A third type of incomplete information is a failure to test for relationships or differences that might be meaningful for understanding the results of the study. The fictional article reports in the results section that age and health rating were both different in students who chose acute versus nonacute fields of practice. One might wonder whether age and rating of health are related. This is a logical question, given what we know about aging and health, and the answer would help us better understand the meaning of the results of this study. However, the author does not test for a relationship between these two variables, so we are left wondering about the possibility of this relationship.

In addition to incomplete information, research reports may present results in a manner that is unclear or unnecessarily confusing. The titles of tables should clearly identify the table's content and should be referenced within the text of the results section. Labels for columns should be consistent with the use of language in the text and with accepted language for reporting statistical results that may be tested and reported about in the results section. Lastly, sometimes a researcher may overinterpret or overgeneralize about results from a study. Similarly, sometimes a researcher actually incorrectly interprets a statistical result. For example, suppose that an author interpreted a correlation between obesity and depression to mean that obesity *causes* depression. A correlation means that there is a connection, but it does not tell us that one of the two connected variables caused the other. These last types of errors are not likely to appear in research reports published in peer-reviewed journals because those types of errors will be found and corrected. However, occasionally, research results in the public sector are overinterpreted or incorrectly interpreted.

CRITICALLY READING THE RESULTS SECTION OF A REPORT FOR USE IN EVIDENCE-BASED NURSING PRACTICE—REVISITED

In Chapter 4, we looked at six questions that can help you to read critically the results section of a research report. These questions are shown again in Box 5.1. Let us revisit some of these questions now that we have talked about inferential statistics. The first question relates to a clearly defined results section. The predictors of postconcussive symptoms article by Ponsford et al. (2012) (Appendix A-5), the literature searching skills to medical students article by Ilic, Tepper, and Misso (2012) (Appendix A-4), the leg length discrepancy article by Peck, Mulhotra, and Kim (2011) (Appendix A-3), the perceptions of caring article by Li, Rukavina, and Foster (2013) (Appendix A-2), and the body satisfaction and behaviors in overweight adolescents by Cromley et al. (2012) (Appendix A-1) all have a specific results or findings section clearly labeled within the articles. The second question to consider asks, "Were the results presented appropriately for the information collected?" As we discussed in the previous section, at times, the results presented are either incomplete or confusing. The authors in the predictors of postconcussive symptoms article provided results in table and descriptive format that is appropriate for the purpose of the study. However, Ponsford et al. (2012) did indicate "more detailed results obtained by the mTBI and TC (control group) participants on each of the variables are detailed in another article" (308–309). The third question listed for critically reading results also addresses a concern with the predictors of postconcussive symptoms report. That question asks about clear identification of descriptive versus inferential results. The authors provide tables with descriptive and inferential results for some of the measures and direct the readers to another article for more detailed results. Our ability to use this research may have improved if all of the findings were provided.

The predictors of postconcussive symptoms study was quantitative, so we cannot use it as an example for answering the fourth question for critically reading results sections.

BOX 5.1
How to Critically Read the Results Sections of Research Reports

Do the results answer the question "Why did the authors reach these conclusions— what did they actually find?"

1. Did the report include a clearly identified results section?
2. Were the results presented appropriately for the information collected?
3. Were descriptive versus inferential results identifiable if this is a quantitative study?
4. Were themes or structure and meaning identifiable if this is a qualitative study?
5. Were the results presented in a clear and logical manner?
6. Did the results include enough information about the final sample for the study?

However, we can decide about the fifth question, which asks how clearly and logically the results were presented. In general, the tables in this report clearly listed descriptive results, and organized the presentation of their results, and clearly indicated this in the readings. Therefore, we might decide that the results are presented clearly and logically. Finally, the last question refers to information about the sample what do you think? The predictors of postconcussive symptoms report provides a table about the characteristics of the final sample in the study and gives us the details about the sample that we might need, such as age and gender, as well as additional information in the results section. We will have to evaluate this aspect of the results further after learning more about samples and sampling.

PUBLISHED REPORT—WHAT WOULD YOU CONCLUDE?

The healthcare team in our clinical case now has an increased understanding of the results and conclusions of the study examining predictors of postconcussive symptoms following an injury. The healthcare team members know that there were several differences in how patients scored on postconcussive symptoms measures. The healthcare team also knows that selected factors, including postinjury anxiety and mTBI, appear to impact PCS occurrences at 3 months post injury. Ponsford et al. (2012) state two limitations of the study: (1) only patients with noncomplex mTBI were included in the sample and (2) age of the sample participants may have influenced the findings. The healthcare team must decide whether the evidence from this study can be used to guide healthcare practice and improve outcomes for patients who have suspected concussions. However, the healthcare team does note that the majority of participants in the study were adults and wonders if some aspect of the approach to sampling led to more adults than adolescents and children being included. Since the healthcare team sees a majority of patients who are between 10 and 22, the healthcare team needs to know more about how this sample was selected before a decision can be made on how useful this evidence is for healthcare practice. Chapter 6 addresses samples and how they affect the conclusions we can draw from research.

OUT-OF-CLASS EXERCISE

What Do you Want to Know About Samples?

The next two chapters focus on the process of sampling and the meanings of different types of samples. In preparation for reading the next chapter, think about your in-class study sample. Write a list of information that you would like to have about the characteristics of the sample for this study, including a rationale for why you would like that information next to each item. Then, think about what you know about the composition of your class and assume that an interesting result that has implications for nursing education was found in the in-class data. If you were writing the conclusions of a report about this finding, how would you describe the group of individuals to whom the results might be applied in the future? Write a short paragraph describing this group, including to whom the results probably apply and to whom they probably do not. If your class did not use an in-class study, you can do this exercise by pretending that a study was conducted using your class group. List what you would want to know about the people in the study and why. Then, given what you do know about those in your course group, write a short paragraph describing to whom the results of a study with this course group probably would apply and to whom they probably would not. After you complete one of these exercises, you are ready to begin Chapter 6.

References

Cromley, T., Knatz, S., Rockwell, R. A., Neumark-Sztainer, D., Story, M., & Boutelle, K. (2012). Relationships between body satisfaction and psychological functioning and weight-related cognitions and behaviors in overweight adolescents. *Journal of Adolescent Health*, *50*, 651–653. doi:10.1016/j.jaohealth.2011.10.252

Ilic, D., Tepper, K., & Misso, M. (2012). Teaching evidence-based medicine literature searching skills to medical students during the clinical years: a randomized controlled trial. *Journal of the Medical Library Association*, *100*(3), 190–196. doi:10.3163/1536-5050.100.3.009

Li, W., Rukavina, P. B., & Foster, C. (2013). Overweight or obese students' perceptions of caring in urban physical education programs. *Journal of Sports Behavior*, *36*(2), 189–208.

Peck, C. N., Malhotra, K., & Kim, W. Y. (2011). Leg length discrepancy in cementless total hip arthroplasty. *Surgical Science*, *2*, e183–e187. doi:10.4236/ss.2011.24040

Ponsford, J., Cameron, P., Fitzgerald, M., Grant, M., & Mikocka-Walus, A. (2012). Predictors of postconcussive symptoms 3 months after mild traumatic brain injury. *Neuropsychology*, *26*(3), 304–313. doi:10.1037/a0027888

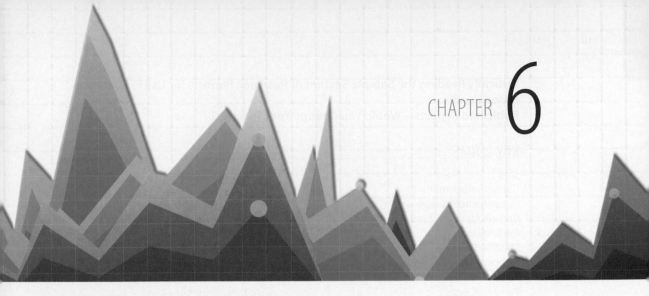

CHAPTER 6

Samples

To What Types of Patients Do These Research Conclusions Apply—Who Was in the Study?

> **LEARNING OBJECTIVE** The student will relate the sampling methods and study sample to results, conclusions, and clinical meaningfulness of the study.

Samples Versus Populations

Does the Population for This Study Reflect the Types of Patients or Situations of Interest?

Does the Sample in the Study Reflect the Population of Interest?

Does the Approach for Choosing the Sample Limit the Usefulness of the Study Results?

Sampling in Qualitative Research

Strengths and Weaknesses of Qualitative Sampling Approaches

Sample Size in Qualitative Research

Summary of Qualitative Sampling

Sampling in Quantitative Research

Strengths and Weaknesses of Quantitative Sampling Approaches

Sample Size in Quantitative Research

Summary of Quantitative Sampling

Differences in Qualitative and Quantitative Sampling
Problems With the Sampling Process
Problems With Sampling Outcomes
Common Errors in Reports of Samples
Connecting Sampling to the Study Results and Conclusions

Critically Reading the Sample Section of Research Reports for Use in Evidence-Based Practice
Published Reports—Would You Change Your Practice?

KEY TERMS

Bias	Random assignment
Cluster sampling	Randomly selected
Convenience sample	Response rate
Criteria for participation	Sample
Generalizability	Sampling frame
Matched sample	Sampling unit
Nonprobability sampling	Saturation
Population	Selectivity
Power analysis	Simple random sampling
Probability sampling	Snowball sampling
Purposive sampling	Stratified random sampling
Quota sampling	Systematic sample

Each of the healthcare providers in the clinical cases discussed in previous chapters had an EBP clinical question and sought an answer through evidence in research-related publications. As we reviewed what each could conclude regarding their questions, we had to wonder whether the results and conclusions of the study could be applied to the patient or patients of concern to the healthcare provider in the clinical cases. Specifically, we wondered

1. What THA implant approach (cemented or cementless) can decrease postsurgical leg length differences in patients undergoing THA surgery?

2. What strategies assist medical students in performing evidence-based literature searching skills during clinical practice?

In exploring the topic of research samples, we will revisit the previous clinical cases as well as the research found by our healthcare providers.

Regardless of whether we are using EBP strategies to answer questions related to using research to guide discharge planning or to direct the planning of care, education, or programs, it is important to answer the question "To what types of patients do these research conclusions apply?" We must consider this question because a study may address a clinical problem of interest to you, but it may not have used a sample that reflects your patients. As a healthcare provider, you will need to understand the implications of different sample types to your ability to use study results as evidence in EBP to address clinical practice effectively. One of the first things that you will need to understand is the difference between a sample and a population.

SAMPLES VERSUS POPULATIONS

As discussed, research is rarely able to include in one study all the cases that might be affected by the research question. A study of cardiovascular risk factors in children with insulin-dependent diabetes mellitus (IDDM), for example, could not possibly study every child with diabetes. A study of male patients with trauma resulting from combat is a smaller group, but it is still impossible to include all of these men in one study. All of the studies discussed so far were interested in understanding something about a larger group of patients than those included in their actual studies. The larger group, called the study **population**, is all of the individuals that the researchers are interested in studying. The population for any particular study is defined by specific common characteristics. For example, the population of interest in the "Predictors of Postconcussive Symptoms 3 Months After Mild Traumatic Brain Injury" (Ponsford, Fitzgerald, Grant, and Mikocka-Walus, 2012) study (Appendix A-5) had four common characteristics: they (1) were adults above the age of 18, (2) had some type of physical injury, (3) were medically treated in Australia, and (4) had a minimum of 9 years of education (p. 308). The population of interest in the study by Ilic, Tepper, and Misso (2012), "Teaching Evidence-Based Medicine Literature Searching Skills to Medical Student During the Clinical Years: A Randomized Controlled Trial" (Appendix A-4), shared characteristics of (1) being medical students, (2) being a 3rd-year Monash student, (3) being in a 5-year undergraduate course of study, and (4) participating in medicine information sessions using PICO frameworks. The population of interest in the "Leg Length Discrepancy in Cementless Total Hip Arthroplasty" by Peck, Malhotra, and Kim (Appendix A-3) shared population characteristics of (1) "undergoing an elective total hip arthroplasty between June 2007 and May 2008" (p. 183), (2) first time in receiving a hip replacement, and (3) were treated at a specific hospital in England. In the "Overweight or Obese Students' Perceptions of Caring in Urban Physical Education Programs" study (Li, Rukavina, & Foster, 2013) (Appendix A-2), the population shared characteristics of (1) being overweight, (2) being between 11 and 18 years of age, (3) attending school in an urban district, and (4) participating in a physical education program. Notice that it is possible to clearly identify the common characteristics that comprise each population. Authors using descriptive statistics in tables or in text provide valuable information regarding the population of interest.

Of course, none of these studies included every member of the population of interest. There are thousands of children who are overweight. There are thousands of adults who have minor brain injuries, so the research will select a smaller, more workable group for conducting their study. This subset of the overall population that is included in a study is called a **sample**. To understand whether a study applies to your clinical situation, you can start by considering three general questions about the study sample and the related population: (1) Does the population for this study reflect the types of patients or situations that I am interested in understanding? (2) Does the sample in the study reflect or fit with the population of interest? (3) Does the approach taken to choosing the sample limit how much I can use the results of the study?

Most of this chapter addresses the third question, but the first and second questions are also essential to answer in order to understand and use research in clinical practice.

Does the Population for This Study Reflect the Types of Patients or Situations of Interest?

As we have discussed many times, EBP is a process of decision making regarding clinical questions that looks at available evidence to answer a clinical question. If research-based evidence is to be meaningfully considered in your EBP strategy, you will need to decide whether a study addresses a population that is relevant or clinically similar to the patient group you are interested in understanding. To do this, you will need to identify the common characteristics of your patient population. One of the ways to identify clearly the population that fits your clinical question is to use the *Who, What, When, Where* approach to forming an EBP clinical question. As you use this approach, you are, in essence, listing characteristics of the population in which you are interested. This will then give you a comparison of those characteristics of the identified sample within a research report.

Healthcare providers occasionally have a problem using research because they look for studies that exactly fit the specific patients with whom they are working. In the clinical case in Chapter 1, if the healthcare provider caring for M.D., the 17-year-old female adolescent who is medically obese, had searched the Cumulative Index to Nursing and Allied

Health (CINAHL) or other health-related databases for a study that specifically addressed needs of 17-year-old female teenagers, who were obese, had specific health issues and self-image/esteem issues, the healthcare provider would have had difficulty finding studies matched to such a narrow population. Or if the healthcare provider had searched for a single study that included all of those characteristics, the healthcare provider would have likely found little or nothing. The combination of gender, age, obesity, health, and self-image/esteem issues associated with obesity as patient characteristics is so specific that no one may have implemented a study focusing on that narrow a population. By broadening the characteristics that define the population to only adolescents with obesity or obesity and self-image/esteem, however, the RN found two studies. When these two studies are taken together, they cover several of the characteristics that could potentially apply to the healthcare provider's specific patient care situation. Yet, too broad a definition of the population might have found studies with populations that were too different from M.D., making them useless in planning care for her. For example, a literature search that used only the term *obesity* would yield a large number of studies, many without any attention to adolescents. Although there may be some overlap between the concerns of the population of adolescents with obesity and adolescents with self-image/esteem issues, clearly there are some important differences that affect how useful these studies will be to understanding M.D.'s case.

How do you learn what the population of a study may be? Several places in a research report should identify the population for the study, but in this chapter, we focus on the section of most reports that is labeled "Sample," "Sampling Methods," or something similar. In this section of the report, the author identifies how individuals were selected for the study and lists its **criteria for participation**. Remember our definition of a sample—that it is a subset of the population; therefore, the criteria for participation in the study should be the common characteristics that define the population of interest. In the study report used in Chapter 4 from Appendix A-4 on literature searching skills to medical students (Ilic et al., 2012), the authors state that "participants were required to be a third year Monash MBBS [bachelor of medicine/bachelor of surgery] student at the time of the study" (p. 191). This tells us that the target population was college students in an MBBS program willing to participate but does not tell us their grade point averages or previous experiences. In some cases, such as a meta-synthesis study, where the findings of several studies are examined, the actual identification of the sample may be more difficult to find. Also, reports may not have a specific section called *sample*, but the description of the sample may be located under the method or results sections. The statements of sample characteristics above supply us with information that we can compare with the population of interest to the healthcare providers in our clinical cases. In summary, it is important to identify the criteria for study participation in order to understand the targeted research study population and to decide on its applicability to your clinical practice.

Does the Sample in the Study Reflect the Population of Interest?

At first glance, this question may appear to be the same as the first question, but it is not. Once a study defines the population of interest—that is, the larger group we are interested in gaining knowledge about—the researcher must find a way to recruit or get a sample of individuals who are members of that population. This is sometimes more difficult than it might seem. Occasionally, it is not ethical to ask members of the population to submit to the study, and it might be difficult to get members of the population to agree to be in a study. As well, there may occasionally be limits inherent to a setting that make it difficult to get members from the population of interest. We discuss each of these potential problems in getting study samples later in this chapter. For now, it is important to realize that a researcher may define the population of interest for a study one way and end up with a sample that does not fit that planned population.

If you have discovered a lack of fit between the sample and the population of interest in a research article, this should be considered a limitation to the study and may limit your ability to apply the evidence to your clinical concerns. To read intelligently and to use research, it is important to identify (1) the population of interest, (2) the population for a particular research study, and (3) whether the sample reflects that population of interest.

⬤ CORE CONCEPT 6.1

A researcher may define the population of interest in one way but end up with a sample that differs from that defined population.

Does the Approach for Choosing the Sample Limit the Usefulness of the Study Results?

Our third broad question considers how the researcher obtained his or her sample and whether that approach limits how you can use the study conclusions in clinical practice. To address this, we must first discuss some of the unique language used in research to describe samples.

The language used differs between qualitative and quantitative studies because the general purposes of the two types of research differ in two broad areas: (1) constraining versus enriching the complexity of samples and (2) rigidity or flexibility in sampling. In general, qualitative research neither tries to predict future occurrences of the phenomena nor attempts to control any aspects of the phenomena as it is studied. Therefore, samples in qualitative research try to derive what is called *rich* samples. These samples contain as many of the complex aspects of the phenomena as possible. Qualitative research samples are also flexible. As researchers begin to understand more about what they are studying, the sample may change. These approaches to sampling can be contrasted to quantitative research, where the researcher will often attempt to constrain aspects of the phenomena when studying it and the sample is generally rigid, not changing after it is selected. We will now discuss these significant differences between qualitative and quantitative research in more detail.

SAMPLING IN QUALITATIVE RESEARCH

When reading qualitative research, understanding whether the sample fits the population of interest is essential because the subjective experiences of the sample are at the heart of the study. Suppose that a researcher studies homeless patients' satisfaction with health care. The population of interest in such a study would have the characteristics of (1) being homeless and (2) having had experiences with healthcare. If the researcher enrolls subjects who have been homeless in the past but are now in some type of housing, even temporary housing, this might alter the fit. The meaning of the experiences for formerly homeless individuals is likely to be different from the meanings for those who are currently homeless. Because the goal of this hypothetical research would be to inform our practice by increasing our knowledge about the overall satisfaction with the experience of receiving primary healthcare as a homeless person, a sample of formerly homeless individuals would not have been appropriate and would have entirely changed the population for the study.

In the clinical case in Chapter 2, the healthcare provider is interested in developing a plan of action to assist adolescents in becoming healthier and having a higher self-esteem. In looking for research-based evidence to support EBP, the healthcare provider finds the perceptions of caring report (Li et al., 2013) (Appendix A-2). A qualitative study such as this has a goal of broadly increasing our understanding of the population of interest, recognizing that each piece of the picture that we collect gives us a better sense of the whole phenomenon. In order to accomplish this, the sample must then be composed of individuals who have knowledge of the phenomena. In our example of the researcher looking at homeless patients' satisfaction with primary healthcare, the phenomenon of interest to the research is satisfaction with care. So, to find a sample of this population, the researcher would need to select individuals who are homeless and who, while homeless, had received primary care services.

As the researcher plans to find such a group of individuals, we will notice one of the first obvious things that differentiate a qualitative sample from a quantitative sample. In qualitative research, the individuals who comprise a sample are most often called *participants*, *volunteers*, *members*, or *informants* rather than being called *subjects*. Use of these terms reflects the perspective seen in qualitative research that the individuals are an active part of the research process and are sharing their knowledge and experiences with the researcher.

The qualitative researcher is looking for the most content and the most contextually rich sources of data available to understand the meaning of the experiences of interest. Immersion in the experience with as much complexity as possible is critical in understanding these realities and experiences. Therefore, the qualitative researcher wants each participant or informant to be different so as to lend additional insight, or richness, about a particular phenomenon. The researcher will intentionally seek ways to find individuals who are deeply involved and a part of the phenomenon being studied. In the study of perceptions of caring (Li et al., 2013), the researcher searched for overweight students who were involved in a physical education program. In this sense, they could be assured that they were finding students who were deeply involved in the phenomenon of interest and who were overweight. Think about how the sample would have been less rich if they used a small community school for students of any weight. Under the "Participants" heading (pp. 192–193), the authors list the inclusion criteria for obtaining their sample. This criteria identifies the characteristics of the sample, and therefore, of the population. They identify that (1) participants had a BMI (body mass index) of >85th percentile and (2) students were from a specific city school district. Reading this, we know that the participant sample was composed of overweight students who were in a physical education program. The sample was delimited to "overweight and obese students" (p. 192). This type of sampling, used in qualitative research, is **purposive sampling**. A purposive sample consists of participants who are intentionally or purposefully selected because they have certain characteristics related to the purpose of the research. The characteristics sought in the sample will vary, depending on the approach taken by the researcher. Occasionally, a researcher's goal is to obtain as much diversity as possible in the sample, but sometimes the goal is to focus intently on a particular aspect of the phenomenon under study. If researchers are interested in understanding smoking cessation, they may wish to look at a purposive sample of individuals who have quit smoking in the last month. In this approach, they will purposefully not recruit individuals who are still smoking or who have been tobacco free for over a year. But the researchers may also take a different approach and purposefully recruit individuals who have tried three or more times to quit but who are still smoking. From these examples, we can see that different experiences with a phenomenon may be used by researchers to select the sample purposefully.

Another type of sample used in qualitative (and quantitative) research studies is called a **convenience sample** because it includes members of the population who can be readily found and recruited and are "convenient" for the researcher to recruit. There is no attempt to limit the sample. Participants are selected on the first-come-first-served basis.

Qualitative research may also use an approach called **snowball sampling**. A snowball sample is just as the name implies. The researcher will start with one participant or member of the population and will then use that member's contacts to identify other potential participants for the study. The next few participants will share other contacts who may have experiences of interest, thus ever increasing the sample. Snowball sampling is most commonly used when the researcher would have difficulty in finding participants who might otherwise not be identified easily. Snowball sampling often allows the inclusion of several views or experiences.

Strengths and Weaknesses of Qualitative Sampling Approaches

A convenience sample for a qualitative study has the advantages of being relatively easy and inexpensive to acquire but may have the disadvantage of yielding a group of participants that is not as diverse and cannot provide as rich a detail about the phenomenon of interest. For example, a convenience sample of homeless people from just one shelter may yield individuals who have been homeless for only a short time because of the location of the shelter or the type of services offered at that shelter.

Similarly, purposive sampling has its advantages and disadvantages. A purposive sample in a qualitative study actively seeks to enrich the data by including participants who have a particular type of experience, characteristic, or understanding to share. The potential disadvantage to this type of sampling is the possibility of prematurely focusing the data collection on one experience or understanding and missing the broader range of data that may come from a convenience sample.

Sample Size in Qualitative Research

Qualitative sampling strategies are fluid and flexible and are intentionally and thoughtfully revised as the data analysis suggests new avenues to explore or aspects that need additional focus. These strategies are used to seek a detailed and rich understanding of the aspect under study. This process continues until the information shared by participants has become redundant and no new information is being added; at this point, the researcher identifies that **saturation** has occurred. Saturation of data is the point in data collection at which the data become repetitive and no new information or participants is being added.

Sample size is usually dictated by the process of data analysis in qualitative research; data saturation is an example. The size of the sample in a qualitative study is dictated by the method of study and the complexity of the phenomenon of interest. Because the data-collection methods in qualitative research yield much data from each participant, the sample sizes in this type of research are usually smaller than in quantitative research. The composition and richness of the setting and participants, rather than the sample size, tell us how useful the results of a qualitative study may be with our own patients. In general, qualitative samples tend to use fewer than 50 participants. Some methods might only require two to five participants. The sampling strategy and the complexity of the phenomenon of interest also dictate sample size in qualitative research.

Summary of Qualitative Sampling

In general, sampling strategies in qualitative research seek to identify participants who have experience with the phenomenon of interest to the researcher and who will bring detail and complexity to the study. Even when a researcher uses a purposive sample to focus on a particular type of experience, the goal remains to have as much depth and detail as possible. As a result, sampling in qualitative research is usually driven by the data being collected and may change as the study progresses. In our above example of smoking-cessation research, if the researcher used purposive sampling, he or she might have a sample of participants who have quit smoking in the last 6 months. In collecting data from this sample, the researcher begins to understand that all of the participants had a significant stressor in their lives in the month before they quit. The researcher at this point may begin to seek out new participants who are smokers and who have experienced a significant stress in the last week so that the process of making the decision to quit can be more fully examined. The example highlights how qualitative researchers collect data and analyze it concurrently as well as how they can use insights from the data to guide further participant recruitment.

SAMPLING IN QUANTITATIVE RESEARCH

The sampling approaches in quantitative research focus on acquiring subjects who match the population of interest as closely as possible. To accomplish this goal, sampling strategies in quantitative research either attempt to remove extraneous variation from the study subjects or to use strategies that prevent the sample from being limited to any particular group or characteristic. In general, quantitative studies that seek to describe and understand some aspect related to health and healthcare use sampling strategies that lead to a sample that closely resembles the target population. Studies that seek to predict or to test predictions use sampling strategies focused on eliminating factors that might confuse the results of the study. For example, a quantitative descriptive study of the process of smoking cessation should include subjects who have different economic, educational, racial, and gender backgrounds found in the community of interest. We saw in the qualitative section above that these were not issues of concern to the qualitative researcher. In contrast, a study of the effectiveness of a smoking-cessation program that compares a group using the intervention to a group not using it should ensure that the groups are similar in factors such as race or education. If these factors differ, they might affect quitting success and make it difficult to determine whether the intervention itself made a difference.

In either case, one of the goals in sampling is to avoid bias. **Bias** occurs when some unintended factor confuses or changes the results in a way that can lead to incorrect conclusions. We say that a bias distorts or confounds the findings, making it difficult or impossible to interpret the results.

The goal of limiting or avoiding the introduction of bias into the study sample is reflected in the consistent use of the term *subjects* to describe the members of the quantitative sample. By using this term, it conveys that the researcher is separate and as removed as possible from those in the sample. The distance and impersonal tone implied by using *subject* are intended to help the researcher to avoid introducing any of the researcher's expectations or interests into the study findings. Just as we saw several different approaches to selecting the qualitative sample, there are many ways to select the quantitative sample. Next, we will look at a few of these approaches.

Nonprobability Sampling

Quantitative studies usually use nonprobability samples. **Nonprobability sampling** uses approaches that do not necessarily ensure that everyone in the population of interest has an equal chance of being included in the study. These types of sampling strategies are usually used because they are easier or less costly or because it is not possible to identify everyone in the population. Some of the types of nonprobability samples may sound familiar, as they include convenience samples, purposive sampling, quota sampling, and matched samples.

The same processes are used to obtain a convenience sample in quantitative research as in qualitative research. This type of sample consists of subjects who meet the participation criteria and who can be readily identified and recruited into the study. The pool of all potential subjects for a study is also called a **sampling frame**—that is, the pool of all individuals who meet the criteria for the study and, therefore, can be included in the sample. When the study tells us that the sample was one of convenience, we know that subjects from the sampling frame were included because they could be conveniently accessed, often on a first-come-first-served basis. This means that those who heard about the study first, or were most open to being in a study or happened to be nearby when the researcher came to recruit the subjects, were the ones in the study. If there is not an equal chance for every subject to participate in the study, the sample would be considered a nonprobability sample.

Purposive sampling is used in quantitative research as well, particularly when the population of interest is unusual or difficult to access. Remember that purposive sampling is the careful and intentional selection of subjects for a study based on specified characteristics. Although purposive sampling is used frequently in qualitative research, it is used less often in quantitative research because the potential for introducing unintended bias into the sample can be high. This type of sample might be used in quantitative research if the researcher were interested in describing family adaptation when a member survives a lethal health problem. The researcher might intentionally seek out the families of individuals who have survived ovarian and pancreatic cancers because they are two of the most lethal types of cancer. Clearly, other lethal conditions occur in healthcare, but the categories of ovarian and pancreatic cancer are readily identifiable and consistently have low survival odds. Therefore, the researcher might purposely select families with survivors of these two conditions.

Quota sampling is another type of nonprobability sampling in which every member of the population does not have an equal chance of being included in the study. In a quota sample, one or more characteristics are identified that are important to the study, and they are used to establish limits on or quotas for the number of subjects who will be included. The goal is to make the sample more representative of the population in a situation where all members of the population cannot be identified. For example, the researcher studying nursing students' choices of field of practice might have decided that gender would be an important factor to consider. After discerning that the known percentage of male nursing students in the state was 16%, the researcher might have used quota sampling to ensure that the sample would have a similar gender composition. This may have been done by setting a goal of recruiting 21 female nursing students and 4 male nursing students so that 16% of the sample would be male.

The last type of nonprobability sample often used is a **matched sample**. In a matched sample, the researcher plans to compare two groups to explain or understand something that differentiates them but knows that some other important characteristics could confuse or bias understanding. To prevent the other important characteristic(s) from making comparison difficult, the researcher intentionally selects subjects whose important characteristics are the same, or matched. An example of this approach might be found in a study of urinary retention care. Suppose the researcher indicates that the original sample for the study comprised 102 long-term care patients who had a permanent indwelling urinary catheter and 102 long-term residents who were intermittently catheterized. The researcher wants to compare indwelling and episodic catheter patients in terms of how often the patients developed infections and did not want the groups to differ on their risk for bedsores, which can also cause infection. Therefore, the specific factors that put a patient at risk for bedsores such as decreased mobilization, poor nutrition, and the presence of skin tears were identified before the study, and subjects were recruited who were similar on those characteristics but differed on whether they had indwelling catheters or were episodically catheterized. This matched the subjects—that is, they had the same risk factors for infections within each group. Again, all acutely ill patients did not have an equal chance of being in the study because they were included only if they had risk factors for urinary infections that were similar to those of other subjects who differed from them in terms of catheter status. Thus, at the beginning of the study, for each subject in the indwelling catheter group, there was a subject who matched him or her in risks for infection in the noncatheterized group.

Probability Sampling

Quantitative studies that intentionally try to predict some aspect of health are more likely to use probability sampling strategies than nonprobability strategies. **Probability sampling** strategies ensure that every member of a population has an equal opportunity to be in the study. The most common types of probability sampling strategies are simple random sampling and several variations on that sampling: stratified random sampling, cluster sampling, and systematic sampling.

Although **simple random sampling** is familiar to most people, the principles involved in this type of sampling are important to understand. Here, all the members of a population of interest must be identified and listed, and each member of the population is assigned a number. Therefore, to select a random sample, all members of the population must be part of the sampling frame. After deciding how many members of the population will be in the study, the researcher uses some device, such as a random number table (Fig. 6.1) or a computer program, to select who will be in the study. Box 6.1 discusses the use of a random number table to identify a random sample. Researchers arbitrarily pick a number from a random number table, which consists of rows and columns of numbers, and then continue in any direction in the table to select numbers. Because all possible numbers are represented in the table, it is by chance alone that the number of any particular member of the population is chosen.

In **stratified random sampling**, the population of interest is first divided into two or more groups based on characteristics that are important to the study, and then members within each group are **randomly selected**. If a researcher were interested in studying some aspect of respiratory care students in Wyoming that may be significantly different for undergraduate and graduate students, the population of all respiratory care students could be stratified—that is, divided according to level of study. Then, the students in each stratum

79	75	64	48	5	70	28	68	79	66	64	40	6	59	30	11	42	29	97	9
65	25	22	58	19	27	80	36	63	16	25	20	12	93	47	1	38	42	19	79
58	13	92	29	56	10	51	38	16	0	97	76	65	40	67	34	20	39	86	79
18	97	73	96	28	54	85	80	9	77	43	47	89	13	24	61	6	63	86	99
91	70	17	84	26	21	82	24	42	32	51	94	89	35	93	10	15	28	71	98
81	78	61	93	75	27	17	39	20	18	66	98	12	73	96	88	31	3	57	72
9	7	49	77	38	53	87	86	52	42	12	14	37	5	50	68	80	4	90	15
50	28	27	49	31	67	53	91	15	48	23	83	90	65	25	69	31	14	79	82
72	66	0	83	52	25	93	26	39	23	10	73	44	58	13	85	21	24	22	79
59	27	90	21	52	41	73	40	83	49	93	97	81	40	49	51	7	44	56	39

FIGURE 6.1   Random number table of 200 numbers between 0 and 99.

> ### BOX 6.1
> #### Using a Random Number Table to Identify a Random Sample
>
> In order to identify a random sample, the researcher must enumerate the entire population. Then, the researcher arbitrarily picks a number from a random number table, which consists of rows and columns of numbers, and continues in any direction in the table to select numbers. Because all possible numbers are represented in the table, it is by chance alone that the number of any particular member of the population is chosen. Therefore, to obtain a random sample of nursing students in Wyoming, a researcher must identify and list all nursing students in the state. If the researcher wants a sample size of 100 nursing students, he or she will assign numbers to each student, pick a number in the random number table, and continue to read off numbers going down, up, or diagonally through the table, until the numbers of 100 students have been picked. Because the goal of quantitative research is to generalize and to avoid bias, a simple random sample is considered the best type of sample because the only factors that should bias the sample would be present by chance alone, making it highly likely that the sample will be similar to the population of interest.

would be listed and assigned a number, and the selection of a random sample would be carried out twice, first with the undergraduate students and then with the graduate students. This strategy is similar to the nonprobability sampling strategy of quota sampling, except that in stratified sampling, members in each stratum have an equal opportunity to be in the sample.

Cluster sampling is a third type of probability sampling that can make it easier to acquire a random sample. This type of sample occurs in stages, starting with selecting groups of subjects who are part of a larger element that relates to the population and then sampling smaller groups until eventually individual subjects are selected. A cluster sample of respiratory care students in Wyoming might start by listing every undergraduate program in Wyoming. A random sample of 10 of these programs might be selected, and then a random sample of 200 students might be chosen from a list of every respiratory care student in those 10 programs. Every respiratory care student in Wyoming had an equal opportunity to be selected for the sample, but the researcher did not have to identify and list every student to select that sample. Instead, the larger element of colleges and universities with accredited respiratory care programs was sampled, followed by sampling from those colleges and universities.

The last type of probability sample that may be used in healthcare research is a **systematic sample**. This strategy is similar to the random sample because the members of the population are identified and listed. However, rather than using a random digit table to select members of the population, the members are selected at a fixed interval from the list. The selected interval may be every tenth member, every fifth member, or any other interval that will lead to a sample of the size desired. When using a systematic sample, it is important to ensure that the members are not listed in some order that creates bias in the sample. For example, the students from every program of respiratory care in Wyoming might always be listed starting with undergraduate students. If the researcher were using systematic sampling, taking every fifth student for a total of five subjects from each program, the students selected might all be undergraduates because only the top part of each list would be included in the sample. If, on the other hand, the students in each program were listed alphabetically, selecting the fifth student for up to five subjects would lead to a sample that was likely to consist of undergraduate students in the proportion that exists in the population as a whole. Table 6.1 summarizes the types of samples used in qualitative and quantitative research. The same strategy is described using slightly different language, depending on whether it is used in a qualitative or quantitative study.

| TABLE 6.1 | Sampling Strategies for Qualitative and Quantitative Research |

QUALITATIVE RESEARCH	QUANTITATIVE RESEARCH
Convenience sample: Participants who are readily available and represent the phenomenon of interest are included in the sample	**Convenience sample:** Members of the population who are easily identified and readily available are included in the sample; a nonprobability sample
Snowball sample: Participants who are known to and recommended by current participants are identified and included, building the sample from a few participants to as many as are needed	**Quota sample:** One or more criteria are used to ensure that a previously established number of subjects who fit those criteria are included in the sample; a nonprobability sample
Purposive sample: Participants who are intentionally selected because they have certain characteristics that are related to the purpose of the research are included in the sample	**Purposive sample:** Subjects in the sample are limited to those who have certain characteristics that are related to the purpose of the research; a nonprobability sample
	Simple random sample: Subjects are selected by enumerating all members of the population, and a completely random process is used to identify who will be included; a probability sample
	Stratified random sample: Members of the population are grouped by one or more characteristics, and subjects are selected from each group using a completely random process; a probability sample
	Cluster sample: Groups of the population are enumerated and selected by a completely random process, then individual subjects from within these groups are randomly selected; a probability sample
	Systematic sample: The members of a population are enumerated and every kth member at a fixed interval is selected as a subject; a probability sample

Strengths and Weaknesses of Quantitative Sampling Approaches

As with qualitative methods, a convenience sample for a quantitative study also has the advantages of being easy and inexpensive, but it has the disadvantage of not having control over factors that may prejudice the study. A convenience sample consists of those subjects who happen to be at the right place at the right time to be included in the sample. What brings those people to the "right" place and time may have to do with their age, economic status, education, illness, or history—factors that may then prejudice the results of the study. In addition, because a convenience sample takes those who are readily available, often on a first-come basis, participants who willingly and readily volunteer may differ in significant ways from those people who would be more reluctant to participate.

In quantitative research, purposive sampling is used to identify a sample that has certain characteristics relevant to the population of interest. The advantage is that selected factors are clearly defined and identified in the sample, but the disadvantage is that the greater a sample is limited and defined by selected characteristics, the less likely it is to reflect the population at large. In the example of a purposive sampling of families with a member who has survived ovarian or pancreatic cancer, for example, both of these cancers occur in relatively young individuals, leading to their families being relatively young and making the results less applicable to older families. A second bias that may be introduced in this sample is that cancer may make unique demands on families that other highly lethal conditions, such as a severe closed head injury or acute pancreatitis, do not.

In quantitative research, nonprobability sampling strategies are usually more likely to allow bias to enter a sample and make it less likely to be representative of the population of interest. This is because all nonprobability samples have the potential for some outside unidentified factor directing who is and who is not included in the study. By definition, probability samples eliminate the potential of some outside factor systematically entering into the sample because all of the members of the population have an equal chance of being included. However, probability sampling strategies have the disadvantage of being complex, costly, or not feasible, given the population of interest. For example, it would not be possible to enumerate all of the homeless individuals in any particular state as one might enumerate all of the respiratory care students, making a probability sample more difficult. However, it might be possible to enumerate all homeless shelters in a state, use cluster sampling to randomly select shelters, and then randomly select residents of these shelters. This would yield a probability sample of homeless people who are housed in shelters within the state—but not of all homeless people because many homeless individuals do not use traditional shelters.

One approach that is taken to decrease the potential for a bias in a sample using quantitative methods is to assign subjects randomly to different groups. This is not truly a sampling strategy, but more of a research method that is used to offset a potential problem that can occur from nonprobability sampling. **Random assignment** ensures that all subjects have an equal chance of being in any particular group within the study. The sample may be one of convenience or purposive, so there may be some bias influencing the results. However, because that bias is evenly distributed among different groups, the bias will not unduly affect the outcomes of the study.

Obviously, random assignment is only an option when a study is going to include more than one group of subjects because the process requires giving each subject in the sample an equal chance to be in any particular group. If a researcher were interested in studying HIV prevention for homeless individuals, he or she might use random assignment of different shelters to try to decrease any bias rather than using a convenience sample of one homeless women's shelter. Often random assignment is desirable but not feasible. In our example, if the researcher wanted to test the usefulness of an HIV prevention program for homeless women, there might be great difficulty in creating two groups and in giving such an intervention to some women in a shelter and not to others. Table 6.2 summarizes the advantages and disadvantages of different sampling strategies.

TABLE 6.2	Advantages and Disadvantages of Sampling Strategies in Qualitative and Quantitative Research			
SAMPLING STRATEGY	QUALITATIVE RESEARCH		QUANTITATIVE RESEARCH	
	Advantages	Disadvantages	Advantages	Disadvantages
Convenience sample	Easier to identify participants; often provides a breadth of information	May "miss" a source of information that is not readily available	Inexpensive; easier to recruit subjects	Most likely to include biases that make it difficult to generalize
Purposive sample	Focuses research on the potentially richest sources of information	Only likely to become a disadvantage if the sampling becomes too narrowed	Locates a sample that is hard to recruit or identify	Likely to include many unique characteristics that limit the ability to generalize
Snowball sample	Allows the researcher to locate sources of information that might otherwise not be identified or available	Could lead to focusing the research and understanding prematurely		

(Continued)

TABLE 6.2	Advantages and Disadvantages of Sampling Strategies in Qualitative and Quantitative Research (*Continued*)			
SAMPLING STRATEGY	QUALITATIVE RESEARCH		QUANTITATIVE RESEARCH	
	Advantages	Disadvantages	Advantages	Disadvantages
Quota sample			Allows the researcher to control the sample on selected characteristics, so that it more closely resembles the population of interest	Open to systematic variations that can bias the sample
Simple random sample and stratified random sample			Eliminates likelihood of a systematic bias in the sample so that results are more readily generalized	Time-consuming, costly, and may not be feasible to enumerate the population
Cluster sample			Same advantages as a simple random sample, but more efficient	Population of interest may not be readily grouped or the groups identified may narrow the population
Systematic sample			Can be easy to implement	May introduce a bias if there is some systematic factor embedded into the list that occurs at regular intervals

Not all samples consist of individuals. A **sampling unit** is the element of the population that will be selected and analyzed in the study. The unit depends on the population of interest and can comprise individuals, but it can also be hospitals, families, communities, or outpatient prenatal care programs. Occasionally, samples consist of more than one sampling unit. If we continue with our example of a researcher interested in HIV prevention in homeless women, the researcher might use shelters as the sampling unit and compare two or more types of shelters. Then, the researcher might move to the level of individuals in the shelters. When the sampling unit is shelters, there may be only six or eight in the sample; whereas when the unit becomes the individual residents of the shelters, there may be 75 to 100 in the sample.

Sample Size in Quantitative Research

In addition to understanding how the approach taken to sampling will affect to which patients the results of the study will apply, it is important to understand how the sample size affects the ability to draw conclusions from a study. In quantitative research, the goal of **generalizability** drives the sample size. Probability samples often can be smaller than nonprobability samples because probability samples control for bias through the random selection process. Nonprobability samples must be larger in general so that any unusual or systematic factors that could bias the study will be canceled out by the number of subjects. For example, if the study "Predictors of Postconcussive Symptoms 3 Months After Mild Traumatic Brain Injury" (Ponsford et al., 2012) (Appendix A-5) had only included 10 patients with mild traumatic brain injuries instead of the 100 used, there would be a good chance that some of those patients would have unusual circumstances, such as having significant personal problems prior to the injury or having undiagnosed medical conditions impacting cognition, that might bias the results. Even 1 or 2 of the 10 patients having unusual circumstances or characteristics could have had a significant impact on the study's results. However, with 100 in the sample, the impact of only 1 or 2 individuals with unusual circumstances will not be as great. Therefore, in general, the larger the sample size in a quantitative study, the more likely the sample will be representative of the population of interest, and the more likely the study will apply to our clinical situations.

In addition to the logic inherent in obtaining larger samples to eliminate the effects of odd or unique cases, sample sizes in quantitative research are determined by the goal of having a reasonable likelihood that the inferential statistics applied to the data will yield statistical significance. Remember that inferential statistics are used to calculate a test statistic that is then compared with a distribution for test statistics occurring by chance alone for that particular sample size. The larger the sample size, the more likely we are to get results that are statistically significant—that is, that did not happen by chance alone. However, it is always costly to recruit and implement a study with many subjects, so it is useful for the researcher to know how large a sample is likely to be needed to be able to apply inferential statistics accurately to the data. Quantitative researchers often use a process called **power analysis** to determine how large a sample they will need. This allows the researcher to compute the sample size needed to detect a real relationship or difference in the phenomenon under study, if it exists. You may see a written statement of power analysis indicating that a specified sample size was adequate. Some authors may provide the actual results of the power analysis in the "sample" section. In this way, the authors are telling you why they used the selected sample size and how it may have impacted the study results.

Summary of Quantitative Sampling

The goal of quantitative sampling strategies is to acquire a sample that is as representative as possible of the population of interest so that the findings from the study can be generalized. To accomplish this, quantitative studies control and limit differences in the sample that may bias or distort the results. Quantitative research does not necessarily want everyone in the study to be exactly alike, but only that the sample is similar to the population of interest.

Nonprobability approaches, such as quota sampling and matched sampling, limit variations that may bias a study. For example, it is generally recognized that the people who are most likely to agree to participate in research studies are white and educated. There are several social and historical reasons for this, but as a result, researchers may implement sampling strategies that specifically target underrepresented groups using a quota or matched sample approach.

The goal of probability sampling is to ensure that every member of a population can be in the study so that no systematic factor defines the sample and makes it different from the population.

Quantitative sampling often limits or controls the variety that qualitative sampling seeks. Researchers in quantitative studies remove themselves from the selection of subjects to eliminate personal bias. Therefore, in quantitative research, a sampling plan is identified and strictly followed, and analysis of data usually is not started until the entire sample is identified and recruited. If the sampling plan includes stratifying or matching, then selected characteristics of the sample are identified and analyzed throughout the selection process, but the findings regarding the variables of interest are not examined until the entire sample is in place. While qualitative studies will thoughtfully change sampling strategies in response to data analysis, a quantitative study will usually follow a clearly identified plan that is determined before sampling has started and that is not modified during the sampling process.

DIFFERENCES IN QUALITATIVE AND QUANTITATIVE SAMPLING

Earlier, we stated that qualitative and quantitative sampling differ in overall goal and approach. Because these goals are different, the strengths and weaknesses of the different strategies for each approach differ as well. This is important to understand because it allows

TABLE 6.3	Differences in Sampling Approaches Between Quantitative and Qualitative Research	
SAMPLING APPROACH	**QUALITATIVE RESEARCH**	**QUANTITATIVE RESEARCH**
General goal of sampling	To include as many sources as possible that add to the richness, depth, and variety of the data	To ensure that only the variables of interest influence the results of the study by limiting extraneous variations in the sample
Approach to sampling	Usually driven by the data as it is collected; therefore, flexible and evolving as the study develops	Established before beginning the process of sampling and followed strictly to avoid introducing bias into the sample
Language for those in the sample	Participants, volunteers, and informants	Subjects

you to understand better how a sample and the approach taken to obtain that sample affect the usefulness of the research for your EBP. A summary of the differences in sampling approaches between qualitative and quantitative research is provided in Table 6.3.

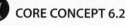 **CORE CONCEPT 6.2**

Sampling strategies in qualitative and quantitative research differ in their goals and approaches, even when they are using a similar strategy.

 # PROBLEMS WITH THE SAMPLING PROCESS

As we discussed sampling, it may have crossed your mind that many patients are intimidated by or distrustful of the research process and may decline to participate. This reluctance is a hard reality of research with human subjects: The goal of finding a representative sample might jeopardize the goal of maintaining the rights of individuals. Chapter 7 will discuss in detail the rights of human subjects, but we will mention here that researchers know that the process of seeking informed consent can bias a sample because of some systematic characteristic that causes certain individuals to decline to be in a study. Studies that examine who generally agrees to participate in research studies show that those who are more educated are more likely to participate than those who are less educated. Thus, in research, the sample may have more highly educated patients than those with less education simply because the consent process is intimidating or because research is not viewed as valuable by those with less education. Clearly, the obligation to ensure that the basic human rights of potential subjects are protected supersedes the concern that consent processes may limit study enrollment, but researchers must consider this factor as they examine the results of their studies.

An associated problem that can occur in sampling is the withdrawal of subjects partway through a study. Individuals who agree to participate may withdraw for a number of reasons, such as personal problems, lack of time, or even physically moving out of an area. A researcher will usually plan for subject withdrawal by attempting to include more subjects in a research study than are actually needed. However, if there is some consistent reason why subjects withdraw, then the ability to generalize results of the study is limited. Withdrawal from a study is an active statement of a decision to no longer participate in that study. Sometimes subjects do not formally withdraw but simply drop out without notification or are lost to follow-up. In this case, the subject simply cannot be found to complete a study or does not return study materials. For example, in studies of smoking cessation, there is always a concern that the subjects who do not succeed in quitting may drop out of the study due to discouragement. This can lead to the final sample including a higher proportion of successful quitters than is really the case, biasing the results by yielding an artificially inflated success rate.

Whether a potential subject declined to be in a study, withdrew, or was lost to follow-up, it is important to know as much as possible about what happened during the sampling process in order to make informed decisions about the use of the results in clinical practice. Therefore, as an intelligent user of research, you should expect that the sampling section of a research report will tell you enough about the process of acquiring the sample so that you can judge how that process affected the results. Often, that information includes a statement about the number of potential subjects who declined to be in a study, withdrew, or dropped out. When subjects withdraw or drop out of a study, some information is usually given about them. Researchers can use this information to compare the subjects who stayed in the study with those who did not, and they may be able to tell us whether there is some important difference between those who did and did not stay in a study.

In addition to concern about who agrees to be in a study and who stays in a study, another problem that can affect the sampling process is the exclusion and inclusion criteria. As discussed earlier, sample criteria define a study's population. A criterion for exclusion is a characteristic that makes the potential subject ineligible for the study, and a criterion for inclusion is a characteristic that makes the subject eligible for the study. Researchers choose to focus on inclusion or exclusion, depending on the nature of the desired sample. In a convenience sample in which numerous subjects are being sought, a researcher will generally discuss exclusion because most individuals will be eligible to participate, and only a few will be excluded. A study that aims for a tightly controlled sample will more likely describe criteria for inclusion because the focus is on who can enter the study. The predictors of postconcussive symptoms (Ponsford, et al., 2012) study describes the inclusion and exclusion criteria in the "Participants" section (Appendix A-5). These criteria define the study's population and may limit how the results can be used in practice.

The last problem with the sampling process is having incomplete data. This is a problem of data collection, but it is closely linked to how a sample may be changed or limited, which affects how useful it is for clinical practice. *Incomplete data* refers to partial information about the variables in a study. Although the specific problems that can lead to incomplete data are addressed in Chapter 8, the effect of this is that the researcher may drop data about selected subjects from the analysis of the results. This raises the question of whether those subjects had some characteristic or characteristics that led to their incomplete data. If so, then a systematic bias will be introduced into the final sample.

Suppose, for example, that some of the subjects in a smoking-cessation study completed only part of a questionnaire used by the researcher and did not answer questions about how much they were smoking after they completed a smoking-cessation program. If the researcher drops these subjects from the analysis (because the amount of smoking after the program is a major variable in the study, and there are no data available for these subjects), then it is likely that the sample is biased in the direction of subjects who were successful and, therefore, willing to report their smoking status. We do not know why the data were incomplete, but we must be concerned that the reason is connected to the variables under study.

In summary, several aspects of the sampling process can lead to problems with the final study sample. The criteria used to identify who will be included or excluded from a study may narrow the sample to the point that the population represented no longer reflects the characteristics of real patient populations. Subjects may withdraw or fail to follow up for some consistent reason that is related to the purposes of the study itself, thus limiting what we can learn from the study. Incomplete information may be collected because of some factor that relates to the study, causing some data about subjects to be dropped from the data analysis and changing the actual sample. As intelligent readers and users of research, healthcare providers must understand not only the strengths and weaknesses of different sampling strategies

TABLE 6.4	Potential Problems With the Sampling Process
PROBLEM	**EXAMPLE**
Subject withdrawal from study	After starting in a study, subjects may decide that they do not want to continue to participate. If some aspect related to the study leads to withdrawal, it can bias the sample.
Lost to follow-up	After agreeing to be in a study, subjects become unavailable to be in it. This may include not returning questionnaires, missing appointments, moving, or having a change in telephone number. If the subjects lost to follow-up represent a particular characteristic related to the study (perhaps high income), then the final sample may have a bias.
Exclusion/inclusion criteria applicability of the sample	If a sample is tightly controlled or restricted to make the research successful, it may lead to the population being so specific that clinical meaningfulness is limited.
Incomplete data	Data are not provided, are skipped, or are missed, causing the researcher to drop subjects from the analysis of the results. If there is some systematic reason for the data being incomplete, dropping subjects can bias the results.

discussed in this chapter, but also what can go wrong with the sampling process and how that affects the meaning of the study. Table 6.4 summarizes the problems discussed in this section. Other factors that can lead to problems with samples are discussed in the next section.

PROBLEMS WITH SAMPLING OUTCOMES

In addition to problems with the sampling process, some problems can occur with the sampling outcomes—that is, the final sample—that are only indirectly related to the strategy used and problems that can occur in the sampling process. Previously, we discussed the importance of avoiding bias, an unintended factor that confounds the findings of a study, in a sample. Some sampling strategies, such as nonprobability sampling, are more open to a bias, whereas others, such as probability sampling, are less open to it. When a researcher uses a nonprobability sampling strategy, the process may be implemented correctly, but the resulting sample may still be biased.

One type of bias that can be introduced in a nonprobability sample occurs when a researcher fails to recognize or consider subjective factors or approaches that could influence participation in the study. For example, a researcher may be more comfortable approaching either men or women when trying to recruit subjects, thus unconsciously biasing a study in the direction of one gender. In addition, a researcher may collect data only at a certain time of the day, such as Monday through Friday, between 8 AM and 5 PM, preventing anyone who works 12-hour shifts or night shifts from being in the study. If type of work and hours worked are related in some way to what is under study, then a bias has been introduced.

Another kind of bias may occur as a result of the unique characteristics or perspectives of the person who is actually recruiting subjects. For example, because a healthcare provider's main role is to provide care for patients, he or she may not be particularly motivated to provide a patient with information about the potential to participate in a study or may conclude that a patient does not need to be bothered with a study. An example of this introduction of bias into a sample might be a study that is conducted in a clinic that cares for both physical and mental health problems. If the person recruiting subjects primarily works with the mental health patients and recruits familiar patients, then the subjects in the study are more likely to have mental illness than the overall population of the clinic.

A second problem that can occur with samples is **selectivity**. Selectivity is the tendency of certain population segments to agree to participate in studies. In this case, the bias is not introduced by the researcher but by those people who are willing and interested in being in a study. We have already discussed one kind of general selectivity that occurs in all research: the tendency of more educated individuals to agree to participate compared with less educated individuals. However, selectivity can occur that is more specific to the purposes of a particular study. A particular study may attract people who are worried about the problem under study or those who are lonely and want someone with whom they can talk. It may be that mostly women are willing to participate in a particular study or, perhaps, only people with family members who have experienced a particular problem will return a mailed questionnaire. The difficulty for the researcher and for the user of research is to determine whether some aspect of the study may have led to selectivity in the sample and how this, in turn, affects the knowledge gained from the study.

Limited response rates can be another problem with samples. **Response rate** is the proportion of individuals who participate in a study divided by the number who agreed to be in a study but did not participate in it. Response rate is not a significant problem when the study occurs in a controlled setting, such as a hospital, because those who agree to participate are essentially a captive group. However, in almost any research survey in which subjects are recruited and asked to return a questionnaire or provide data by appointment, some individuals do not return the questionnaire or keep the appointment. As with the other problems that affect samples, we need to know who the nonresponders are and why they did not respond. Their lack of a response caused by a factor related in some way to the study could bias the sample. In these types of situations, the research report should tell you the response rate so that you have an idea of whether a large or small number of possible subjects did not participate in the study. Withdrawal and dropping out of a study are two reasons why response rates can be low.

All of the problems in samples that we have discussed occur in recruiting subjects for any type of study, but they will cause more problems in nonprobability samples than in probability samples. Although the potential bias of a low response rate can affect a random sample, the effects of selectivity and researcher bias are mostly offset in a random sample because the entire population is enumerated, and all members of the population have a chance of being included in the study. Therefore, it is common to find more detail describing the sampling process and the final sample when nonprobability sampling is used because the researcher wants to ensure to the reader that steps were taken to prevent the potential biases that may be present in the final sample.

In summary, three factors are related to both sampling strategy and the sampling process that can lead to problems in samples. The first is bias *introduced by the researcher* or the individual recruiting the sample that reflects the beliefs or characteristics of that researcher or recruiter. The second is *self-selection by individuals* within the population that can lead to a bias. The third is a *limited response rate* that makes us wonder about the characteristics of those who did not respond and how they differ from those who did. Table 6.5 summarizes these three types of problems with samples.

TABLE 6.5	General Potential Problems With Sampling Outcomes
PROBLEM	**EXAMPLE**
Bias in subject recruitment	Some aspect of the recruitment process allows an unidentified factor to enter into the identification of subjects requested to participate in the study. Examples include time of day of sampling or recruiter comfort level with selected subjects.
	Selectivity: Certain subjects volunteer to be in the study due to some characteristic that could relate to the problem being studied. Examples include subjects who are older and lonely being more available or subjects who care about a particular problem volunteering. This can lead to overrepresentation of one segment of the population in the sample.
Response rate	Many potential subjects or actual subjects do not participate in the study. If a study has a low response rate, then the ability to generalize the results of the study to the entire population of interest is limited.

COMMON ERRORS IN REPORTS OF SAMPLES

The most common error that occurs in study reports of sampling is a lack of adequate detail, leading to the inability to decide whether the types of subjects or participants allow us to apply the results of the study to our clinical situation. In qualitative research, this error will most likely take the form of an inadequate description of the study setting and participants. We have been using the example of a researcher examining a study pertaining to homeless individuals' satisfaction with health care. In order to determine whether the results of such a study are useful to our clinical practice, we must have information about the environment of the participants. If this research had only used participants who were housed in substance-free shelters, the understanding gained from the study would be less complete than the understanding gained from a study of participants from several settings, including a clinic, a soup kitchen, and different shelters.

In quantitative studies, the information that may be missing or inadequate in a research report usually involves the process of acquiring the sample. To judge either the representativeness of a sample or whether the sample reflects the clinical population of interest requires knowing the sampling strategy and the sampling criteria as well as how the strategy was implemented. For example, a convenience sample of dental students exiting a school of dental building at lunchtime is more likely to be representative of the dental students in that college than a convenience sample of students from any one particular classroom. This is because students who exit the building are more likely to reflect a range of levels of study, whereas a single class will mostly consist of students at the same level.

Similarly, a random sample of homeless shelters that then takes a convenience sample of homeless individuals is less likely to yield a representative sample of homeless persons than a random sample of those staying at all shelters on a particular night. To use information about sampling intelligently, we must know the setting where the study occurred and the process of implementing the sampling plan. We also must be given the descriptive statistics that relate the characteristics of the final sample acquired.

CONNECTING SAMPLING TO THE STUDY RESULTS AND CONCLUSIONS

We started this chapter by asking whether the results and conclusions from the five different studies used so far could be used to guide practice in the different clinical situations described in previous clinical cases. Sampling strategies connect to the results of a study in several ways. In both qualitative and quantitative studies, the characteristics of the sample affect the meaning of the results. The appropriateness and focus of sampling in a qualitative study both are driven by and drive data collection, and the detail and complexity of the resulting themes or theory will reflect that sampling. In quantitative studies, the sampling strategy dictates how certain we can be that the results found represent what exists in the real population. Along with sample strategy, sample size also affects the believability of study results. In the clearest connection between sampling and the potential results, some studies require a certain sample size to use certain inferential statistical procedures.

Sampling should also be connected to the conclusions of a study. The nature of the sample and the sampling strategies used may be either a limitation of the study or an aspect that needs further evaluation. For example, let us take the study we introduced in Chapter 5, predictors of postconcussive symptoms (Ponsford et al., 2012) (Appendix A-5). In this study, the authors obtained participants from the "Alfred Emergency and Trauma Centre in Melbourne, Australia" (p. 306). In the discussion section, the authors state, "This sample represents the very mildest end of the mTBI for whom predictors of outcome may differ" (p. 306). This conclusion fits with the sample used. If the authors had stated that their conclusion applied to patients with complex or severe traumatic brain injuries, we would have had to question the connection made.

CRITICALLY READING THE SAMPLE SECTION OF RESEARCH REPORTS FOR USE IN EVIDENCE-BASED NURSING PRACTICE

Box 6.2 provides us with questions to ask when critically reading the sample section of a research report. The first question is "Did the report include a clearly identified section or paragraphs about sampling?" This is fairly straightforward, yet it is surprising that sometimes we have to hunt to find the information about sampling. In the report predictors of postconcussive symptoms (Ponsford et al., 2012) (Appendix A-5), we can easily find the sample information on page 306 under the heading "Participants." However, in some articles it is more difficult to find information on the sample. Part of this is reflective of the different types of research methods used, and some may be the style of the authors' writing or the format of the journal in which the report is published.

Our second question is "Did the report give me enough information to understand how and why this sample was chosen?" The report found by the healthcare provider in the clinical case for Chapter 5, predictors of postconcussive symptoms (Ponsford et al., 2012) (Appendix A-5), is a good example to look at to answer this question. It gives us a sense of who the sample represented—patients with mTBI who presented to the Emergency and Trauma Center—and identifies further specific population characteristics. The article gives a clear sense of who were included in the sample, but do we know why they were chosen? In order to understand this, we will need to read the literature review section, which will be discussed in Chapter 10.

Our third question is "Is there enough information about the sample to tell me if the research is relevant for my clinical population?" This is an important topic in evidence-based healthcare practice. If you plan to use research-based evidence in order to answer clinical questions, you need to critically examine whether the sample is similar to the population in which you are interested. The first part of answering this is based on how well you have formed your clinical question. As you remember from Chapter 1, your question

---

BOX 6.2
How to Critically Read the Sample Section of a Research Report?

Does the report answer the question "To what types of patients do these research conclusions apply—who was in the study?"

1. Did the report include a clearly identified section or paragraphs about sampling?
2. Did the report give me enough information to understand how and why this sample was chosen?
3. Is there enough information about the sample to tell me whether the research is relevant for my clinical population?
4. Was enough information given for me to understand how rights of human subjects were protected?
5. Would my patient population have been placed at risk if they had participated in this study?
6. Can I identify how information was collected about the sample?

gives a "Who, What, Where, When" that establishes who and what makes up your clinical population. A PICO or PICOT formatted question can also provide information about your population of interest. Once you know whom you are interested in, you then need to see what the report tells you about the sample. The clinical case for Chapter 3 yielded a clinical question of "What THA implant approach (cemented or cementless) can decrease postsurgical leg length differences in patients undergoing THA surgery?" This clinical question tells the healthcare provider in our case that the researchers are looking for evidence about a population that includes (1) patients who had a total hip arthroplasty, (2) patients who had either a cemented or cementless implant, and (3) patients who had leg length differences following a THA surgical procedure. If we then check the report, we can see whether there is a variation between the healthcare provider's clinical population of interest (our clinical case) and the sample (from the study) in that the sample included only participants meeting the study's criteria. The healthcare provider will need to know information about the population of interest within their own practice setting to make the decision of whether the sample's results from the study can be applied to practice.

As we continue to critically read the sample section of a research report, we come to our fourth question, "Was enough information given for me to understand how rights of human subjects were protected?" The issue of using human subjects will be discussed in detail in Chapter 7, but we probably have some awareness now that sample subjects can be vulnerable and have rights even if they agree to participate in research. All subjects need to know the risks of any research and to have the right not to be coerced into participation. In the predictors of postconcussive symptoms (Ponsford et al., 2012) (Appendix A-5), the authors tell us about the rights of human subjects. They state, "After providing informed consent and demographic information, participants completed the acute assessment . . . within 48 hours of injury" (pp. 306–307). We will see in Chapter 7 that this may not be enough information to constitute a thorough statement regarding the protections of subjects' rights. We see similar but perhaps more clear statements in other reports that we have read. The fifth question we can ask is "Would my patient population have been placed at risk if they had participated in this study?" In order to answer this, you need to be clear of who your patient population is. Much like we stated in addressing the third question, a strong clinical question needs to be formed with a clear *Who, What, Where*, and *When* or PICO/PICOT format in order to answer this. As a healthcare provider using research to find answers to practice questions, you will need to think about what the sample was asked to do while participating in the study. The subject may have been asked to participate in interviews to discuss the researcher's questions. As we think about it, there is usually not much risk to the sample when participating in interviews. But what if the researcher had decided to take blood specimens to measure serum cortisol and track the stress level of family members in that manner? We can now see a little more risk is present. The subject may bleed from the site of the blood draw, or the site might become infected. While unlikely, it is not risk free. Finally, what if the researcher in this study had decided to include brain scans using the injection of a contrast dye prior to the scan in order to measure activity in the stress-related areas of the family members' brains as they experienced having a family member in the ICU? We can now see a considerable increase in the risk to the sample. The injection of a dye prior to the brain scan will give the best results, but the dye can be dangerous, people can be allergic to it, and the injection might be the source of significant complications. Thus, to answer our fifth critical question, we need to look at what our sample was asked to do and then decide whether our population could, and would, be willing to do the same procedure.

Our final question is "Can I identify how information was collected about the sample?" This is very important because it begins to speak to your ability to implement an evidence-based change in patient care based on the study. The healthcare provider in our Chapter 5 clinical case about patients with mTBI is interested in patients at risk for postconcussion syndrome. The healthcare provider will want to see whether the information collected during the study could reasonably be collected in his or her population. Ponsford et al. (2012) of the predictors of postconcussive symptoms study (Appendix A-5) report that they collected information in the form of interviews and physical and mental assessment tests. They also state how the assessment tests were conducted and how long the assessment tests lasted. What is not clear is how demographic information was collected and who conducted the interviews and assessment tests.

PUBLISHED REPORTS—WOULD YOU CHANGE YOUR PRACTICE?

The importance of being able to critically read something like the sample section of a report is to allow you to become comfortable in deciding which evidence you should use in EBP. As your skill at reading research-based evidence improves, the overarching question becomes "Should I change my practice based on this published report?"

In this chapter, we have concentrated on critically reading the sample section as part of reaching a conclusion about EBP. We have seen thus far that sampling strategies discussed in a report are directly connected to results and conclusions and that understanding the language and meaning of sampling in research adds one more piece to the puzzle of reading and comprehending research for use in EBP practice. Once you have decided whether the population for the study reflects the type of patients or situations that are of interest to you, the subjects' rights were protected, the sample reflects your population, and the approach taken to choosing the sample limits the meaning of the study, you are well on your way to knowing whether the study results can be applied to your clinical question.

As we review the reports that we have examined so far, you may be starting to see that the healthcare providers in our clinical cases have not so much changed their minds about practice as much as they have acquired a better sense of how useful these research studies will be for their practice. They have received insight into other issues to consider, and they have raised other questions. EBP provides information, but it will never directly tell you what to do. As the healthcare provider, you will always need to think through the evidence before considering whether to or how to apply it to your practice in the best way.

In summary, information about the sampling strategy and the actual sample are important in understanding which results of a study may apply to your clinical question. Unique language is associated with the sampling process for both qualitative and quantitative research. Sampling in qualitative research gathers as rich and complete a set of data as possible, and sampling strategies are guided by and may change based on the concurrent data analysis. Sampling in quantitative research eliminates potential bias and gathers information from a subset of the population that closely resembles the actual population. Sampling strategies in this type of research are carefully planned, with important characteristics defined and used to limit or control the subjects. Probability samples are considered to be better than nonprobability samples in quantitative research because these types of samples eliminate systematic bias, but they are also more difficult and costly than nonprobability sampling. Sample size depends on the strategy and methods used, with qualitative samples generally being smaller than samples for quantitative studies.

Understanding the language of sampling and the meaning of the sampling strategies helps to make the relationship clear between the sample and the results and conclusions of the study. This chapter focused entirely on the language and process of sampling in quantitative and qualitative research. What we have not discussed is the important subject of the rights of individuals who participate in research. This topic is discussed in the next chapter.

OUT-OF-CLASS EXERCISE

Free Write

Before you move on to the next chapter, take a moment to think about the in-class questionnaire that you may have completed or about some past occasion when you were asked to participate in some type of research. Write a paragraph describing how the study or questionnaire was explained to you and what you were told with regard to filling it out. Then, write your thoughts about whether your rights, safety, and privacy were protected. Finally, write down types of individuals or situations that you feel should be excluded from participating in research. What makes you believe that these individuals or situations should or should not be included in research? Refer to these paragraphs as you read Chapter 7.

References

Ilic, D., Tepper, K., & Misso, M. (2012). Teaching evidence-based medicine literature searching skills to medical students during the clinical years: A randomized controlled trial. *Journal of the Medical Library Association, 100*(3), 190–196. doi:10.3163/1536-5050.100.3.009

Li, W., Rukavina, P. B., & Foster, C. (2013). Overweight or obese students' perceptions of caring in urban physical education programs. *Journal of Sports Behavior, 36*(2), 189–208.

Peck, C. N., Malhotra, K., & Kim, W. Y. (2011). Leg length discrepancy in cementless total hop arthroplasty. *Surgical Science, 2*, e183–e187. doi:10.4236/ss.2011.24040

Ponsford, J., Cameron, P., Fitzgerald, M., Grant, M., & Mikocka-Walus, A. (2012). Predictors of postconcussive symptoms 3 months after mild traumatic brain injury. *Neuropsychology, 26*(3), 304–313. doi:10.1037/a0027888

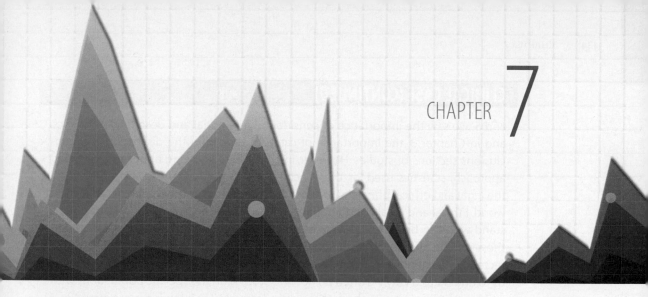

CHAPTER 7

Ethics

What Can Go Wrong?

LEARNING OBJECTIVE The student will evaluate legal and ethical principles, and potential problems as they apply to research.

Which Healthcare Team Member Actions Are Research and Require Special Ethical Consideration?
Informed Consent
When Research Is Exempt
Critically Reading Reports of Sampling and Recognizing Common Errors
Published Reports—What Do They Say About Consent and the Sampling Process?

KEY TERMS

Anonymous
Assent
Coercion
Confidentiality
Exempt
Five human rights in research

Informed consent
Institutional review board (IRB)
Practice
Risk–benefit ratio
Withdrawal

CLINICAL CASE

We have thus far looked at several aspects of the process of research as we have followed the healthcare team member in the cases discussed in earlier chapters. As you can see, there is much to consider as a healthcare team member draws conclusions about clinical questions that are based on research studies before using information in evidence based practice. For example, in Chapter 6, we saw the importance of considering the sampling approaches used in studies. In Chapters 4

(Continued)

CLINICAL CASE (CONTINUED)

and 5, we saw the importance of considering inferential and descriptive statistics, and in Chapter 3, the importance of carefully critiquing the discussion and conclusions sections of studies. However, in addition to knowing about the sampling approach, statistics used, or the conclusions reached, we must also understand the legal and ethical principles that guide the conduct of the researcher in today's world. Ethical and legal considerations are important because they help us understand who can be recruited into research studies, how the researcher can recruit these people, and how the studies are to be conducted so that the people are protected. Understanding the ethical and legal issues surrounding research also helps us to understand why we often do not find studies on the specific populations with which we are working, or those that we are interested in knowing more about.

To better understand the connections between legal and ethical principles and the research process, consider the sampling process in "The Affects of a Single Bout of Exercise on Mood and Self-Esteem in Clinically Diagnosed Mental Health Patients" (Ellis, Randall, & Punnett, 2013) (Appendix A-6). In this study, ethical approval was sought and given by the Staffordshire University Faculty of Health Sciences Ethics Board, and the NHS Research Ethics Committee (a Special Health Authority established by the Government of the United Kingdom) was notified, although the NHS approval was not needed because this was a service evaluation. This type of ethical approval would be similar to that obtained via an **Institutional Review Board (IRB)** in the United States. More information about the function of IRB's is located later within this chapter.

As you will notice, the researchers are deliberate in stating that potential participants were initially approached by staff members and given an explanation about the study. They were then given 7 additional days to determine whether they would like to participate in the study, which allowed them time to think about the risks and benefits, and whether they wished to involve themselves in physical activity. It is noted that participants were required to sign written informed consent if they elected to be part of the study. The researchers also clarify that participants had to meet inclusion criteria on the day of physical activity by stating that they had to be "well enough on the day to complete the questionnaire" (Ellis et al., 2013, p. 82). Participants were also offered a private room to complete the questionnaires, and assistance with this if needed (Ellis et al.).

WHICH HEALTHCARE TEAM MEMBER ACTIONS ARE RESEARCH AND REQUIRE SPECIAL ETHICAL CONSIDERATION?

One important notion regarding research ethics is being able to understand when a particular healthcare team member action is considered to be research, versus when it is a standard care practice. Research actions require full patient consent and IRB authorization (concepts we will discuss shortly). However, practice actions are held to a different standard. Sometimes healthcare team members may be asked to collect new data or to perform their care actions in a different manner. It is important for the healthcare team member to be able to determine whether the new action is research or whether it is new care practice in order to safeguard the patient.

While both research and practice can often look alike and can actually occur together, they are different primarily in the purpose and expected outcome. The Belmont Commission Report (1979) defined ethical principles for the protection of human subjects of research and in doing so provided guidelines for deciding whether an action is research or whether it is practice. **Practice** is composed of actions that are planned and implemented exclusively for the enhancement of health and the improvement of the well-being of an individual. Research, on the other hand, is composed of systematic actions that are planned and implemented exclusively to test a hypothesis, to examine a phenomenon, to allow for conclusions to be drawn, or to generate new knowledge or confirm past knowledge. Research does not have any outcome that specifically improves the patients' health or well-being.

Depending on the specific discipline, certain professional documents exist to help healthcare team members make decisions regarding the ethics of research. For example, in the profession of nursing, the American Nurses Association (ANA) and the International Council of Nurses (ICN) have published Codes of Ethics. The ANA's Code of Ethics for Nurses was approved by the ANA House of Delegates in 2001 and provides details on the ethical standards of RNs (ANA, 2001). In 2005, the ANA released Interpretive Statements to accompany the 2001 Code of Ethics for Nurses, which can be found on their Web site (http://www.nursingworld.org/MainMenuCategories/EthicsStandards/CodeofEthicsforNurses/Code-of-Ethics.pdf). The ANA states that the Code of Ethics for Nurses with Interpretive Statements provides nurses with a framework to use in ethical analysis and decision making (ANA, 2005). The ICN Code of Ethics for Nurses (ICN, 2012) is an international code of ethics for nurses and was first adopted by the ICN in 1953, revised and reaffirmed at various times since, and most recently revised in 2012. Both of these documents assert that nurses have fundamental responsibilities to promote health, prevent illness, restore health, and alleviate suffering. Inherent in these ethical statements is the belief that nursing is integrally involved with respecting human rights, including the right to life, to dignity, and to be treated with respect. Similarly, healthcare research, as an action in which healthcare team members are involved, carries the need to safeguard these rights of patients. Healthcare professionals are urged to seek out their specific profession's Code of Ethics, or ethical position.

The two mentioned nursing documents are predicated on three ethical principles important to research. These are applicable within all healthcare professions, as they focus on autonomy, beneficence, and justice. Autonomy, as it pertains to research, is a fundamental ethical principle that underpins both self-determination and the right of every person to give clear and knowledgeable informed consent. If autonomy is not safeguarded, a healthcare team member has failed to uphold the ethical standards of the profession. Remember that a patient may, appropriately, be asked to participate in research that carries great risk. The research is not inherently unethical as long as the person's autonomy rights have been addressed and the person's decision to be involved in research is a fully informed decision. There is no requirement that researchers only propose studies that involve no risk. Researchers and the healthcare team member involved must, however, fully reveal any potential risk and assist patients to be fully informed so that patients can make unencumbered decisions about whether or not to enter the study.

The second ethical principle, beneficence, is the basis of the ability of the healthcare team member to act in the best interest of the research subject and to always function in an advocacy role as patients consider becoming research subjects. The third principle, justice, is fundamental in research and identifies how subjects should be recruited and treated during the research study. Justice assumes that the healthcare team member will ensure that research subjects are always selected from a wide array of the population and are not recruited in coercive ways.

INFORMED CONSENT

When considering how informed consent is obtained, you must be mindful of your specific professional roles and your scope of practice. Certain members of the healthcare team may operate within a scope where they are able to obtain informed consent from a participant, while others may operate within a scope where they are able to witness (observe) a participant giving informed consent. Review your specific profession's parameters and roles, as well as your State's laws regarding your profession's scope, as they apply to informed consent. For purposes of examples within this chapter, we will assume that the healthcare team member practices within a scope where they are permitted to obtain informed consent.

Suppose that the healthcare team member is involved in a replica study of the research regarding "The Affects of a Single Bout of Exercise on Mood and Self-Esteem in Clinically Diagnosed Mental Health Patients" (Ellis et al., 2013). It is important that the healthcare team member recognizes that a patient's consent to participate is essential; the healthcare team member also knows that, as a professional, he or she is ethically obligated to follow the three ethical principles of autonomy, beneficence, and justice. The healthcare team member decides to review the consent form so that he or she can plan how to respond to any questions that a potential participant in the study might have. Upon review, the healthcare team member realizes that there are three distinct components to the consent form: (1) a description of the study, including specifically what the subject will be asked to do as a research participant; (2) a description of any potential risks and any potential benefits to participating in the study; and (3) a description of the subject's rights if he or she chooses to participate. As an example of how these categories may be aligned with a professional organization's ethical stance, each of these sections of an informed consent relates to at least one of the **five human rights in research** that have been identified by the ANA guidelines for nurses working with patient information that may require interpretation. They are

1. Right to self-determination
2. Right to privacy and dignity
3. Right to anonymity and confidentiality
4. Right to fair treatment
5. Right to protection from discomfort and harm (ANA, 1985, 2001)

Table 7.1 defines these rights, and we discuss them as they relate to the process of research.

TABLE 7.1	Definitions of the Five Rights of Human Subjects in Research (ANA, 1985)
RIGHT	**DEFINITION/DESCRIPTION**
Right to self-determination	Individuals are autonomous and have the right to make a knowledgeable, voluntary decision that is free from coercion as to whether or not to participate in research or to withdraw from a study.
Right to privacy and dignity	Individuals have the right to the respect of choosing what they do and what is done to them and to control when and how information about them is shared with others.
Right to anonymity and confidentiality	Individuals should be afforded the respect of having information they share or that is gathered about them kept in a manner that does not connect them to the individual information and the respect of choosing for themselves who knows that they are participating in a research study.
Right to fair treatment	Individuals have the right to nondiscriminatory selection of participants in a study, to nonjudgmental treatment that honors all agreements established in the consent, and to resources to address any concerns or problems that should arise during participation in the research.
Right to protection from discomfort and harm	Individuals have the right to be protected from exploitation and to be assured that every effort is made to minimize any potential harm from a study, while maximizing the potential benefits of the study.

Informed consent is the legal principle that an individual or his or her authorized representative can make a decision about participation in a research study only after being given all the relevant information pertaining to the study as well as being given a reasonable amount of time to consider the decision to participate. The written consent form is a legal document indicating that the principle of informed consent has been adhered to. This document, along with a relatively detailed description of the study, is generated by a researcher before beginning a study and is reviewed and approved by an entity called an **IRB**. An IRB is a board created for the explicit purpose of reviewing any proposed research study to be implemented within an institution or by employees of an institution. Most hospitals have an internal IRB, whereas small clinics may share one or use one associated with a local hospital or university. The individuals who sit on the IRB always represent a variety of backgrounds and interests and usually include members who are researchers, one or two lay members from the community, and individuals, such as ministers, who have a special knowledge and interest in ethics. The diversity of the members' backgrounds helps to ensure that a proposed research study is evaluated from numerous perspectives. The IRB does not examine the scientific merit of the proposed study, but only the ethics of what is being proposed and what is being asked of the study participant.

The establishment of IRBs occurred in response to incidences of unethical and dishonest research practices in the past. Best known examples include the Nazi medical experiments brought to light during the Nuremberg War Crimes Trial following World War II and the Tuskegee Syphilis "Study" that withheld treatment for syphilis from men from a poor black community in the South without their knowledge in order to study the progression of the disease. To address the concern of ethics in research, the National Research Act, Public Law 93-348, was signed on July 12, 1974. This law created the National Commission for the Protection of Human Subjects of Biomedical and Behavioral Research. This federal commission was empowered to identify the ethical principles that should be included in the planning and conduct of all research involving human subjects. They further were empowered to develop guidelines to ensure that research is conducted in accordance with those principles. The results of this commission still impact research today and include (1) identifying the differences between research and activities that are routine care practices; (2) establishing the importance of reviewing the risk–benefit ratio to determine the ethical nature of planned research; (3) establishing guidelines for the selection of human subjects for participation in research; and (4) identifying what is required in the informed consent process for various types of research. The findings of this commission were released in the previously mentioned *Belmont Report* (1979).

The Belmont Report's name was derived from the Smithsonian Institution's Belmont Conference Center, where the commission met to finalize the report. It remains the most important modern document that identifies basic ethical principles and guidelines that should be applied to all research involving human subjects. The report was published in the *Federal Register* and is still the guiding document whose principles are used by IRBs as they consider research proposals. Although the majority of researchers are honest and ethical, there have been continued occasions when researchers have falsified data, failed to disclose risks, or failed to report adverse events that have occurred during their research. IRBs exist to guard against these types of unethical and dishonest practices.

The function of an IRB is to ensure that the research project includes procedures to protect the rights of its participants. It is also charged with deciding whether the research is basically sound to ensure that the time and potential risk to the participant is outweighed by the potential scientific gain that could come from the study. A research study that asks anything of individuals is, at a minimum, using their time. A study that is not well planned or has a major flaw will make the results meaningless and wastes its participants' time and effort. It is the IRB's responsibility to make sure, as best can be determined, that this is unlikely to happen.

Beyond ensuring the soundness of a research study, an IRB also looks at the balance between the risks and benefits of the study. This evaluation of the risk–benefit ratio (read as "risk to benefit" ratio) is integral to protecting a study subject from discomfort and harm. A **risk–benefit ratio** is a comparison of the level of risk present for participants compared with the level of benefit. A study that proposes to ask healthy college-age students to take an experimental acne drug that has a high potential of causing kidney failure has a very poor risk–benefit ratio and would not be approved. But a study that asks terminal cancer patients to take an experimental cancer drug that may cause kidney failure has a much better risk–benefit ratio and would likely be approved.

Researchers are obligated to identify any potential risks to participation in their study and describe how they will try to prevent these risks, how they will monitor for their occurrence, and what they will do if they occur. If the researcher's plan is considered inadequate, the proposed research will not be approved. Some studies entail risks to life or health that simply are too great, regardless of their potential benefit and despite efforts made to minimize those risks.

CORE CONCEPT 7.1 _____

It is unethical and illegal to implement a research study that uses animal or human subjects without IRB approval.

_____

One potential risk to research participants is considered so important that it is viewed as a separate right. This is the risk of a breach in anonymity, confidentiality, or both. A participant in research is considered **anonymous** when no one, including the researcher, can link the study data from a particular individual to that individual. **Confidentiality** is related to anonymity because although the researcher knows the identity of the participant, it ensures that neither the identities of participants nor any information that participants provide individually will be revealed to anyone. Because many research studies examine sensitive areas such as abusive relationships, HIV status, sexual function, anxiety, and substance use, merely being identified as a participant in a study can reveal personal and private information about an individual. A study that follows subjects over time cannot ensure anonymity until the study is complete because the researcher must know who the participants are to stay in touch with them throughout the study. However, researchers can guarantee that participation in and responses of individuals in the study are kept confidential and that only the researcher(s) has access to the data. Once a study is completed, all links between individuals and specific data can be destroyed; this ensures that future work with the research data will be anonymous. As with any potential risks in a study, a researcher must tell the IRB in writing how the confidentiality and anonymity of subjects in the study will be achieved and how the security of any collected data will be maintained.

The IRB members address the subject's right to fair treatment by reviewing the researcher's plan for recruiting subjects. A subject recruitment plan must give all the members of the population of interest an opportunity to participate and may not target vulnerable groups simply because it is "easier" to get their participation. Vulnerable populations include groups such as (1) prisoners, as they are available and may feel compelled to participate as a show of good behavior; (2) the homeless, who may be unduly influenced to participate because of such incentives as payment rather than from a true desire to participate; or (3) the mentally ill, who may be less able to fully consent to treatment or who may feel coerced to participate. Additionally, researchers cannot avoid inclusion of individuals who are more difficult to recruit or who have more risk considerations. An example of this would be women. Women, especially during reproductive years, always carry an increased need to consider risks, as they may become pregnant and may be unaware of this during their early participation in a study. Because women have been actively avoided in past research, new studies must now include women and children as well as men, if at all appropriate to the research question, and must include individuals with diverse economic and racial characteristics. Additionally, the researcher must make the IRB aware of the location for data collection, the strategies used to recruit subjects, and any criteria for participation.

In Chapter 6, we discussed that the criteria for participation define the population and are used to either purposely seek diversity or to limit and control for factors that may confound the study findings. In the study by Ellis et al. (2013), male and female participants with a mean age of 44.6, who were of white British, black British, or "other" ethnicity, with a mean inpatient length of stay of 59.22 days, with a primary diagnosis of anxiety, were included. Whatever the criteria for inclusion in a study, the IRB will review them carefully to be sure that they are fair.

CORE CONCEPT 7.2

The goal of the research with human subjects is always to minimize the risks and maximize the benefits.

Ensuring the right to self-determination as well as the right to privacy and dignity are also the IRB's responsibility. These rights are reflected in the informed consent document by providing a clear explanation of the study, what will be required of individuals who participate, and the actual or potential risks and benefits of participation. The intent is that a potential research subject can make a knowledgeable decision based on the information provided in the consent form. In addition, respect for the potential subject is indicated through allowing them the freedom to decide what they will or will not do or share. Self-determination is also included as a direct right within any study consent form in a statement that says that the subject has the right of **withdrawal** from the study at any time, without penalty, until the study is completed. Once a study is complete, all data become anonymous, and it is no longer possible to withdraw information received from any specific individual. All research consent forms are expected to clarify with subjects that if they start in a study and later change their mind about participating, for any reason, they retain the right to self-determination and are free to withdraw.

Another aspect of self-determination is the right to decline participation in a study without consequences. A researcher must assure the IRB that individuals who either decline to participate in research or later withdraw after initial consent will not be punished. This is particularly relevant if the study is being conducted in a health care setting where it is possible that a patient might feel direct or indirect coercion to participate. **Coercion** involves some element of controlling or forcing someone to do something. In the case of research, coercion would occur if a patient felt forced to participate in order to receive a particular test, service, or treatment; to "please" a healthcare team member or provider of care; or to receive the best quality of care. Even if not forced to agree to participate in a study, a potential subject still experiences coercion if he or she feels that the best possible care will not be given if the choice is made not to participate. Therefore, any consent form for research where withholding or modifying treatment would be possible will include a clear statement that treatment and care will not be influenced by whether the individual participates in the study. Of course, the researcher is responsible for conducting the study in keeping with that statement, ensuring that action is taken so that treatment and care are not influenced by the individual's decision about whether to participate or not.

The right to privacy and dignity is also related to the right to anonymity and confidentiality. A researcher must inform a potential subject whether participation in a study will involve invasive questions or procedures, again ensuring the respect of being in charge of deciding what will or will not be shared or exposed without the subject's approval. This reflects the participant's right to privacy. Clearly, once data become anonymous, there is no longer a risk of breaching privacy, but until that point, it is the responsibility of the researcher to ensure the right to privacy.

The last aspect of informed consent is a statement about the rights of the participant to care whether some untoward effect should occur from participating in the research, and the provision of the specific names and telephone numbers of the researcher(s) and an IRB representative. These sections of the form give the potential participant access to both the researcher and an independent resource, usually the IRB representative, if he or she has questions or problems. Individuals who agree to participate must be given a copy of the consent form so that they can contact the researcher or IRB representative as needed throughout the research and after it is completed.

Throughout this section, we have discussed the responsibilities of IRBs, which are in place to guarantee an organization that any research carried out within that organization or by its employees conforms with, protects, and respects the rights of their subjects. Although IRBs have the responsibility for review, it is always the primary responsibility of the researcher to plan for and guarantee the protection of subjects.

Let us return to the healthcare team member in our clinical case. Box 7.1 shows a sample informed consent form that might have been developed had a researcher chosen to perform a replication of a study concerning "The Affects of a Single Bout of Exercise on Mood and Self-Esteem in Clinically Diagnosed Mental Health Patients" (Ellis et al., 2013). As discussed in Chapter 2, a replication study essentially repeats an earlier study with a different sample to see whether the same results are found. Having reviewed the informed consent form that will be presented to potential participants, the healthcare team member recalls that for this study to have been approved by the institution's IRB, the board must have reviewed the basic soundness of the study in addition to its risk–benefit ratio. This provides the healthcare team member with some assurance that an individual's participation would not be a waste of time or effort. It also provides some assurance that the risks to the participant are probably reasonable, given the potential benefits from the study.

BOX 7.1
Fictional Informed Consent Form for Participation in a Study of The Affects of a Single Bout of Exercise on Mood and Self-Esteem in Clinically Diagnosed Mental Health Patients

Prison Hospital XYZ

INFORMED CONSENT

PRINCIPAL INVESTIGATOR: Jane J. Doe, PhD & Bob L. Smith, PhD

TITLE OF PROJECT: The Affects of a Single Bout of Exercise on Mood and Self-Esteem in Clinically Diagnosed Mental Health Patients

PURPOSE: The purpose of this study is to understand the impact of a single bout of exercise on mood and self-esteem in patients with a wider clinical mental health diagnosis.

DURATION: Volunteering for this study will involve being screened, participating in one 45-minute aerobic exercise of moderate intensity, and completing preactivity and postactivity questionnaires. The preactivity questionnaire will take 10 to 15 minutes preexercise, and the postactivity questionnaire will take 5 minutes postexercise. Participation in this study is entirely voluntary, and deciding not to participate will not affect your care now or in the future in any way.

PROCEDURES: Participation in the study means allowing the staff to meet with you in person to distribute and collect preactivity and postactivity questionnaires as outlined in the "Duration" section and participating in one 45-minute aerobic exercise of moderate intensity. These observations and interactions with the staff will be provided to you at no cost. In addition, participation in this study means that the researcher will collect some information from you about your diagnoses, medications, and general health.

POSSIBLE RISKS/DISCOMFORTS: Depending on your comfort level with participating in an episode of exercise, answering questions about exercise, or participating in this activity may be embarrassing or upsetting to you. As with any type of exercise, there is risk of physical injury that may occur as a result of participating in this exercise activity. There are no other known risks to participation in this study.

POSSIBLE BENEFITS: A possible benefit to participation in this study is experiencing a positive effect on your mood and/or self-esteem after an episode of exercise. Other possible benefits include gaining the knowledge that you are contributing to a study that may help people like yourself in the future.

CONTACT FOR QUESTIONS: If you have any questions or problems, you may call Jane J. Doe at 555-555-0811 or Bob L. Smith at 555-555-0912. You may call the Chairman of the Institutional Review Board at 555-555-7777 for any questions you may have about your rights as a research subject.

CONFIDENTIALITY: Every attempt will be made to see that your study results are kept confidential. A copy of the records from this study will be stored in the Department of Research, Room 100, at ABC University for at least 10 years after the end of this research. Your conversations with the healthcare team member may be tape recorded, but all reasonable efforts will be made to protect the confidentially of your information. The results of this study may be published and/or presented at meetings without naming you as a subject. Although your rights and privacy will be maintained, the Secretary of the Department of Health and Human Subjects, the ABC University Institutional Review Board, the Food and Drug Administration, and the Department of Research will have access to the study records. Your records will be kept completely confidential according to current legal requirements.

COMPENSATION FOR MEDICAL TREATMENT: ABC University will pay the cost of emergency first aid for any injury that may happen as a result of your participation in this study. It will not pay for other medical treatment.

VOLUNTARY PARTICIPATION: The nature, risks, and benefits of the project have been explained to me as are known and available. I understand what my participation involves. Furthermore, I understand that I am free to ask questions and withdraw myself from the project at any time, without penalty. I have read and fully understood the consent form. I sign it freely and voluntarily. A signed copy has been given to me.

Your study record will be maintained in strictest confidence according to current legal requirements and will not be revealed unless required by law or as noted.

_____

SIGNATURE OF VOLUNTEER OR LEGAL REPRESENTATIVE & DATE

_____

SIGNATURE OF INVESTIGATOR & DATE

When reviewing the first section of the informed consent, the healthcare team members sees a description of the purpose of the study, duration of the study, and procedures. The first thing the healthcare team member notes is that the consent clearly states under the section of "duration" that participation in the study is voluntary and will not be connected to a participant's care in any way. The healthcare team member knows that this is an important point to convey so that a participant does not feel coerced to participate in the study. The healthcare team member knows that it is important to read all of the language within the consent form and be prepared to use more common language when talking with a participant, if need be. The healthcare team member also knows that the idea of discussing mood, self-esteem, and/or exercise may be uncomfortable to some patients. The healthcare team member must find an approach to explaining the use of procedures that gives a fair and impartial explanation but also allays any unreasonable fears that a participant may have.

By considering these aspects of explaining the consent form, the healthcare team member is honoring the rights to self-determination, dignity, and protection from discomfort. Only by fully and correctly understanding the purpose and procedures of the study can a participant make a knowledgeable decision with regard to participation, ensuring self-determination. By being sure that a participant fully understands the nature of the procedure that may be performed and the reasons for that procedure, his or her rights to dignity and protection from discomfort will be ensured as well.

CORE CONCEPT 7.3

The five human rights in research are first and foremost the responsibility of the researcher(s) and are linked to the three ethical principles of autonomy, beneficence, and justice.

When the healthcare team member reviews the sections describing the possible risks/discomforts and benefits, he or she can see that these are clearly stated and include an explicit acknowledgment that personal disclosure is difficult. The consent form seems neither to exaggerate nor to minimize the risks and benefits of this study for the participant. The next two sections of the consent form directly address the participant's rights by providing him or her with the names and telephone numbers of the researchers and of an independent source of information, the chairman of the IRB. The consent form also tells the participant that his or her records will be kept confidential, the location of those records, and for how long they will be kept.

Finally, the consent form tells the participant that he or she has a right to compensation for any emergency care that might be needed because of his or her participation in the study. This statement may cause alarm for the participant because nothing in the form has suggested that there could be a need for emergency care. The healthcare team member knows that he or she must explain that this is a legally required statement that may have limited applicability for this particular study. It should be noted that if there are risks involved, the participant has a right to know about those in detail. The primary researcher should be the one to conduct this discussion with the participant.

The last paragraph of the consent form confirms that the participant has read and understands the study and that he or she will always have the right to withdraw from the study, if he or she chooses to do so. The right to withdrawal without any consequences is as important as the right to decline to participate and assures the patient the right to self-determination and fair treatment throughout participation. Table 7.2 summarizes the links between the five human rights in research and the specific sections of the consent form that we have discussed. After a careful and thoughtful review of the consent form, the healthcare team member is prepared to approach the participant professionally for his or her consent to participate in the study.

One last point must be understood about informed consent. So far, we have been discussing informed consent to participate in a study, meaning agreement based on a full understanding that assumes the ability to understand and make rational decisions. Occasionally, in research, the potential subject is not able to understand fully and make rational decisions regarding participation, as is often the case for children and persons with cognitive disorders or severe mental or physical illness. Under those circumstances, a researcher is obligated

TABLE 7.2	Five Basic Rights and Relevant Components of the Informed Consent Form	
BASIC RIGHT	**COMPONENTS OF INFORMED CONSENT**
Right to self-determination	Description of purpose of study
	Description of procedures in study
	Description of possible risks/discomforts
	Description of possible benefits
	Statement of right to withdraw from study
	Statement of voluntary nature of participation without consequences if person chooses not to participate
	Information about contacts for questions
Right to privacy and dignity	Description of possible risk/discomfort
	Description of confidentiality
Right to anonymity and confidentiality	Description of confidentiality
Right to fair treatment	Description of purpose of study
	Description of procedures in study
	Description of any compensation for medical treatment
Right to protection from discomfort and harm	Description of procedures
	Description of potential risks/discomforts
	Description of potential benefits

to seek consent from a designated legal representative of the potential subject, such as a parent, guardian, or other relative. The researcher must be cautious to ensure that the legal representative is indeed the correct person who is able to provide consent, meaning that they must be the legal guardian of the potential subject. Researchers must also ascertain that the legal representative not only understands the implications of consent, but also do not have a personal stake in the interest of their loved one's participation in the research.

However, the subject may have a level of function that allows the researcher to seek his or her assent. To **assent** means to agree or concur and, in the case of research, reflects a lower level of understanding about the meaning of participation in a study than consent. Assent is often sought in studies that involve older children or individuals who have a level of impairment that limits their ability but does not preclude their understanding of some aspects of the study. If a study included a participant who is a minor, his or her legal guardian is legally designated as the participant's representative, so the healthcare team member would explain the study and review the consent form with both the minor and the legal guardian. The legal guardian's signature would be needed to include the minor in the study. However, the healthcare team member and the minor's legal guardian could seek the minor's assent to be in the study by asking him or her briefly if he or she would mind helping in a study and then explaining what the study is about in terms that the minor can understand. If the minor agrees, we would consider that he or she has assented to participate in the study: He or she has agreed without completely understanding all the aspects of the study, and it will be his or her legal guardian who will make the knowledgeable decision, assuring the minor's full rights.

WHEN RESEARCH IS EXEMPT

There are some instances in which research that is submitted to an IRB will be considered **exempt**, which essentially means that the study falls under a category of research that is free from the some of the constraints that are normally imposed upon research involving human subjects (U.S. Department of Health & Human Services, 2009). Some examples of research that may be considered exempt include, but are not limited to, research on educational curriculum efficacy, research involving observation of human behavior (without contact with the individuals observed), and research involving collection of publically available data where subjects cannot be identified. It is of critical importance to understand that proposals for any kind of research, even research that is likely to be considered exempt, be forwarded to the appropriate IRB for consideration. The IRB is responsible for determining exempt status, not the researcher. Once approval has been secured from the IRB, then the researcher may continue his or her study.

There are numerous questions that IRB reviewers must consider when determining whether a study is exempt. The Office for Human Research Protections (OHRP) has designed graphic aids to assist IRBs in their processes when determining whether an activity is considered research that must be reviewed by an IRB, whether the review can be performed in an expedited fashion, and whether informed consent may be waived (OHRP, 2004). An example of one of these algorithms is included in Figure 7.1.

CRITICALLY READING REPORTS OF SAMPLING AND RECOGNIZING COMMON ERRORS

Informed consent, as well as the problems that can arise in samples described in Chapter 6, can affect the answer to the question "To what types of patients do these research conclusions apply—who was in the study?" The most common error found in a sampling report related to the ethics of a study is the failure to tell us enough to let us judge the occurrence of potential problems. Almost every study report will include some descriptive information about the sample, and most will indicate the source of the subjects or the location of the study subjects. However, this information may not be adequate for evaluating the sampling process for ethical principles.

As you critically read reports of research, there are two questions to ask that directly address ethical considerations in sampling. These are the fourth and fifth questions listed in Box 6.2 in Chapter 6. The fourth question asks, "Was enough information given for me to understand how rights of human subjects were protected?" and the fifth question asks, "Would my patient population have been placed at risk if they had participated in this study?"

PUBLISHED REPORTS—WHAT DO THEY SAY ABOUT CONSENT AND THE SAMPLING PROCESS?

As we look at the research, it is important to realize that when considering sampling as a factor in implementing evidence-based practice, the clinical healthcare team member often is the expert. We have discussed the meaning of several terms used in research to describe sampling strategies and actual samples, and these are important for understanding the conclusions of a research study. What we have not discussed is that often it is the practicing healthcare team member who most readily recognizes the limits to IRB protection and sampling process because those in practice understand their patients' needs, functionality, and characteristics. If the healthcare team member researcher is not directly involved in patient care with the population of interest, he or she may not realize that a certain segment of the population is not represented in the sample or has special ethical needs. Once a healthcare team member understands the sampling language and the IRB process, they are likely to be the best judges of whether a study sample reflects real patient populations and is appropriate to a particular research question. It is also important that the healthcare team member recognizes that all samples have strengths as well as some limitations.

The next challenge for the healthcare team member is to reach a better understanding of why and how data were collected from the individuals in these samples. Just as the sample affects the meaningfulness of a study for practice, the measures used and approach taken to procuring data can affect the knowledge gained.

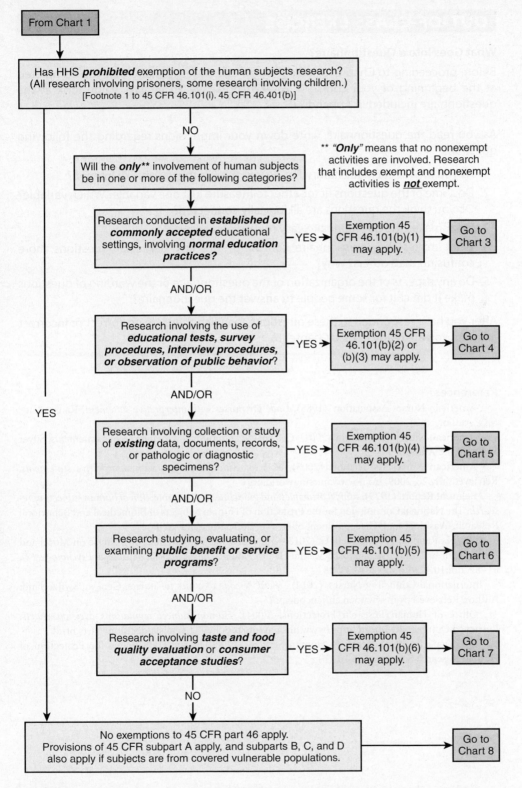

FIGURE 7.1   Chart 2: Is the research involving human subjects eligible for exemption under 45 CFR 46.101(b) (From Office for Human Research Protections. [2004, September 24]. *Human subject regulations decision charts.* Retrieved October 2013 from http://www.hhs.gov/ohrp/policy/checklists/decisioncharts.html.)

OUT-OF-CLASS EXERCISE

What Goes Into a Questionnaire?

Before proceeding to Chapter 8, look at the in-class questionnaire that you completed at the beginning of your course. If you did not have an in-class study, look at the questionnaire included in Appendix C.

As you read the questionnaire, write down your impressions regarding the following questions:

1. As you look at each question, what do you think is the variable of interest?
2. Do some of the questions fit together to measure just one variable? Which variable? Do you think the questions are all logically connected?
3. What makes the questionnaire easy to read and answer?
4. What makes the questionnaire confusing? Are any particular questions more confusing than others? Why?
5. Do any aspects of the organization of the questionnaire or the wording of questions make it difficult for some people to answer the questionnaire?

After you have responded to these questions, to which there are no correct or incorrect answers, you are ready to read Chapter 8.

References

*American Nurses Association. (1985). *Code for nurses with interpretive statement*. Kansas City, MO: Author.

*American Nurses Association. (2001). *Code of ethics for nurses with interpretive statements*. Silver Spring, MD: Author.

*American Nurses Association. (2005). *Code of ethics for nurses with interpretive statements*. Retrieved July 26, 2009, from www.nursingworld.org

*Belmont Report. (1979). *Ethical principles and guidelines for the protection of human subjects of research*. The National Commission for the Protection of Human Subjects of Biomedical and Behavioral Research. Washington, DC: Department of Health, Education, and Welfare.

Ellis, N., Randall, J., & Punnett, G. (2013). The Affects of a Single Bout of Exercise on Mood and Self-Esteem in Clinically Diagnosed Mental Health Patients. *Open Journal of Medical Psychology*, *(2)*, 81–85. doi:10.4236/ojmp.2013.23013

International Council of Nurses. (2012). *The ICN code of ethics for nurses*. Geneva, Switzerland: Author. Retrieved from www.icn.ch/icncode.pdf

*Office of Human Research Protections. (2004). *Human subject regulations decision charts*. Retrieved October 2013 from http://www.hhs.gov/ohrp/policy/checklists/decisioncharts.html

*U.S. Department of Health & Human Services. (2009). Basic HHS Policy for Protection of Human Research Subjects, §46.101(b).

indicates a definitive or classic work or publication regarding this subject matter.

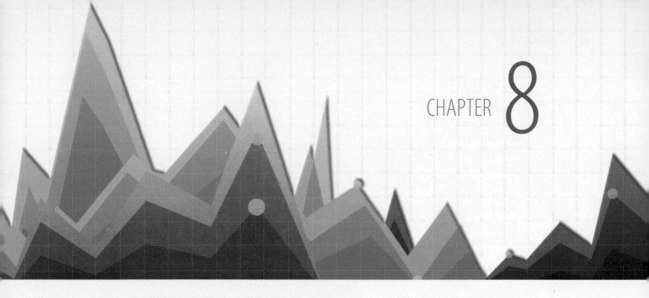

CHAPTER 8

Data Collection Methods

How Were Those People Studied—Why Was the Study Performed That Way?

> **LEARNING OBJECTIVE** The student will relate the data collection methods of a study to the meaning of its results and conclusions.

Revisiting Study Variables

Methods for Constructing the Meaning of Variables in Qualitative Research

Errors in Data Collection in Qualitative Research

Trustworthiness
Confirmability
Transferability
Credibility

Methods to Measure Variables in Quantitative Research

Errors in Data Collection in Quantitative Research

The Quality of Measures—Reliability and Validity
Errors in Implementation of Quantitative Data Collection

Common Errors in Written Reports of Data Collection Methods

Critically Reading Methods Sections of Research Reports

Connecting Data Collection Methods to Sampling, Results, and Discussion/Conclusion

Published Reports—Would You Use These Studies in Clinical Practice?

KEY TERMS

Audit trail
Confirmability
Construct validity
Content validity
Credibility
Criterion-related validity
Error
Field notes
Group interviews
Instrument
Internal consistency reliability
Interrater reliability
Items
Likert-type response scale
Member checks
Operational definition

Participant observation
Questionnaire
Reliability
Rigor
Scale
Semistructured
    questions
Structured questions
Test–retest reliability
Theoretical definition
Transferability
Triangulation
Trustworthiness
Unstructured interviews
Validity
Visual analog

CLINICAL CASE

A nurse is caring for Mindy, a 12-week-old girl who is undergoing repair for a cleft lip. The nurse recognizes that postoperative complications can arise if the suture line is disrupted, particularly if the infant places her fingers into her mouth. For this reason, elbow restraints have been routinely used to prevent this from happening. The nurse is curious about whether this is considered best practice, and searches for evidence to guide decision making about the use of restraints in infants who have undergone cleft lip repair. As you will see in Table 8.1, the results of the literature search shows one research report that seems particularly relevant titled "The Use of Postoperative Restraints in Children after Cleft lip or Cleft Palate Repair: A Preliminary Report" (Huth, Petersen, & Lehman, 2013).

TABLE 8.1	Statement of Clinical Question from the Clinical Case
DO THE USE OF POSTOPERATIVE RESTRAINTS IN CHILDREN WHO HAVE HAD CLEFT LIP OR CLEFT PALATE REPAIR HAVE A RELATIONSHIP TO POSTOPERATIVE COMPLICATIONS?	
The *Who*	Children below the age of 2 years undergoing repair of a cleft lip or a cleft palate by a single surgeon
The *What*	Use of postoperative restraints
The *When*	After cleft lip or cleft palate repair
The *Where*	Akron Children's Hospital
Key search terms to find research-based evidence for practice	• Postoperative restraints • Cleft lip • Cleft palate • Repair • Children • Pediatric

REVISITING STUDY VARIABLES

The unique language of research associated with data collection is extensive, as a quick glance at the key terms listed at the beginning of this chapter shows. The purpose of the article found by the nurse indicates that this study tested whether the use of elbow restraints after cleft lip (or cleft palate) repair has a relationship to postoperative complication in patients who are like Mindy. After reading the article, however, the nurse realizes that understanding how complex aspects of health, such as the concept of "use," were measured is essential to understanding the results and conclusions of the study. The nurse begins to read the methods section to help achieve this understanding.

To examine the measurement approaches taken, the nurse first has to identify the variables in the study. We discussed variables in Chapters 4 and 5, defining them as some aspect of interest that differs in a variety of groups or situations. Both qualitative and quantitative studies have variables, but only quantitative studies use the categories of independent and dependent variables. Independent variables are factors in the study that are used to explain or predict the outcome of interest and are sometimes called *predictor variables* because they are used to predict the dependent variable. Dependent variables are those that depend on other variables in a study, or are the outcome variables of interest. In the article the nurse from our clinical case read, the independent variable was use of postoperative restraints in children after cleft lip or cleft palate repair, and the dependent variable was postoperative complications.

As a review, remember that it is not the variable itself but how it is used that makes it either independent or dependent. For example, in one study, the purpose might be to describe the effects of chemotherapy on patients' levels of stress. In such a study, the outcome or dependent variable is stress. Another study might seek to understand how factors such as education, stress, and perceived benefits lead to nonadherence of diet restrictions. In such a study, we also see the variable "stress," but now it is an independent variable because it is being used to predict the outcome of adherence.

Before we continue, let us look at how we determine the variables in a study. Although it is logical that variables differ across groups or situations, many research reports will not explicitly identify or list the study variables. Obviously, variables should reflect the topic of interest, which, in turn, should be described in the purpose, background, and research questions, sections of a research report discussed in depth in Chapter 10. Because a qualitative study usually begins with one or more broad questions and uses open-ended approaches to collecting data, the variables of interest are often clearly identified within the research questions. In contrast, reports of quantitative studies should clearly describe the variables even if they are not explicitly labeled as such because the data collection methods in quantitative research are specifically aimed at measuring study variables as objectively as possible.

The data collection section of a report of a quantitative study should describe how each variable was measured and identify each variable. The nurse in our clinical case found the outcome variables identified under the opening "overview" section in a line entitled "Purpose." The study design was described in the same opening section in a line called "Methods." These topics are described fully in their respective subsections under the general heading of "Methods."

Variables also can be identified and discussed in terms of their definitions rather than whether they are independent or dependent. Variables can be defined at two levels: the theoretical level and the operational level. A **theoretical definition** is one that is described and understood conceptually, not concretely. Because it is stated conceptually, this definition is not always clearly measurable. Therefore, a second type of definition called the *operational definition* is needed. An **operational definition** is one that is defined in specific, concrete terms that allows us to see how we might actually measure the variable. If researchers do not have a clear understanding of the theoretical meaning of a concept, then they may be inconsistent in their measurement of that concept, leading to disagreement about what was actually measured and questions about the overall meaning of the study.

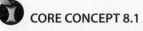

CORE CONCEPT 8.1

The measures in a quantitative study should reflect the specific variables under study.
        For example, the variable "stress" can be defined as an individual's perceptions that an event is threatening and that he or she has no way to manage the threat. This definition is conceptual, giving the reader a clearer idea of what is meant by the word *stress*, but it does not tell us how that variable might actually be measured. An operational definition of stress might be an individual's summed score regarding his or her ratings on a four-point scale of the perceived level of threat from 40 life events. Or, still using the same theoretical definition, stress could be operationally defined as the number of beats per minute that the heart rate increases when a person looks at pictures of negative events. These two definitions are concrete and tell the reader exactly how the variable "stress" will be measured.

Although some variables such as temperature or heart rate are concrete and may only be defined operationally, many variables of interest to healthcare are relatively abstract and may need both a theoretical and an operational definition if they are going to be used in a quantitative study. Examples of these types of variables include mood and cognitive status. If a researcher believed that we had a theoretical understanding of the mood variable, he or she might break it down into one or more concrete components that would then comprise an operational definition. For example, he or she might operationally define, or operationalize, mood as scores on the Structured Clinical Interview for Axis I DSM-IV Disorders (SCID) scale (First, Spitzer, Gibbon, & Williams, 1996). Alternatively, a researcher might operationalize quality of life (QOL) as a single item rated on a 10-point scale. Almost any variable can be operationalized, but the correctness and accuracy of that operationalization must be evaluated. You can think of an operational definition, or the operationalization, of a variable as a form of translation: The researcher is translating an abstract theoretical idea into a concrete set of measures.

CORE CONCEPT 8.2

Operationalizing variables is like translating a phrase from one language to another. The researcher is translating an abstract, theoretical variable into a concrete measure or set of measures.

When a variable is not measured with 100% accuracy, we say that there is error in the measurement. In research, **error** refers to the difference between what is true and the answer we obtained from our data collection. If we operationalized gender as the data collectors' assessment of gender based on observation, that observation might be wrong probably only 1 in 1,000 times. Think about that: If we had a data collector sit in a hospital waiting room and record the gender of each person walking in the room, occasionally he or she might misperceive or be confused by odd dress or appearance. In almost all measurement, there could still be some error because an observational assessment would be wrong occasionally. The difference between the gender of 1,000 people and the measurement of gender through observation would be the error in the measurement of that variable.

Remember that we said measurement is about translation. If you have experienced having someone translate your words into another language, you know that translation is open to interpretation and even error. Qualitative research does not operationalize variables because it does not presume to know enough about the variables of interest to be able to select appropriate and accurate concrete measures. Yet, qualitative research does translate specific experiences or observations into theoretical concepts or descriptions of variables during the process of data collection and analysis. Therefore, qualitative research is open to errors in interpretation during the data collection process. For example, a researcher may get focused on an idea that one or two participants who are trying to quit smoking discuss, such as "fear of failure," and start looking for that theme in other interviews. The researcher may then hear statements about discouragement as well as about disappointing significant others as variations of the fear of failing when, in fact, discouragement and disappointment are important and different themes that warrant exploration.

Because quantitative research often examines abstract variables that require both a theoretical and an operational definition, the opportunities for error in measurement can be even greater. Error can occur in the translation from theoretical to operational, and it can occur in the operationalized measurement process. Therefore, both qualitative research and quantitative research are open to problems in the translation of variables. We will discuss how those potential problems with translation can affect the meaning of the results of a study for practice later in this chapter.

Before looking at specific approaches used to collect data for studies, let us apply the ideas of theoretical variables and operational definitions to the fictional article in Appendix B about nursing students' choices of field of practice. The author of the article tells us in the first paragraph, under the heading of "Measures," that the questionnaire used in this study had three sections: one that asked about demographic characteristics; one that asked about education, well-being, and career choice; and one that asked about automobile preferences. Demographic variables are usually fairly concrete and commonly understood, so the author does not offer theoretical definitions of them. However, the author does tell us indirectly that these variables were measured by self-report because they were measured through a questionnaire that was completed by the students. Therefore, the operational definition of age in this study is the actual reported age. The variable age then might be translated to be "the subject's report of his or her age in years." Age also could have been operationally defined by asking for the subject's birth date, which the researcher could then have used to compute age to the day using a computer calculation that subtracts date of birth from the current date. The fictional article does not tell us whether the questionnaire asked for age in years or for birth date, so we do not know exactly how the age variable was operationalized.

The second section of the questionnaire was used to operationalize several variables in the study, including educational background, well-being, and student preference for clinical practice after graduation. Educational background was operationalized by the answers to two questions: (1) if the student was currently licensed to practice as an RN or a licensed practical nurse (LPN) and (2) the total number of years of the student's postsecondary education. Well-being was operationally defined as the student's rating of his or her health on a four-point scale. Anticipated field of choice was operationally defined as choice from a list of career options. In each case, a variable has been translated into a specific measure or measures, and alternate translations could have been used. Equally important, there is room for error both in the translation of a variable to a measure and in the measuring process itself. The remainder of this chapter discusses the measurement process and how error may occur.

Finally, the researcher in the fictional article included in the questionnaire an open-ended question regarding life experiences that led to choice of field of practice. In this last question, the researcher does not concretely translate a variable but asks the subjects to share experiences that may help his or her to develop a definition of the variable "life experiences affecting choice of field." Because this variable is not concrete, the researcher will have to start by developing a theoretical translation or definition before considering an operational definition. The fictional article provides several examples of operationally defined variables but includes no theoretical definitions.

METHODS FOR CONSTRUCTING THE MEANING OF VARIABLES IN QUALITATIVE RESEARCH

A study that is using a qualitative approach should examine variables and increase understanding of something that is abstract and unknown by asking for, or looking for, specific examples, experiences, or perceptions. However, because a qualitative study does not attempt to measure variables concretely, we do not expect to find operational definitions included in a report of the study methods. The primary purpose of many qualitative studies is to develop a clear theoretical definition of a variable so that it might eventually be operationally defined and concretely measured. For example, let us assume that we plan to conduct a qualitative study about the unique needs of a family caring for a loved one who has dementia. Because the purpose of that study would be to increase our understanding of what "family needs" actually are, a definition of "family needs" should not exist prior to the research. A concrete definition would presume that we already had a relatively clear understanding of "family needs" and could concretely measure it. In actuality, by doing the research, the researchers would be trying to construct a theoretical definition of "family needs" that then could be translated into an operational definition.

In qualitative research, the study methods used to collect data are intended to allow the researcher to construct a description of the meaning of the variable(s) under study. Remember that a qualitative approach assumes that truth is a moving target. The more we can know, feel, or understand about a variable of interest, the closer we will come to a full and complete meaning, but that meaning will always be context laden and, therefore, changing and evolving. A qualitative method for data collection, then, does not aim to measure specifically or make concrete a variable of interest. Rather, these data collection methods aim to expand our understanding about a variable or variables on as many levels as possible.

Qualitative methods of data collection depend on the participants' open sharing of their thoughts, feelings, and experiences verbally, visually, in writing, with music, and within life activities. Although it may not be surprising that participants can share through speaking and writing, other means of expression, such as music or cooking a meal, are probably less frequently considered but can be meaningful avenues for understanding a participant's experiences or feelings. Therefore, the data methods include interviews, journaling, participant observation, and art analysis. Interviews are commonly used methods for collecting data in qualitative research, with two broad categories of interviews used: those that are unstructured and those that use groups.

Unstructured interviews involve asking questions in an informal and open fashion, without a previously established set of categories or assumed answers, to gain understanding about a phenomenon or variable of interest. Unstructured interviews in qualitative research assume that the product of the interview reflects the interactions among the interviewer, participant, and interview environment or setting. Depending on the type of qualitative study, the researcher may identify and purposely set aside or bracket his or her knowledge, beliefs, or expectations about the variable, or he or she may not bracket and instead may carefully document and incorporate his or her knowledge, beliefs, and perspectives into the data collection process. In any case, data collection using an unstructured interview includes not only the actual words of the participant but also notes the participant's tone, expressions, and associated actions and what is occurring in the setting. These notes are often called **field notes** because they are a record of the researcher's observations about the overall setting and experience of the data collection process while in that setting or field. Field notes are used to enrich and build a data set that is thick and dense with information to define the variables and illuminate the phenomenon.

Not all interviewing techniques are unstructured. However, qualitative research does not generally use either semistructured or structured interviews because these types of interviews assume and control options for answers to questions. As such, semistructured and structured interviews do not fit with the perspective of a qualitative researcher that it is the participant's own ideas and language that extend our knowledge and understanding of a phenomenon.

Unstructured interviews may take several forms, including in-depth interviews, oral histories, storytelling, and life reviews. In all forms, the intent is to openly explore the understanding and experiences of the study participants. Unstructured interviews usually are tape-recorded or videotaped, then transcribed verbatim into a written form that will include notes on pauses; vocalizations that are not actual words, such as sighs; and even voice tone at times.

A related method of data collection is **participant observation**. In this type of observation, the researcher intentionally imbeds himself or herself into the environment from which data will be collected and becomes a participant. From the perspective of active participation in the experiences and lives of those studied, the researcher/participant records observations, feelings, conversations, and experiences regarding the phenomenon of interest.

Group interviews are also used to collect data in qualitative research and involve collection of data by interviewing more than one participant at a time. The data collected, then, are not just the participant's responses but are also the responses that occur due to the interaction of the participants as they hear and respond to each other. Group interviews may take the form of focus groups, in which a preset topic is addressed in an open-ended fashion and the researcher keeps the focus of the group on that topic. Another form of group interview is brainstorming, in which no particular focus or direction is established, and group dialogues about a broad topic in an unstructured discussion. Group interviews may occur spontaneously in a setting where a researcher finds or facilitates two or more participants in naturally dialoguing about a phenomenon of interest. For example, a researcher studying the experience of receiving government assistance and observing a group of women waiting for their food stamps might see several women talking about what it is like to shop with the stamps. The researcher might introduce himself or herself, obtain consent, and join the discussion, asking a few questions and listening to what the women have to say. In general, group interviews are rich in data and can be a relatively inexpensive method of data collection. However, use of group interviews may limit hearing and knowing unique perspectives or ideas because groups limit some individual expression.

Use of journals is another approach that can be used to collect data in qualitative studies. In journaling, a researcher can ask participants to describe, in writing, their ongoing experiences with a phenomenon of interest. This type of data collection can provide continuous and evolving information from an individual perspective that cannot be collected in face-to-face interviews. However, it clearly depends on the participant's ability and willingness to write on a regular and detailed basis. The researcher also depends on the participant's own description of the setting and interactions related to an experience under study because he or she is not present during the journaling. A more limited form of written data can be collected by directly asking participants to write a response or description about a phenomenon on the occasion of data collection. This approach is often called a *free write*. The fictional article in Appendix B about students' choices of fields of nursing used a limited version of written data collection by asking an open-ended question about students' experiences that had affected their choices of field in nursing. This can be considered to be a form of qualitative data collection because it does not constrain or limit the responses that students can give and lends itself to providing data about the meaning of life experiences for future life choices.

A similar form of data collection involves the use of expressional media or art forms such as art, music, or poetry. Here, data such as drawings or photography are collected, as it is assumed that they reflect the participant's perception and interpretation of certain experiences. When art is used, an interview often is included so that the participant can share or interpret his or her art to the researcher. For example, homeless individuals might be given disposable cameras and asked to take photographs that reflect their experiences of being homeless. The researcher might then analyze the photographs for common subjects or common reflected moods.

Another form of data collected in qualitative research is documents and records. These types of data are used in historical research and may include personal and business letters, logs, contracts, accounts, and other written records. These data are compiled and examined to create a clear picture of some past aspect and are particularly useful when the phenomenon of interest has evolved over time, such as the elimination of wearing nursing caps in the clinical setting.

In all of these methods, the researcher is not collecting discrete, clearly defined, and limited information. Qualitative data are used to develop theoretical meaning by creating a verbal, a visual, or an auditory picture of a variable of interest. Although data collection in qualitative research is not structured and objectified, it is carefully planned and thought through, and it involves clearly identified methods for the overlapping processes of collecting, handling, and analysis.

ERRORS IN DATA COLLECTION IN QUALITATIVE RESEARCH

In qualitative research, error can be introduced into a study in two major ways. Problems can occur with the processes of data collection and analysis, or both. When considering the aspects that can create error, qualitative researchers aim to ensure the rigor of both processes. **Rigor** is a strict process of data collection and analysis as well as a term that reflects the overall quality of that process in qualitative research. It is reflected in the consistency of data analysis and interpretation, the trustworthiness of the data collected, the transferability of the themes, and the credibility of the data. Qualitative researchers use several tools and processes to guarantee that each of these aspects of rigor is ensured.

Trustworthiness

Trustworthiness refers to the honesty of the data collected from or about the participants (Lincoln & Guba, 1985). To collect trustworthy data, the researcher must have a meaningful relationship with the participants, which may require time to develop. Participants also must want to share information so that they can communicate their feelings, insights, and experiences without feeling pressured or wanting to censor what they share (Lincoln & Guba). People who participate in research studies are not as likely to share their experiences and perceptions honestly and openly unless they believe that the researcher has a real interest in their perceptions and an acceptance of them and their life experiences. Participants do not develop such openness without first getting to know the researcher, at least to some extent. Trust and a respectful relationship must be established early in the study process.

Trustworthiness of data collection may also be supported by using a consistent protocol in data collection. Use of a protocol may seem contradictory to the open-ended nature of most qualitative data collection methods. However, a protocol can provide a broad framework for data collection and ensure a similar setting and interaction, without structuring the data collected.

Confirmability

A second aspect of ensuring rigor in qualitative data collection is **confirmability**—that is, the consistency and repeatability of the decision making about the process of data collection and data analysis (Lincoln & Guba, 1985). One approach taken to ensure confirmability of data in qualitative research is developing and maintaining an audit trail. An **audit trail** is an ongoing documentation regarding the researcher's decisions about the data analysis and collection processes. Documentation from the audit trail may include field notes about the process of data collection, theoretical notes about the working hypotheses or developing ideas during the analysis, or methods notes regarding approaches to categorizing or organizing the data. The audit trail can be used to assist the researcher in being consistent as well as to demonstrate the presence of consistency when sharing the data.

Qualitative researchers often use computer software programs, such as ATLAS.ti, QDA. miner, NU.DIST, and N.VIVO, to help them to organize and analyze data. These programs do not perform the thinking and conceptualizing that is at the heart of qualitative data analysis, but they can be used to examine the data efficiently, to organize it around themes and dimensions as they are identified in the data, and to synthesize large volumes of data. As the researcher begins to identify a data theme, different units of language or observations can be categorized under this theme. As new themes arise, the software can reorganize the data consistently. In addition, a record of the evolving decisions about themes and the classification of data are maintained, ensuring that the researcher is consistent in the analysis of all the data and assisting the qualitative researcher in maintaining an audit trail.

Taking a simple example, suppose that the researcher for the choice of field study reported in the fictional article (Appendix B) had broken down the students' written answers describing experiences that contributed to their choices of field into units that were the individual sentences and then stored them within a computer program. The researcher might decide that whenever students described some kind of experience with fiction about health care, such as a novel or television series, that this reflected a theme. The researcher now must explore the data to decide what are and are not examples of experiences with fiction about healthcare. For example, novels, plays, movies, and television series may all clearly fit into the theme of fiction, but are advertisements that depict healthcare also part of this category? As the researcher decides and tells the program that references to television, radio, literature, film, and theater all reflect exposure to media, the computer will find and place into a category any sentences with those references. When the researcher later adds some additional data from another class of students, it might also be decided that identification with selected actors or actresses is a separate theme from the broader media exposure. The computer can be told to reorganize the data, looking for references to particular actors or actresses, but it will also retain the information about how the original category was formed. This provides the researcher with a powerful ongoing record of decisions, enhances the ability to work with large data sets, and decreases the possibility of the researcher defining or describing a category inconsistently from one time to another.

Transferability

A third aspect of rigor in a qualitative study is the transferability of the concepts, themes, or dimensions identified. **Transferability** refers to the extent to which the findings of a study are confirmed by or are applicable to a different group or in a different setting from where the data were collected (Lincoln & Guba, 1985). Transferability is different from generalizability because the focus is not on predicting specific outcomes in a general population. Rather, the focus is on confirming that what was meaningful in one specific setting or with one specific group is also meaningful and accurate in a different setting or group. One of the methods used to ensure transferability is to describe themes that have been identified in one sample to a group of similar participants who did not contribute to the initial data collection to determine if the second group agrees with the themes. This procedure is sometimes called *external checks*. Transferability also can be ensured if the researcher actively seeks sources of data that contradict the ideas that are emerging from the data. If disconfirming data are found, they can be used to modify or reinterpret the total body of data to develop more comprehensive and credible findings. Findings that reflect the breadth of experiences or ideas will then be more easily transferred or related to different groups.

Credibility

Credibility, the fourth aspect of rigor of concern to qualitative researchers, overlaps with transferability and trustworthiness. **Credibility** refers to the confidence that the researcher and user of the research can have in the truth of the findings of the study. Lincoln and Guba (1985) suggest that the credibility of qualitative data can be supported by a researcher performing several actions, including seeking feedback from participants regarding evolving findings and interpretations and seeking participants whose perceptions differ from those already included in the study. The former activity is often referred to as *member checks*. **Member checks** means just what it sounds like—that the data and findings from data analysis are brought back to the original participants to seek their input concerning the accuracy, completeness, and interpretation of the data.

Credibility also is ensured through processes that guarantee trustworthiness and transferability, such as spending time with the participants and maintaining thorough phenomenon-focused observations. It can be further ensured through the use of triangulation. **Triangulation** is the process of using more than one approach or source to include different views or to look at the phenomenon from different angles (Lincoln & Guba, 1985). This process focuses on the data, seeking different types of sources of information regarding a phenomenon, or it can focus on the use of more than one investigator, the use of several theories, or the use of numerous methods in the study (Denzin, 2001). When multiple sources of data all lead to the same conclusions, the credibility of those findings is increased.

Table 8.2 summarizes the aspects of rigor that we have discussed. As we read and consider using results from qualitative research in practice, we must consider the rigor of the data collection methods and analysis. The greater the rigor in the study, the more we can be confident that the findings are meaningful truths that we can use to understand our patients. What helps us to be confident includes the use of processes to ensure the trustworthiness of the data, such as the researcher's establishment of meaningful interactions and maintenance of ongoing contact with participants. That the data are confirmable can be indicated by the researcher stating that an audit trail was maintained or that selected software was used to assist in data analysis. Use of approaches such as external checks and searching for participants who differ or have dissenting views can help to ensure us of the transferability of the data. The credibility of the data can be supported by member checks and triangulation.

TABLE 8.2	Aspects of Rigor	
ASPECT	**DEFINITION**	**METHODS**
Trustworthiness	The honesty of the data collected from and about participants	• Establishment of ongoing or meaningful interactions • Use of a protocol
Confirmability	The consistent repeatable nature of the data collection and analysis	• Use of computer software to organize and analyze data • Audit trails
Transferability	The extent to which findings relate to other settings or groups	• External checks • Seeking disconfirming cases or outliers
Credibility	The confidence in the truth of the findings	• Triangulation • Member checks

METHODS TO MEASURE VARIABLES IN QUANTITATIVE RESEARCH

In quantitative research, the methods used for data collection aim to clearly, specifically, and accurately measure the variables of interest. Earlier, we said that an operational definition of a variable is a description of how it will be measured and that a researcher doing a quantitative study almost always must decide how to measure the variable of interest, even when it is as concrete as a subject's gender. Remember also that the goal in quantitative research is to measure variables numerically so that they can be statistically described and analyzed. Therefore, the methods used for data collection in quantitative research include physiologic measurements, chemical laboratory tests, systematic observations, and written measures containing carefully defined questions, questionnaires, and/or scales.

In quantitative studies, variables often are discussed and defined at theoretical and operational levels because the goal in a quantitative study is to examine discrete factors as concretely as possible. Imagine that we were reviewing a study in which there were variables called *mood, anhedonia*, and *suicidal ideation*. Because these variables can have many conceptual meanings, the researchers would have to provide a theoretical definition clarifying "mood" (e.g., sad, hopeless, depressed, stable mood, euthymic), anhedonia (e.g., diminished interest in activities, lack of motivation or pleasure), and suicide ideation (e.g., thoughts of death, thoughts of suicide). These types of definitions are included in the "Measures" section of a research report.

Although all variables in a quantitative study should have an operational definition, not all variables in quantitative research will have a theoretical definition. Concrete variables, such as gender, weight, platelet count, or oxygen saturation, do not have or need a theoretical definition. There is a common understanding of the conceptual meaning of "gender," so it does not need a theoretical definition. But even concrete variables need an operational definition when they are being examined in research because several approaches can be taken to measure them. For example, we can operationally define gender in at least three different ways (1) the presence or absence of a Y chromosome, (2) a self-reported characteristic, or (3) an observed characteristic. In most cases, we will get the same result no matter which way we define and measure gender. However, in rare cases, some people perceive themselves to be the opposite gender from that indicated in their chromosomal composition, and some people are androgynous enough that a superficial observation might lead to incorrect categorization. Therefore, even a variable as concrete as gender must be operationally defined so that we can understand exactly what was measured.

CORE CONCEPT 8.3

In a quantitative study, every variable should have an operational definition that specifies how the variable was measured.

Physiologic measurement is arguably the most concrete type of data collection in quantitative research and may include anything from a simple measurement of blood pressure to the calculation of pulmonary function values. As was pointed out with the gender variable, physiologic measures must still be defined operationally because most of them can be measured in several different fashions and with different levels of accuracy. A research study that examines a physiologic variable should report specifically how the physiologic parameter was measured so that the accuracy and appropriateness of that measure can be evaluated. Similarly, a study that includes a variable measured by a laboratory test should specify the actual test or procedure used to arrive at the study values. For example, if blood sugar were measured in a study, the report should indicate whether it used a capillary sample or a venous sample and what type of control and calibration measures were used to ensure consistency and accuracy.

A second method of measuring variables in quantitative research involves systematic observation of the variable of interest. Measurement by systematic observation differs from the observation data collection methods used in qualitative research because it is structured and defined to ensure that each measurement is accurate and comparable to earlier or later measures. As a result, systematic observation does not try to collect as much detail and variation as possible but has a narrow focus on specific components of the variable under study.

For example, in a study that was trying to describe factors affecting fecal incontinence, the researchers would need to operationalize the variable fecal incontinence, perhaps by stating that the specific observation required to indicate the presence of fecal incontinence is the presence of uncontrolled release of stool and/or soiled clothing. Thus, the variable is clearly defined, and the data collection focuses on the specific components of the definition. Therefore, data collectors would not be interested in factors such as urinary incontinence, skin condition, type of bedpan, staffing ratio, or the subject's ability to use the call button. Data collectors will look for and record reports by the staff or the client of involuntary release of stool, and they will count the presence or absence of the defined components to give each subject a value of "yes" or "no" for the variable fecal incontinence.

A third method for measurement in quantitative research is use of an instrument. The word **instrument** is used in research to refer to a device that specifies and objectifies the data collecting process. Instruments are usually written and may be given directly to the subject to collect data or may provide objective description of the collection of certain types of data. The Structured Clinical Interview for DSM-IV Disorders (SCID) is an example of a written instrument (First, Spitzer, Gibbon, & Williams, 1996). Some instruments provide directions for observations, and the measure depends on observers noting certain specified and defined types of behaviors, counting the presence or absence of those behaviors, and converting them into a final numeric score. For example, in the study regarding postoperative restraint use after cleft lip or cleft palate repair (Huth, Petersen, & Lehman, 2013), the researchers might have chosen to use an observational measure of postoperative complications that required a healthcare team member to objectively make note of specific factors, such as disruption in the suture line or development or postoperative fever. When a researcher uses this type of observational measurement, the components that define the variable have been specified before data collection begins, and the study does not seek to expand the understanding of the components of that variable, as would a qualitative approach, but seeks to count the extent to which they are present.

We have said that instruments are devices that define and objectify the data collection. Some quantitative studies collect data using **semistructured questions** (Box 8.1) in order to collect data that specifically target objective factors of interest. For example, telephone surveys often consist of semistructured questions, such as "tell me how you use television to relax in the evening." Phenomenologic (qualitative) research continues this questioning process by asking further flexible questions, such as probes and inquiries; the answers given help the researcher to broaden the scope of information received from the participants, in an effort to understand a complete picture of their lived experience. For example, in Box 8.1, the researcher is studying the lived experience of students who have chosen to earn their baccalaureate degree from an accredited online college or university, rather than from a brick-and-mortar college or university. The initial semistructured questions allow the researcher to gain an initial impression of the participants' perspective about this way of attending school, while the probes and inquiries provide an avenue to understand, in a broader fashion, how students truly have experienced this online program. If this study had been conducted quantitatively, the researcher may have used a **structured question** that

BOX 8.1
Examples of Semistructured Questions, Probes, and Inquiries

Questions

1. How do you feel about your experience with your classmates in the online environment, in terms of how much you sensed an atmosphere of camaraderie?
2. How do you feel about your experience with your facilitator in the online environment in terms of how much he or she promoted an atmosphere of camaraderie?
3. How would you describe the social immediacy you experienced in the online environment?
4. To what extent did you fear psychological distance in the online environment?
5. How would you describe the atmosphere of "caring" that you feel that your facilitator in the course had for you?
6. To what degree do you feel that the facilitator created a sense of community for you and your classmates?
7. To what degree do you feel that your classmates interacted with you and respected your feelings?
8. To what degree do you feel that your facilitator interacted with you and respected your feelings?

Probes

1. To what degree do you feel that the sense of community and relationships you experienced with your classmates in this course contributes to your success in this course?
2. To what degree do you feel that the sense of community and relationships you experienced with your facilitator in this course contributes to your success in this course?
3. To what degree do you feel that the sense of community and relationships you experience with classmates will ultimately contribute to your success in your online degree program?
4. To what degree do you feel that the sense of community and relationships you experience with facilitators will ultimately contribute to your success in your online degree program?
5. How important is the sense of community to you in an online degree program environment?

Inquiries

1. What was your incentive for moving into an online degree program as opposed to a brick-and-mortar program?
2. What factors do you feel would improve connections (psychological distance and social immediacy) in the online environment?

provides measureable choices of answers to questions, such as "how many online colleges or universities did you explore before choosing one to attend."

Many instruments used in research collect data in a written form, provided directly by the subjects in the study. These instruments are also called *instruments*, *questionnaires*, or *scales*, and can include interview questions, directed observations, or written collection of data. A **questionnaire** is an instrument used to collect specific written data, and a **scale** is a set of written questions or statements that, in combination, are intended to measure a specified variable. The questions or statements included on a scale are often called **items**. Box 8.2 summarizes and gives an example of frequently used terms in quantitative measurement.

> **BOX 8.2**
> **Definitions and Relationships among an Instrument, Questionnaire, Scale, and Item**
>
> *Instrument*—a device that specifies (describes) and objectifies (clarifies) the process of data collection
> *Example:* Written instructions for a focused observation of behaviors indicating pain
> ↓
> *Questionnaire*—an instrument that is completed by the study subjects
> Example: Three-page written form that asks subjects about their personal characteristics, medications, past medical history, and pain
> ↓
> *Scale*—a set of written questions or statements that measures a specified variable
> *Example:* Three questions that ask the subjects to rate how often they experience pain in different situations (e.g., "How often do you experience pain when walking?" "How often do you experience pain when sitting still?" and "How often do you experience pain when playing sports?").
> ↓
> *Item*—the individual question or statement that comprises a scale
> *Example:* How often do you wake up in the night because of your pain?
>
> | 0 | 1 | 2 | 3 |
> |---|---|---|---|
> | Never | Rarely | Occasionally | Frequently |

Many of the abstract concepts that we want to measure in research are operationalized by using written scales of one type or another. Because the concepts are abstract, it is not logical or reasonable that we could measure them with a single question. For example, suppose we want to measure the concept of "stress." One could simply ask subjects "Are you stressed—yes or no?" However, answers to this question alone will not capture levels of stress, negative versus positive stress, sense of managing or not managing stress, or the nature of the stresses. To collect a fuller and more complex measure of stress, one needs more than one simple question, hence the use of scales that consist of several statements or items related to the concept being measured.

The first step in developing a scale to measure an abstract concept is to identify items or questions that are relevant to the concept. Identification of items may be based on previous research about the concept, theory related to the concept, experts' knowledge regarding the concept, or individuals' experiences with the concept. Often, items for a scale are created based on several of the sources described. For example, a list of items to measure stress might first be developed based on a theory of stress and coping, then reviewed by experts in the field of stress and coping for suggestions, and finally, reviewed or tested with small groups of individuals who are experiencing stress to see what they think about the items. The result might be five items such as those listed in Box 8.3. (*Note:* This is not an existing and established stress scale; it is simply intended to be an example.)

> **BOX 8.3**
> **Sample Stress Measurement Items**
>
> 1. How often do you feel anxious?
> 2. How often do you have difficulty sleeping at night?
> 3. How often do you feel overwhelmed?
> 4. How often do you feel tired, even after a good night's sleep?
> 5. How often do you feel angry for no identifiable reason?

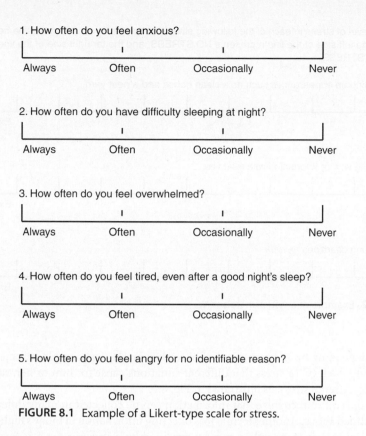

1. How often do you feel anxious?

Always   Often   Occasionally   Never

2. How often do you have difficulty sleeping at night?

Always   Often   Occasionally   Never

3. How often do you feel overwhelmed?

Always   Often   Occasionally   Never

4. How often do you feel tired, even after a good night's sleep?

Always   Often   Occasionally   Never

5. How often do you feel angry for no identifiable reason?

Always   Often   Occasionally   Never

FIGURE 8.1 Example of a Likert-type scale for stress.

In addition to developing items that all are intended to address the same abstract concept or variable, scale development requires deciding how subjects will be asked to respond to the items. One type of response asks subjects to respond whether an item is true or false. A second approach to responding is called a **Likert-type response scale**. This type of response asks for a rating of the item on a continuum that is anchored at either end by opposite responses. For example, a Likert-type response scale that asks subjects to rate the frequency with which they experience what is described in each item that reflects stress from Box 8.3 might range from "always" at one end to "never" on the other end, as illustrated in Fig. 8.1. Another example that could be used with the same items intended to measure stress could ask about frequency of experiencing what is described in the item with four options: 0 = never, 1 = once a week, 2 = two to three times a week, and 3 = daily. Likert-type scales may include from three to as many as eight or more choices, although the usual number of responses ranges from four to six. Notice that the answers to these questions are structured so that the subject cannot answer anything that he or she wishes such as "once every other week" or "sometimes." Use of this scale to measure stress would result in a number between 0 and 15, which is a sum of the number for each item. The score on the scale could be considered to reflect the stress of the individual subject with subjects who answered "never" for all items, getting a score of 0, and subjects who answered "daily" for all items, getting a score of 15.

Visual analog is another response format that can be used in scales that differs from true/false, yes/no, and Likert-type scale responses. A visual analog consists of a straight line of a specific length that has extremes of responses at either end but does not have any other responses noted at points along the line. Subjects are asked to mark the line to indicate where they fall between the two extreme points. Often, the line is 100 mm because a line of that length fits easily on a standard piece of paper, and the subject's response is scored from

Rate your level of stress in each of the following situations by placing an "X" on the line below each situation. The left side of the line represents NO STRESS, and the far right side of the line represents EXTREME STRESS.

1. Keeping up appearances such as a clean house and a neat yard.

No stress   Extreme stress

2. Visiting with or interacting with relatives.

No stress   Extreme stress

3. Meeting deadlines at work.

No stress   Extreme stress

FIGURE 8.2 Example of a visual analog scale.

1 to 100, depending on the placement of his or her mark. For example, a subject might be asked to rate the level of stress that different situations cause for him or her, ranging from no stress to extreme stress, as illustrated in Fig. 8.2.

It is important to recognize that information can be collected in many different capacities, as outlined above. Another format for collecting information in today's highly advanced technological society is via online surveys provided by companies such as SurveyMonkey and Zoomerang. Their products provide the user with different survey formats and include survey wizards that will walk the user, step by step, through the creation of a tool. In addition to the creation of a survey instrument for data collection, they also provide services for analysis. Information can be gathered quickly, with data presented in real time. Some of these companies also provide methodologies for linking survey data to other sources, such as integration into kiosks, mergers with professional programs, or incorporation into social networking sites like Twitter or Facebook.

We have now discussed methods to collect data and specific measurement approaches. We also have mentioned that at times error can occur in the methods or in the process of measurement and in the earlier section talked about potential errors in qualitative measurement. The potential for error occurs in both qualitative and quantitative methods of data collection. Understanding how this error can occur is important so that you can consider what that potential error means for understanding and using research in clinical practice.

ERRORS IN DATA COLLECTION IN QUANTITATIVE RESEARCH

In quantitative research, the data analysis process is usually separated from the data collection process. There are two general areas in which error can occur in quantitative data collection (1) in the quality of the measures used to collect data and (2) in the implementation of those measures or the data collection process itself. These two areas are not entirely discrete and do overlap. We start by talking about the quality of the measures used to collect quantitative data.

The Quality of Measures—Reliability and Validity

Accuracy and consistency in measurement are at the heart of successful quantitative research. As an intelligent reader and user of research, you must ask yourself two questions about any measure used in a quantitative study: (1) How consistently does the instrument, questionnaire, or procedure measure what it measures? and (2) Does the instrument, questionnaire, or procedure measure what it is supposed to measure? The first question addresses the reliability of a measure and the second question addresses its validity.

CORE CONCEPT 8.4

Consistent measurement is reliable measurement. Accurate or correct measurement is valid measurement.

Reliability means that a measure can be relied on consistently to give the same result if the aspect being measured has not changed. Consider, for example, measuring the gender of a sample: If three independent observers each record the gender of 1,000 adults as they individually walk into a room, there will be a quite high level of consistency in the final count of the numbers of men and women in the sample. However, if even five or six of the sample are androgynous in their appearance, there may be some small differences in the final counts provided by the three observers. We have already said that this leads to some small error in the measure. If we changed our sample to 1,000 diapered infants all dressed in white, we would expect much more inconsistency in the final totals because gender identification of infants by observation is much more difficult to do consistently. If, instead, three laboratories conducted genetic testings of each of the 1,000 infants, there should be no differences in the final totals for boy and girls (assuming no laboratory error). Thus, the data collection on gender (particularly for infants) using the method of observation is less reliable than the data collection on gender using the method of genetic testing.

The reliability of a measure becomes more difficult to ensure as the measurement process becomes more complicated because complexity allows for more opportunities for error through inconsistency. Several approaches are taken to ensure or examine the reliability of measurement in quantitative research, depending on the type of measurement being used. When data are being collected by observation, a researcher often trains the observers and then tests them with different cases until all the observers agree on their observations the majority of the time. Earlier, we used a hypothetical example of observations to create a score for anxiety. If there were such a measure, the observers might be asked to practice making the observations needed with different "practice patients" to obtain a score on the anxiety scale until they each reached the same score at least 95% of the time.

In addition, when data are being collected by observation, researchers often report an interrater reliability score. **Interrater reliability** is present when two or more independent data collectors agree in the results of their data collection process. So, perhaps, in our hypothetical case of a rating of anxiety, a researcher might report that actual interrater reliability was 97%. This means that in 97% of the occasions, two independent raters got the same score. By this information, the reader of the research would know that this complicated procedure to get a measurement of anxiety was used consistently across the different subjects. That consistency in use decreases the chances that any differences between subjects were due to inconsistent measurement rather than real differences. Assurances of reliability of a measure allow us to be comfortable that little error occurred in the measurement because of inconsistent use of the scale or instrument.

When a measure of a variable in a study is a written questionnaire or scale, two other types of approaches can be taken to ensure that the measure is reliable. The first is to test the measure before it is used in the study by having individuals complete the questionnaire or scale at two or more time points that are close enough together that we would not expect the "real" answers to have changed. This kind of reliability is called **test–retest reliability**; what we hope for is consistency in the answers in the different time points. If a scale or questionnaire is confusing or does not have a lot of meaning for a subject, his or her responses from one time to another are likely to differ. This means that the scores from the measure will not be consistent, and differences found may occur because of a lack of reliability of the measure rather than because of actual differences.

Similarly, one would expect that nursing students' choices of field of practice would not change much during a week. If the author of the fictional article (Appendix B) had administered his or her questionnaire to the students twice, a week apart, and found big differences in choice, we would believe that the questionnaire was not measuring this variable consistently. That inconsistency would then shed significant doubt on the findings of the study because we could not be sure that the study truly measured choice of field.

A second way that reliability is often measured for quantitative measures is by calculating a statistic called an *alpha coefficient*. This statistic reflects a computation of how closely the answers to different questions or items within a scale are related and is, therefore, often called the *internal consistency reliability coefficient*. **Internal consistency reliability** is the extent to which responses to a scale are similar and related. Remember that we said that many abstract concepts in healthcare are measured using scales consisting of several items or questions that all relate to the same aspect being studied. If, in fact, all the items or questions address the same aspect or variable, we would expect a consistent pattern in how subjects respond to or answer the items.

Let us go back to the five items that we are pretending were developed to measure stress (Box 8.3). We would expect that a highly stressed person would indicate that most of the experiences listed were happening regularly. If, instead, we found that subjects indicated that one or two of the items were occurring regularly but that others were not occurring at all, there would be a low internal consistency among the items. Alpha coefficients, often called the *Cronbach alpha* after the statistician who developed the test, can range from 0 to 1.0, with a value of 0 indicating that there are absolutely no relationships among the responses to the different items in a scale and a value of 1.0 meaning that the answers to the items were all completely connected or related to each other. In general, researchers hope for an alpha coefficient of greater than 0.7, indicating a relatively strong relationship or connection among the responses to the different items on any particular scale.

To summarize, the reliability of a measure reflects how definite we can be that the measure will yield the same data consistently if the actual or "real" variable stays the same. When quantitative data are collected using observation, the rate of agreement, or interrater agreement, tells us the consistency of the observational measure. Test–retest reliability can tell us if a measure stays consistent over time when the aspect measured has not changed. Internal consistency reliability or a Cronbach alpha coefficient is a statistic that tells us how consistently subjects responded to a set of items or questions. In all three cases, the goal in quantitative research is to use measures that will most consistently measure the variables of interest.

Validity is the second aspect of measurement that must be considered when deciding on use of research in clinical practice. **Validity** reflects how accurately the measure yields information about the true or real variable being studied. A measure is valid if it measures correctly and accurately what it is intended to measure. Validity becomes more of an issue the more abstract the variable to be measured is; with a concrete variable such as gender, validity is not a great concern. We are generally confident that gender self-report will yield a true measure of gender. However, let us look at another demographic variable

> **BOX 8.4**
> **Please Check the Item Below That Best Describes You**
>
> _____ Black   _____ Asian–not Pacific Islander
> _____ Latino/Latina   _____ Native American
> _____ White–non-Hispanic   _____ Pacific Islander

that may seem as concrete: the variable of race. To measure this variable, researchers might ask subjects to indicate their race by checking one category from a list that looks like the one in Box 8.4. On initial inspection, we might assume that this list is clear and should yield valid results. However, although the use of the term _Native American_ traditionally represents the indigenous peoples of the Americas and is considered politically correct, it also can be interpreted to mean "born in America." If many subjects interpret an item asking about race in this way, then the measure will yield inaccurate information about race.

A second example of an invalid measure might come from Box 8.3, where we listed five fictional items that a researcher might use to measure stress. Looking at those items more closely, one might wonder if they are really measuring stress or if they more accurately measure depression. Certainly, feelings of anxiety and anger, trouble sleeping, and feeling overwhelmed are classic symptoms of depression. Thus, this measure may be an inaccurate measure of stress because it may actually be measuring depression, which is an entirely different concept. The issue of validity of a measure becomes much more complex in scales used to measure variables such as depression, stress, efficacy, motivation, or coping. Scales or written instruments that are developed to measure abstract concepts such as these must find a way to describe or ask about factors that are specific to the concept and are clear enough to avoid confusion with other concepts. Three types of validity are sometimes described within reports of research: content validity, criterion-related validity, and construct validity.

The simplest of the three, and the one that is the easiest for a reader of research to assess, is content validity. **Content validity** asks whether the items or questions on a scale are comprehensive and appropriately reflect the concept that they are supposed to measure. Put simply, the question becomes "Is the _content_ of the scale complete and appropriate?" Researchers who have to develop their own measure of a concept will try to establish the content validity of the measure by asking a group of experts to review the items on the scale for completeness and appropriateness. If researchers are using a measure that has only been used a few times in other research, they may describe what type of assessment was made of the measure when it was developed to ensure content validity. As a user of research, you can assess what is called the _face validity of a measure_, which is simply one person's (perhaps not an expert's) interpretation of content validity. Face validity is a judgment of how clearly the items on a scale reflect the concept they are intended to measure.

As we have said, if we consider the face validity of the items listed in Box 8.3 that were proposed to measure stress, we might begin to question them. In fact, the items listed in that box generally reflect the symptoms that we expect to see when someone is experiencing depression rather than stress. Although depression and stress may be related, we do not necessarily expect everyone who is experiencing significant negative stress to also be depressed. Therefore, the face validity of these items must be questioned. In all likelihood, if a panel of stress experts reviewed these items, they would decide that the items were not valid items for a stress scale.

The second type of validity that may be described in a research report is criterion-related validity. **Criterion-related validity** is the extent to which the results of one measure match those of another measure that is also supposed to reflect the variable under study. The question asked with this type of validity is "Do the results from the scale relate to a known criterion relevant to the variable?" If a researcher were trying to test the criterion-related validity of the five-item "stress" scale in Box 8.3, subjects might be asked to answer those five items and then to rate their stress level on a scale from 1 to 100. If scores from responses on the five items closely matched ratings of stress on the 100-point scale, they might be considered to provide some evidence for the criterion-related validity of the five-item scale. The criterion used in this example is a direct self-rating of stress level, and the example is one of a test for concurrent criterion-related validity. That is, the test looked for a relationship between two measures concurrently, or at the same time.

A second type of criterion-related validity looks for a relationship between the scale being tested and some measure that should be closely related that occurs in the future. This type of validity is called *predictive validity*.

The last type of validity that is sometimes discussed in a report of research is construct validity. **Construct validity** is the broadest type of validity and can encompass both content and criterion-related validity because it is the extent to which a scale or an instrument measures what it is supposed to measure. The construct validity of a scale or an instrument is supported with time if results using the measure support theory about how the construct (variable) being measured is supposed to behave. This may include predictive validity and concurrent validity but also will include other less direct predictions that arise from theory. Several approaches can be taken to measure the construct validity of a scale or an instrument, including use of statistical procedures such as factor analysis or structural equation modeling, comparison of results from the measure to closely related and vastly differing constructs, and the development of hypotheses that are then tested to provide support for the scale. In all cases, the goal is to build evidence that the construct, or abstract variable, is being measured by the scale.

There is a relationship between the validity and reliability of measures: A scale can be reliable but not valid. However, a scale cannot be valid and also not be reliable. A scale may consistently measure something (reliability) but not the something it is supposed to measure (validity). However, if a scale measures what it is supposed to measure (validity), then it will inherently also be consistent (reliable). So a scale must have reliability in order to have the possibility of being valid. For example, we have suggested that the five items in Box 8.3 have questionable validity as a measure of stress, but it is possible that subjects might answer those five questions consistently, giving us reliable data about something— just not about stress.

One last note about reliability and validity is related to data collection from sources such as medical records. In healthcare research, using medical records to collect certain types of data is quite common. However, some unique issues surrounding these data must be considered. As all healthcare team members know, we can be confident that whatever is documented on a patient record is supposed to represent what occurred. Therefore, if we are collecting data about pain level and we find notations regarding the patient's self-reported rating of pain (on a 1–10 scale), we should interpret them to be accurate. However, we cannot be as confident that the absence of a notation about pain means that the patient did not have pain. If a great deal happened during a particular shift and a patient's pain was not exceptional in some way, it is possible that the pain was not charted. Thus, the reliability of certain types of data from medical records—that is, the consistency with which the kinds of data are documented—must be considered when choosing to use medical records to measure study variables.

In summary, the different types of reliability and validity that must be considered when understanding quantitative studies are detailed in Table 8.3. Although reliability focuses on the consistency of a measure, validity focuses on the accuracy or correctness of a measure. Researchers consider three types of validity. Content validity refers to the extent to which

TABLE 8.3	Aspects of Reliability and Validity	
ASPECT	DEFINITION	METHODS
Reliability—how consistent is the measure?		
Interrater reliability	Agreement between two or more independent data collectors about the results of their data collection process	Carefully structured instruments practice until a high level of agreement is reached
Test–retest reliability	Consistency in answers on tests when we would not expect the real answers to have changed	Repeated administration of measures or tests to calculate consistency in responses
Internal consistency reliability	The extent to which responses to a scale are similar and related	Calculation of a Cronbach alpha coefficient
Validity—how accurate is the measure?		
Content validity	The comprehensiveness and appropriateness of the measure to the concept it is intended to measure	• Expert panel review • Face validity
Criterion-related validity	The extent to which results of one measure match those of another measure that examines the same concept	• Concurrent validity • Predictive validity
Construct validity	The extent to which a scale or instrument measures what it is supposed to measure	• Content and criterion-related validity • Hypothesis testing statistical procedures such as factor analysis

the scale or instrument is comprehensive and addresses the concept or variable of interest. Criterion-related validity can be either concurrent or predictive and refers to how closely the results on the measure in question relate to results on other measures of the same concept in the present or future. Construct validity refers to the overall ability of the scale to measure what it is supposed to measure and is established only after the repeated use of a measure yields results that reflect the theoretical expectations for the concept being measured. An instrument of measurement can be reliable but not valid. However, if a measure has been shown to be valid, then it will be reliable; this is reflective of the ideal of evidence-based practice.

Errors in Implementation of Quantitative Data Collection

We said that error can be introduced into the measurement of variables in quantitative research because of problems with either the quality of the measure or the process of implementing the measure. Although reliability and validity speak to the quality of a measure, even a reliable and valid measure can be implemented incorrectly and lead to error. Implementation of data collection requires careful and detailed planning to ensure that the process is consistent and does not invalidate the measures. For example, a researcher could be using a reliable and valid measure of blood sugars, but subjects may fail to understand the dietary restrictions of fasting before samples are collected, thus introducing errors into the data. A procedure that confirms true fasting status would ensure that the measure yielded meaningful data. Another example of an implementation error occurs when a written scale that may have been shown previously to be reliable and valid is administered with incorrect directions, or the subjects are prompted in a way that sways their responses to a measure. Pointing out that the financial support for an agency depends on positive reviews *before* asking subjects to complete a satisfaction survey is an obvious example.

The order in which subjects are asked to complete questionnaires also can affect their responses. For example, if subjects are asked to complete a scale that asks several questions about symptoms of depression and then are asked to rate their level of overall depression, the scale will likely have increased their awareness of how depressed they really are, thus affecting how they rate their overall depression level. Different timing and environments can also affect data collection. For example, asking medical interns about their choices of field when they have just completed an exciting clinical rotation in the emergency department could lead to more of them selecting emergency medicine than would have selected it if they had been asked at some time after that rotation.

Other types of error that can occur in the measurement process include sloppy handling of data, resulting in a loss of some of them. Failure to keep careful records can lead to missed opportunities for repeat measures because subjects' addresses or telephone numbers are misplaced or not accurately recorded. This is a problem, particularly in longitudinal studies in which subjects are asked to complete measures at two different time points.

Finally, the implementation of data collection can introduce error by arbitrarily changing a measure through translating it to another language or administering it in a format other than that which was intended. Measures that are reliable and valid have been successfully translated into other languages, but this requires a careful translation process and then translating the measure back into the original language by independent translators to ensure that the meanings of items on a scale remain intact when the language changes. An issue similar to translation to another language exists when a measure that was developed for reading *by* a subject is instead read *to* a subject. The subject is then hearing the words rather then seeing them, and this can definitely affect his or her understanding and potential response to the items.

In summary, measurement in quantitative research must be carefully planned and controlled. The variables to be measured must be clearly defined. If the variables are abstract, we should expect to see both a theoretical definition and an operational definition so that we can judge both the meaning of the variable and how well that meaning was translated into data through measurement. Errors in measurement can be present because of problems with the measure itself or incorrect implementation of the measure.

Overall, the important points about measurement language in both qualitative and quantitative research are that data collection must be trustworthy, confirmable, and consistent as well as transferable, credible, and accurate. Both the process and actual measures in data collection must be considered as we decide how to use the results of research in practice. To decide how measurement in a study has affected results and conclusions, we must receive complete and clear information about the measures. This leads us to consider what might be some common problems with written reports of data collection.

COMMON ERRORS IN WRITTEN REPORTS OF DATA COLLECTION METHODS

The most common error that occurs in written reports of research studies is provision of incomplete information. For example, the fictional article (Appendix B) leaves several gaps in the information provided about the collection of the data. The author does not give us a clear theoretical or operational definition of the dependent variable in this study—choice of field. Theoretically, "choice" could be defined as what students would really like to do if all options were open to them, or it could be defined as what students expect to do given current openings and other aspects of their personal situations. The results section of this report does give us some idea about how "field of choice" was operationally defined because those categories that were elected by the students are listed. We know that the students were not permitted to write in their choice but were given a list of nursing career options from which to select. However, the author does not tell us what was included in the original list of options, so we do not know if the final categories reported in Table B.1 from the fictional article included all the possible options or if there were options that were not selected or were collapsed into one of the reported categories. In other words, we are not clear about the operational definition for the dependent variable either. This lack of clear information jeopardizes the usefulness of the research for practice because it becomes difficult to be comfortable with conclusions based on measurement that we do not understand or believe was consistent or accurate.

A second common error with written reports of data collection is a failure to organize clearly the information in a manner that makes it understandable. Although numerous studies do not include a written report of the data collection, tables can be very useful to help us visualize the variables and measures used in a study.

A third error that occasionally occurs is a failure to reference the source of measures used in a study. Referencing reports of previous studies that indicated the reliability and validity of a measure is particularly important because it gives the reader the option to learn more about that specific measure and increases one's confidence in the quality of the measure.

CRITICALLY READING METHODS SECTIONS OF RESEARCH REPORTS

There are seven questions you can ask yourself as you read the methods section of a research report (see Box 8.5). The first and simplest question to ask yourself is "Did the report include a clearly identified section describing methods used in this study?" The article about use of postoperative restraints in children after cleft lip or cleft palate repair in Appendix A-7 (Huth, Petersen, & Lehman, 2013) included a methods section with several pertinent subsections. The next question to ask is "Do the methods make this a quantitative or a qualitative study?" In this chapter, more than any up until now, we have been able to clearly separate qualitative and quantitative methods because these two approaches to data collection differ markedly. Thus, if you read that a researcher is planning a qualitative study using a written questionnaire with 25 items that will measure well-being, you will have to immediately wonder about the match between stated approach and actual methods used. You will also be surprised to find a quantitative study report that does not provide information to operationally define the variables in the study. The article may not call the

---

BOX 8.5
How to Critically Read the Methods Section of a Research Report

Does the report answer the question "How were those people studied—why was the study performed that way?"

1. Did the report include a clearly identified section describing methods used in the study?
2. Do the methods make this a quantitative or a qualitative study?
3. Do I understand what my patient population would be doing if they were in this study or a study using similar methods?
4. Do the measures and procedures in this study address my clinical problem?
5. Do I think that the measures used in this study would provide helpful and useful information when used with my patient population?
6. Do I think that the researcher(s) should have planned the study differently in order to answer my clinical question?

description of measurement *operational definitions*, but if no explanation of measurement is present or the measurement is open-ended and unstructured, you may question the fit between approach and methods.

In critically reading the methods section of a research report, you should ask a third question: "Do I understand what my patient population would be doing if they were in this study or a study using a similar method?" If you are not sure what they would be asked to do, or how often they would be asked to do something, then the methods section is not as detailed as needed. Without enough detail about study measurement and procedures, it is impossible to evaluate the usefulness of study results. In particular, if one does not know how a variable was measured, it is not possible to decide whether the measurement was appropriate. A related question is "Do the measures and procedures in this study address my clinical problem?" Again, without enough detail, one cannot answer that question; however, if adequate detail is provided, you will want to ask critically if you think that the methods used address your clinical concern. For example, the nurse in our clinical case is interested in discerning whether evidence indicates that use of postoperative restraints in children after cleft lip or cleft palate repair has a relationship to postoperative complications. Thus, the methods in this study do seem to reflect the nurse's clinical question.

The next two questions to consider address "Do I think that the measures used in this study would provide helpful and useful information when used with my patient population?" and "Do I think what the researcher collected and how it was collected was the best way to address the clinical question?" In a qualitative study, one needs to consider trustworthiness, confirmability, credibility, and transferability of the data based on what is told about the data collection process and the measure used. Similarly, in a quantitative study, reliability and validity of measures used in the study and whether potential error was introduced through the data collection process need to be considered. If the report does not provide enough information for you to answer these questions, then you may not be able to use the findings in your clinical practice.

Finally, you should ask, "How can I use this information as part of my evidence-based practice?" Today's healthcare practice should be grounded in evidence, and the best way to incorporate this into your own professional practice is by reading, understanding, and utilizing the evidence, from credible sources, that is available to you. This last question directly leads you to consider the overall study design, which is the topic of Chapter 9.

CONNECTING DATA COLLECTION METHODS TO SAMPLING, RESULTS, AND DISCUSSION/CONCLUSION

As you learn more about research methods, you will see that sampling and data collection methods are linked in both quantitative and qualitative research. Particularly in qualitative studies, data collection and analysis drive the sampling because additional participants are often sought purposely to focus on aspects of the phenomenon that are emerging from the data. In this chapter, we have also discussed trustworthiness and the use of both member and group checks. These aspects of rigor in data collection require sampling strategies that ensure a trusting and open relationship with the data collector. Further, a researcher may ask the right questions about a phenomenon but may fail to gain access to the right groups to answer those questions; so, as we read about data collection, we must consider the sampling process as well.

In quantitative research, sampling is most connected to data collection in follow-up for repeated measures over time. However, the data collection process can also be affected by the nature of the sample or vice versa. For example, a study of homeless patients that uses measures written in English, yet have no established Spanish version, may exclude a group of Spanish-speaking subjects. Another problem in data collection that is closely related to sampling is the educational level assumed in the measures. A complex written scale that uses language aimed at a ninth-grade reading level may become unreliable when used with subjects who have a reading level of fourth grade. Thus, sampling and data collection can be closely linked in quantitative research as well as in qualitative research.

Throughout this chapter, we have stressed that if variables are not clearly defined or are not consistently and accurately measured, the results of the study must be questioned. Similarly, if rigor is not maintained through both data collection and analysis, the results of qualitative research are jeopardized; the results of a study are only as good as the data that went into those results. Therefore, understanding how data were collected and recognizing how potential sources of error in the data collection were addressed is closely linked to our ability to accept the results of a study, which clearly affects our willingness to accept and adopt the conclusions of a study into our evidence-based practice.

A last link between data collection and the rest of the research process is that between data collection and the section of a research report that speaks to limitations of a study. Despite the best plans and efforts, problems do arise with data collection. These may be mentioned in the write-up of the data collection itself, but the implications of those problems for the conclusions of a study are often addressed when the author discusses limitations. For example, Huth, Petersen, and Lehman (2013) (Appendix A-7) identify the numerical inequality of the control and intervention subgroups as a limitation that may have affected the results of their study. Thus, the conclusions of a study are directly linked back to the measurement process.

PUBLISHED REPORTS—WOULD YOU USE THESE STUDIES IN CLINICAL PRACTICE?

Our nurse was hoping to find information to assist in clinical decision making about postoperative restraint use after Mindy's cleft lip repair. After considering the data collection methods in the article "The Use of Postoperative Restraints in Children after Cleft Lip or Cleft Palate Repair: A Preliminary Report" (Huth, Petersen, & Lehman, 2013), the nurse now understands that the most current evidence does not demonstrate a significant difference in postoperative complications in children between those who had postoperative restraints applied versus those who were intently monitored. The researchers in the study followed a clearly described procedure and used measures that were shown to be reliable and valid. The nurse believes that the outcomes examined—postoperative complications in children who had postoperative restraints applied versus those who did not—are clinically relevant in the nurse's experience with patients like Mindy. Based on this information, the nurse decides that this piece of literature will indeed be helpful in evidence-based clinical decision making. The information in the study has helped raise the nurse's awareness about the need to communicate thoroughly with Mindy's parents, surgeon, and other members of the interdisciplinary team about the best patient-centered methods for decreasing postoperative complications associated with cleft lip repair. The nurse can share the information from this research study and foster professional dialogue about patient-centered care that is designed to produce the desired outcomes following surgery. Utilizing a comprehensive approach targeted toward minimizing risks for postoperative complications following cleft lip repair assists the nurse in creating an effective plan of care for Mindy. The nurse feels confident that the care that Mindy will receive will be based on evidence that is credible and useful in practice.

OUT-OF-CLASS EXERCISE

Free Write

The next chapter continues to address the question of why a study included the people it did and it was done the way it was by talking about research designs. Before reading that chapter, consider the question of whether being in college affects the students' well-being. If you were going to conduct a study to address this question, how would you go about it? What do you think would be the best way to conduct a study to answer this question, and what do you think would be the most realistic approach? Are they the same or different, and why? Think about this, then write in as much detail as possible your ideas about how to conduct a study to determine if and how being a college student affects well-being. Wherever you can, write your rationale for conducting the study in the manner on which you have decided. After you have completed this assignment, you will be ready to move on to read about research designs in Chapter 9.

References

*Denzin, N. K. (2001). *Interpretive interactionism* (2nd ed.). Newbury Park, CA: Sage.

*First, M., Spitzer, R., Gibbon, M., & Williams, J. (1996). *Structured clinical interview for the DSM-IV Axis I disorders.* Retrieved from http://www.ptsd.va.gov/professional/assessment/adult-int/scid-ptsd-module.asp

Huth, J., Peterson, J., & Lehman, J. (2013). The use of postoperative restraints in children after cleft lip or cleft palate repair: a preliminary report. *ISRN Plastic Surgery, 2013,* 1–3. Retrieved from http://dx.doi.org/10.5402/2013/540717

*Lincoln, Y. S., & Guba, E. G. (1985). *Naturalistic inquiry.* Beverly Hills, CA: Sage.

indicates a definitive or classic work or publication regarding this subject matter.

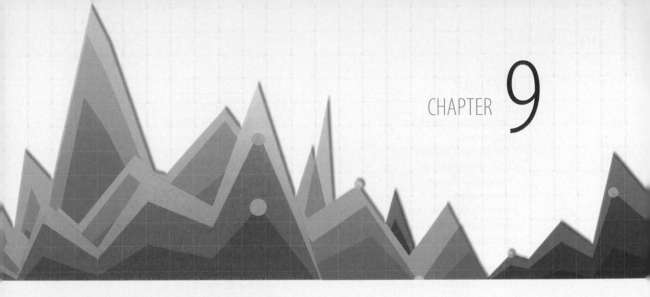

CHAPTER 9

Research Designs: Planning the Study

How Were Those People Studied—Why Was the Study Performed That Way?

LEARNING OBJECTIVE The student will interpret the strengths and weaknesses of research designs in relation to sampling, data collection methods, and the meaning of the results and conclusions.

Research Designs: Why Are They Important?
Answering the Research Question
Ensuring Rigor and Validity

Qualitative Research Designs
Phenomenology
Ethnography
Grounded Theory
Historical

Quantitative Research Designs
Time
Control
Functions of Quantitative Research Designs

How Can One Get the Wrong Design for the Right Question?
Common Errors in Published Reports of Research Designs
Published Reports—Did Design Affect Your Conclusion?
Critically Reading the Description of the Study Design in a Research Report for Use in Evidence-Based Practice

KEY TERMS

Clinical trials
Comparison group(s)
Control group
Correlational studies
Cross-sectional
Descriptive design
Ethnography
Experimental designs
Experimenter effects
External validity
Grounded theory
Hawthorne effect
Historical research method
History
Instrumentation
Internal validity
Longitudinal

Maturation
Measurement effects
Mixed methods
Model
Mortality
Multifactorial
Novelty effects
Phenomenology
Pretest–posttest
Prospective designs
Quasi-experimental designs
Reactivity effects
Repeated measures
Research design
Retrospective designs
Selection bias
Testing

CLINICAL CASE

A psychologist, who works within a small community outpatient facility, has been consulted to see D.M., a patient who is recovering from a serious injury. D.M., a long-distance truck driver, was in an accident 6 months ago when he fell asleep at the wheel and overturned his vehicle, sustaining a crushing injury to his chest. He was in the ditch for 30 mins before help arrived, and it took another 30 mins to extricate him from the cab. The accident took place 1,000 miles from D.M.'s home. Following the accident, D.M. was in critical condition for 2 weeks in an intensive care unit (ICU) at a hospital in the state where the accident occurred. He has since been discharged and has returned home. He is married, has two small children, and used to enjoy coaching his children's soccer teams. He has returned to a desk job at his trucking company, but he has not resumed coaching. D.M. states that he lives with the fear that if he ever returns to driving a truck, he will have another accident that will leave him completely disabled or dead.

D.M.'s psychologist wonders how D.M.'s long-term mental health may be impacted as a result of his accident and hospitalization. The psychologist finds a study entitled "Investigating risk factors for psychological morbidity three months after intensive care: A prospective cohort study" (Wade et al., 2012) that indicates that posttraumatic stress disorder (PTSD), depression, and anxiety are often found in patients who were in intensive care. This article is available in Appendix A-8. Read it before you continue with this chapter so that the examples discussed will be more meaningful. Table 9.1 identifies the clinical question of the psychologist and the key search terms that could be used in a search.

TABLE 9.1	Statement of Clinical Question from the Clinical Case

WHAT PSYCHOLOGICAL CONCERNS MIGHT A PATIENT WHO WAS PREVIOUSLY HOSPITALIZED IN AN ICU HAVE?	
The *Who*	A patient who was previously hospitalized in an ICU
The *What*	Psychological concerns
The *When*	After hospitalization in an ICU
The *Where*	Any setting (implied)
Key search terms to find research-based evidence for practice	ICU
	Intensive care unit
	Psychosocial
	Emotional
	Psychological
	Needs
	Concerns

RESEARCH DESIGNS: WHY ARE THEY IMPORTANT?

As we have considered how to interpret and use research findings in evidence based practice, we have been moving from the end of research reports towards their beginning. We have learned that the conclusions of a report usually do not provide enough information to allow us to fully understand or apply the findings. The usefulness of the study results depends on the sample and the methods used to collect data. We have also learned that various approaches to sampling and data collection have differing strengths and weaknesses. Thus, we need to better understand the overall purpose and nature of research designs because they direct the sampling and data collection processes. This chapter discusses research designs to help explain why a study is planned and implemented using a particular design, and how different designs affect approaches to sampling and data collection, which, in turn, influence the study results and conclusions.

The psychologist in the clinical case reads that the authors used a prospective cohort study model to conduct this research. In reading the abstract, the psychologist notes that evidence shows that although there is increasing concern about status of mental health and quality of life among survivors who have been in ICU settings, there is not yet enough information indicating the root cause that may contribute to mental health concerns in this population (Wade et al., 2012). Life-threatening illness, medication regimens and/or treatments, and patients' psychological reactions during intensive care are all listed as possible factors that may contribute to poor psychosocial outcomes (Wade et al., 2012). The psychologist knows that research can be categorized as qualitative or quantitative, and that some studies are conducted as "mixed methods" studies, which incorporate elements of both types of research. Further, the psychologist understands that there are varying kinds of research that are categorized into the broader category of qualitative or quantitative research. In reviewing the methodology of this study, the psychologist sees that this research is indeed quantitative in nature, and uses the approach of a prospective cohort study. A prospective cohort study is conducted when researchers hope to learn more about outcomes over a period of time that can be related to other conditions or risks (StatsDirect, 2013). The psychologist understands the reasons that Wade et al. (2012) used in this approach, as the researchers stated that their hope was to investigate a larger number of risk factors that contribute to mental health after intensive care than had previously been studied.

A **research design** is the overall plan for acquiring new knowledge or confirming existing knowledge. In Chapter 1, we said that research is characterized by a systematic approach to gathering information to answer questions, which is in contrast to those approaches that use intuition, seek expert advice, or follow tradition. The research design is the plan for that systematic approach, conducted in a way that ensures the answer(s) found will be as meaningful and accurate as possible. The design identifies how subjects will be recruited and incorporated into a study; what will happen during the study, including timing of any treatments and measures; and when the study will end. A research design is selected with two broad purposes: (1) to plan an approach that will best answer the research question and (2) to ensure the rigor and validity of the results. We will discuss each of these purposes in general terms, and then we will look at specific approaches to research design.

Answering the Research Question

The first purpose in selecting a research design is to plan a systematic collection of information that will answer the question of interest. Two considerations are important: (1) the fit of the design to the research question and (2) the functionality of the design for the purpose of the study. Fit refers to how well the design matches the question of interest. It is in considering fit that we begin to address the question the psychologist in our clinical case has asked about understanding the state of long-term mental health that may be impacted as a result of his accident and hospitalization. Depending on what the researcher hopes to learn, it is important to understand that not all research questions can be answered through experiments, because **experimental designs** answer questions requiring that we already know a great deal about the topic in order to set up a meaningful experiment. In the case of the study, the psychologist is reading, the psychologist understands that the study design is put in place to see what kinds of long-term effects (outcomes) materialize. The researchers are not manipulating factors to see if, and how, they affect an outcome; they are simply observing for outcomes that arise. This particular study is not experimental in nature, because an experiment assumes that we know some factors that we want to manipulate in order to see if, and how, they affect an outcome. If we do not know what factors are influencing the outcome of interest, we have nothing to manipulate and therefore, must choose another design to answer our research question!

Research questions can be broadly categorized as questions that seek to describe or understand, questions that seek to connect or relate, and questions that seek to predict or study the effects of manipulation (Box 9.1). Generally, if we do not have adequate knowledge about a phenomenon of interest to healthcare, we have to start by describing and understanding it, and the researcher will select a design that best allows for meeting that need. Once such studies are done and we have some idea of the meaning of the selected aspects of the phenomenon, we can ask questions about connections or relationships among those aspects. To answer those questions, the researcher will need a different form of design. Only after we know something about the connections and relationships can we begin to ask questions that seek to predict or manipulate aspects of the phenomenon, and there are designs specifically matched to this as well.

BOX 9.1
General Types of Research Questions

- Questions that describe
- Questions that connect or link factors or concepts
- Questions that predict or examine effects of manipulation

Now we are more aware that a research design must fit the type of question asked in order to provide appropriate and effective answers. A research design intended to answer questions about prediction will not be useful or appropriate for questions that seek to describe a phenomenon. Similarly, a design meant to allow meaningful description will not answer questions that seek to predict. The fit of a design to a research question depends on the function of the design and on how much is known about the topic of the study. In other words, different research designs serve different functions and, therefore, are particularly well suited to one type of research question, but not to another.

The functions of specific research designs can be broadly categorized, just as types of questions can be categorized. The functions include the following:

1. Designs for describing or understanding.
2. Designs for connecting or relating.
3. Designs for manipulation and prediction.

CORE CONCEPT 9.1

The type of research question being asked affects the type of research design that will and can be used.

Two other important considerations are designs that include timing or time as a factor in the study and designs that seek to control or not to control. Although several other factors differentiate types of research designs, the framework we will use for understanding how research designs influence the meaningfulness of research for practice focuses on three factors: (1) the overall function of the design, (2) how time or timing is incorporated into the design, and (3) whether the design seeks to control or not control study factors. Figure 9.1 depicts these broad factors and how they relate. We will discuss specific designs that fit into each category later in the chapter.

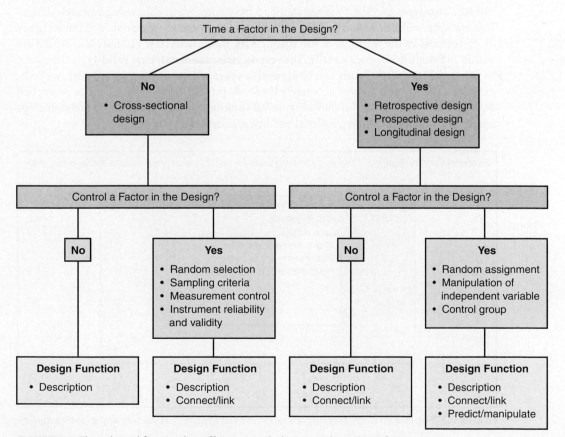

FIGURE 9.1 Three broad factors that affect research design and associated terms.

In summary, when deciding on a design, a researcher must consider several factors, including the functions of a design and the fit of those functions to the purpose of the research. Research designs differ in terms of the type of questions they can answer, whether they include time as a factor, and whether they focus on control within the study. The fit and functionality of a research design significantly influence whether the study can answer the research question of interest.

Ensuring Rigor and Validity

In addition to examining function and fit to answer the research question, the research design has a purpose to ensure the rigor and validity of a study. In Chapter 8, we discussed these concepts in the context of specific strategies for data collection and measurement. The terms *rigor* and *validity* also are used in a broader sense to refer to the overall study. In Chapter 8, we said that rigor is a strict process of data collection and analysis as well as a term that reflects the overall quality of that process in qualitative research. It is in the broader sense of this quality that we consider rigor when discussing study design. Designs in qualitative research usually are more flexible and often are described as "emerging" to indicate that the design may be altered as the study progresses. Nevertheless, the design must still have a function that fits the research question and provides the foundation ensuring the accuracy of the study.

Like the term *rigor*, *validity* is used in research to refer both to specific ways that measures can correctly and accurately reflect their intended variable, and to the accuracy of the overall results. Although use of the word *validity* in reference to measurement and design may be confusing, remember that the validity always has the same general meaning: accuracy or correctness. Content validity, criterion-related validity, and construct validity all refer to aspects of the accuracy of a measure. Validity of a study refers to its accuracy.

Study designs in quantitative research provide the foundation that ensures the overall validity. Two types of validity are mentioned frequently when discussing research design. The first type, called **internal validity**, is the extent to which we can be sure of the accuracy or correctness of the findings of the study. Thus, it refers to how accurate the results are within the study itself, or internally. The second type, called **external validity**, is the extent to which the results of a study can be applied to other groups or situations. In other words, external validity refers to how accurately the study provides knowledge that can be applied outside of, or external to, the study. Figure 9.2 summarizes and illustrates the relationships among measurement validity, internal validity, and external validity.

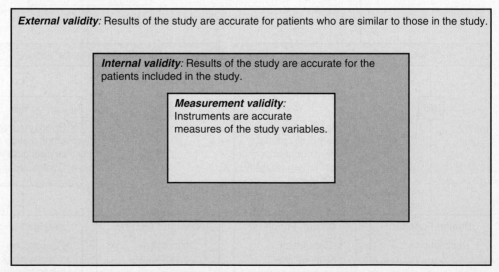

FIGURE 9.2 The relationships among measurement validity, internal validity, and external validity.

Research designs can affect both internal and external validity. Generalizability, discussed in Chapter 6, is a big aspect of external validity because it refers to the ability to infer that findings for a particular sample can be applied to the entire population. External validity also includes the extent to which the findings from a study in one setting can be applied to other similar settings. Logically, if a study lacks internal validity, it automatically lacks external validity: If the results are not accurate within the study, they clearly will not be accurate in other samples or settings. Similarly, if a study lacks measurement validity, it will lack internal validity. However, a study can have measurement validity and not have internal validity, or it can have correct findings and thus be internally valid but not externally valid. That is, the findings of a study may be real and correct to the specific sample and setting of the study, but not applicable to the general population or to other settings. This relationship is illustrated in Figure 9.2 by the nesting of the three boxes representing the three types of validity.

Several aspects of study design can potentially lead to problems with rigor and internal and external validity. These problems are referred to as *threats to validity*, because they threaten the accuracy of internal findings or the ability to apply the findings to other samples or settings. The threats to rigor and internal and external validity often discussed in research literature are listed in Table 9.2.

Threats to the Rigor of a **Qualitative** Study

As was indicated in Chapter 8, the rigor of a qualitative study is reflected in the consistency, trustworthiness, transferability, and credibility of the study. Qualitative designs or methods are based on distinct philosophical perspectives and have clearly defined systematic methods associated with each design. When we talked about these concepts in Chapter 8, we focused on the process of data collection, but in this chapter, we will focus on the process of implementing the entire study. For example, when considering these concepts in reference to the overall rigor of a study, we must consider *consistency* in the application of the study design throughout the study or consider *credibility* given the researchers' accurate use of the study method. Thus, the language used to speak about overall study rigor in qualitative research is essentially the same as that used to discuss the data collection process, but the focus is broadened to the implementation of the study as a whole, and method and standards will differ a little.

Threats to Internal Validity

Threats to internal validity are potential problems that can affect the accuracy or correctness of findings within a study. They include problems of history, maturation, testing, instrumentation, mortality, and selection bias. These threats are summarized in Box 9.2.

TABLE 9.2	Threats to Rigor and Internal and External Validity	
RIGOR—ACCURACY OF FINDINGS OF A QUALITATIVE STUDY	INTERNAL VALIDITY—ACCURACY OF FINDINGS WITHIN A QUANTITATIVE STUDY	EXTERNAL VALIDITY—ACCURACY OF FINDINGS OF A QUANTITATIVE STUDY TO THE SETTINGS AND SAMPLES OUTSIDE OF THE STUDY
Trustworthiness	History	Reactivity effects (Hawthorne effect)
Confirmability	Maturation	Measurement effects
Credibility	Testing	Novelty effects
Consistency	Instrumentation	Experimenter effects
	Mortality	
	Selection bias	

> ## BOX 9.2
> ### Summary of Threats to Internal Validity
>
> Internal validity is threatened because some *outside factor* (**history**) or *time* (**maturation**) affects the dependent variable, because the *measurement process* itself (**testing**) or *changes* in a manner (**instrumentation**) affect results for the dependent variable, or because the sampling process is biased *by loss of subjects* (**mortality**) or *selection of subjects* (**selection bias**).

The threat referred to as **history** is some factor outside those examined in a study affecting the outcome or dependent variable. The term *history* is used because some past event has influenced the dependent variable.

Maturation refers to a change in the dependent variable simply because of the passage of time. Thus, the natural aging process, a type of maturation with time, might lead to decreased daily functioning, regardless of whether the subjects were providing care to a family member. Those studies with a design that did not include a control group would be vulnerable to maturation. We talk more about the role of control groups shortly.

The threat called **testing** refers to changes in a dependent variable that result because it is being measured or because of the measure itself. For example, the mere presence of a nurse asking patients about the amount and quality of their psychosocial supports might increase a patient's anxiety, changing his or her self-report. Another possible example is a study in which a pretest of depression might make a subject more aware of how bad he or she feels, thus increasing the depression. A related threat to internal validity, called **instrumentation**, refers to changing the measures used in a study from one time to another. For example, suppose that the number of injections of pain medication for a postoperative cardiac patient's pain was being examined in a research study. What would happen if the timing of when the researcher collected data on the injections, and the way in which the researcher documented the injections, changed midway through the study? The change in the measurement might lead to different results; thus, values using the first method would not be directly comparable to values from the revised method.

The last types of threats to internal validity frequently considered when selecting a research design are *mortality* and *selection bias*. Selection bias was addressed earlier in Table 6.5. **Mortality** refers to the loss of subjects from a study because of a consistent factor related to the dependent variable. Occasionally, the loss of subjects is from death. At other times, mortality refers to subjects withdrawing from a study.

Selection bias refers to subjects having unique characteristics that in some manner relate to the dependent variable, raising a question whether the findings from the study resulted from the independent variable or the characteristics of the sample. Remember, we examined random assignment in Chapter 6 and learned that the times when we randomly assign subjects; any possible systematic bias in a sample has an equal chance of being present in the subjects of either group. This negates the potential threat of selection bias when comparing two groups.

Suppose that in a study concerning surgical recovery, some patients required additional types of medication. As a result, the researchers might have inadvertently introduced bias into their study by selecting patients who needed additional medication. The bias would occur because additional medications might affect the surgical recovery, thus confounding any differences that might occur solely because of the other variables.

Threats to External Validity

Threats to external validity are potential problems in a study that affect the accuracy of the results for samples and settings other than those of the study itself. As we said earlier, threats to internal and external validity are related, and in fact, overlap exists in the language used to describe the different threats. Because we are discussing the ability to apply the results of a study to other samples and settings, research literature often refers to threats to external validity as the effects of a threat to validity. Several effects are considered when selecting a research study design to ensure external validity. They include the effects of reactivity, measurement, experimenter, and/or novelty.

🏛 CORE CONCEPT 9.2

Studies with problems in internal validity automatically will have problems in external validity. Having internal validity, however, does not guarantee that the study will have external validity.

Reactivity effects refer to the responses of subjects to being studied. Threats to internal validity, such as testing, may cause reactivity. However, reactivity also can occur in a broader sense simply because subjects know that they are being studied. Subjects may be aware that their answers could be scrutinized closely, and although they may not know what specific aspects of their answers the researchers expect, the mere fact of their thinking about how their answers could be perceived might change how the subjects respond.

In another example, let us say that the data being collected were based on observations of interactions between healthcare professionals. Just because the subjects knew that they were being observed, they may have somewhat altered how they usually would interact. If being observed greatly affected their interactions, the results of that study would differ in settings where interactions were not being observed. This would be considered a threat to external validity. Another term sometimes used to describe reactivity is the **Hawthorne effect**. This name was derived from a study at the Hawthorne electric plant in which productivity of workers improved simply because they were being studied, no matter what intervention was applied. Reactivity and the Hawthorne effect are the same concept.

Measurement effects are changes in the results of a study resulting from various data collection procedures. This effect sounds similar to instrumentation and testing (threats to internal validity). Remember that any threat to internal validity automatically affects external validity negatively, and overlaps between internal and external validity can become confusing. Just as there are other forms of reactivity effects besides those inherent in threats to internal validity, there are other forms of measurement effects that are not threats.

The last two effects to consider are novelty effects and experimenter effects. Both involve uncontrolled or unmeasured effects from being in a study. **Novelty effects** occur when the knowledge that what is being done is new and under study somehow affects the outcome, either favorably or unfavorably. Once the independent variable is used outside the context of a study, the enthusiasm or doubts that affected the results are no longer present, so the results are no longer accurate in a setting that is not known to be a study. For example, using a self-help intervention for smoking cessation might be associated with success in quitting smoking, leading the researchers to conclude that the self-help intervention was effective. However, in fact, it was the novelty of the intervention and the subjects' knowledge that it was a new approach that actually led to their success in quitting, and when the intervention was later used in a clinical setting without a study being implemented, the success rate decreased.

Experimenter effects occur when some characteristic of the researcher or data collector influences the study results. For example, subjects may answer the questions the way they believe a researcher wants them to answer, so that results change when subjects are not responding to cues from the researcher.

No matter which threat affects external validity, it reflects some problem with the environment or the research process that may make the study results less valid or accurate for other samples or settings. What is most important for the psychologist in our clinical case is not only to know that research designs are selected for their function and fit to the research question, but also to discern the rigor and validity of the study. Remember, rigor refers to the overall quality of a qualitative study; internal validity refers to the accuracy of the overall results within a quantitative study; and external validity refers to the accuracy of the overall results of a quantitative study in relation to settings and samples that are different or external to that study. Different research designs have varying strengths and weaknesses in relation to rigor and validity. The next two sections of this chapter describe some of these specific designs considering their functions, timing, and efforts at control.

QUALITATIVE RESEARCH DESIGNS

Figure 9.3 places qualitative designs within the framework of the broad factors of function, time, and control. As has been said throughout this book, the goal of qualitative research is to gain knowledge that informs healthcare practice broadly and holistically, understanding that all knowing is evolving and contextual. That means that a design or method for

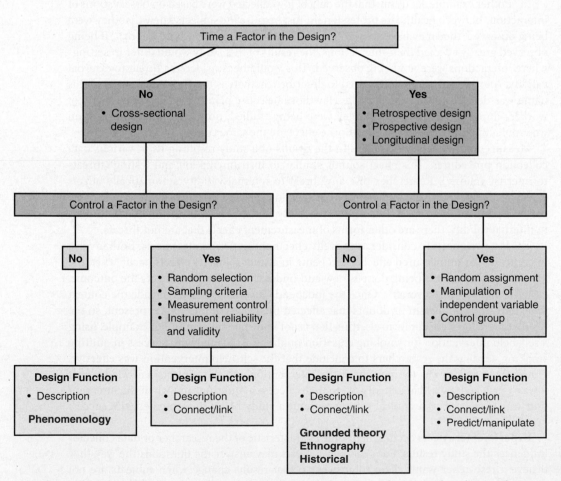

FIGURE 9.3 Three broad factors that affect research design, with associated terms and qualitative designs.

a qualitative study will never focus on controlling factors to isolate specific aspects of a phenomenon. Rather, the methods focus on acquiring the richest possible data—that is, data with the greatest complexity and variety. Therefore, the designs intentionally seek to avoid external control over setting and factors.

Earlier, we said that there are three broad types of research questions: those that seek to describe and understand, those that seek to connect or relate, and those that seek to predict or manipulate. Qualitative research questions seek to describe, understand, and connect or relate, but they do not seek to predict or manipulate. Qualitative studies are most often done when we know the least about the topic of interest. As we gain understanding, the researcher will shift to methods other than qualitative.

There are three broad functions of qualitative research designs, including increasing understanding, promoting participation or immersion, and linking ideas and concepts. Designs that function to facilitate understanding answer **descriptive design** questions. Designs that seek to promote participation or immersion answer questions of both description and connection. Designs that seek to link ideas and concepts answer questions of connection or relationship. We will discuss four general types of designs or methods for qualitative research. Within each method are variations that are often associated with the names of the methodologists who developed them. Some reports of qualitative studies use these specific names rather than the more general method name. It is beyond the scope of this book to describe these variations, but Table 9.3 lists some of the names frequently associated with each of the four methods.

Phenomenology

Phenomenology, or the phenomenologic method, is a qualitative method used to discover and develop understanding of experiences as perceived by those living the experience. There are several variations in the phenomenologic method (Colaizzi, 1973; Giorgi, 1971; Spiegelberg, 1976; van Kaam, 1966), but in general, the method includes identifying the people who are living or have lived the experience of interest and seeking, usually through unstructured interviewing, their perceptions. Thus, you may often hear that phenomenology focuses on the "lived experience." As data are collected, the researcher uses the processes of intuiting, analyzing, and describing to discover essential themes in the experience of the phenomenon (Parse, 2001). Skilled interviewing is needed to promote the most open and rich sharing of experiences as participants lived and perceived them.

TABLE 9.3 Methodologists Commonly Associated with the Major Qualitative Methods	
MAJOR METHOD	**SPECIFIC METHODOLOGISTS**
Phenomenology	Parse
	van Kaam
	Colaizzi
	Giorgi
	Paterson and Zderad
	Munhall and Boyd
	van Manen
Grounded theory	Glasser and Strauss
	Strauss and Corbin
	Stern
Ethnography	Goodenough (ethnoscience)
	Geertz (ethnographic algorithms)
	Sanday (ethnobehavior)
	Leininger (ethnonursing)
History	Bullough
	Hamilton

As presented in Chapter 4, phenomenology uses a spiraling process of data collection and analysis, and detailed field notes of observations during data collection augment the richness and fullness of data. Time is not necessarily a major factor in phenomenologic methods, except as the participants in the study experience it. In fact, the method supports seeking participants who are both currently experiencing the phenomenon of interest and have already experienced it to get a breadth of perceptions of experiences.

In phenomenologic methods, neither the length of time for collecting data nor the number of participants is defined before the study starts. Rather, data are collected until all information is redundant of previously collected data—until saturation occurs. Sampling in phenomenology is best served by a purposive sample because only those who have had the experience of interest are sought, and neither limits nor criteria are placed on who can be a participant, other than the ability to communicate about and having lived the experience. Depending on the specific phenomenologic method used, the researcher often starts by identifying his or her own perceptions or expectations about the phenomenon to be studied and then attempts to consciously bracket them—hold them separate—so that they will not color either the data collection or the analysis process (Spiegelberg, 1976).

Ethnography

The second method commonly used in qualitative research is the ethnographic method, or **ethnography** (Spradley, 1979). This method originated in the discipline of anthropology, and its purpose is for the researcher to participate or to immerse him or herself in a culture to describe a phenomenon or phenomena within the context of that culture. Ethnography assumes that a culture exists, even though it is not visible, and that the only way to know a culture is to get both an insider's view and an outsider's perspective. The insider's view is sometimes called an *emic perspective*.

Again, controlling the environment or aspects of the study is not part of this qualitative method. The researcher tries to become part of the culture studied to acquire an insider's understanding so that he or she can then translate it into a common language understood by those outside the culture (Spradley, 1979). Because cultures are by nature complex, ethnographic methods take time, and the concept of time may be studied within the culture, but there is no set use of time within the method itself. This means that there is no structured plan concerning when data are collected or when the study ends. In general, data are collected as they happen and as opportunities present themselves, although the researcher may seek specific opportunities to interact within the culture. The researcher collects and analyzes data simultaneously so that he or she immediately uses knowledge gained to guide additional data collection. Therefore, there is no structured format for the collection of data.

Grounded Theory

Grounded theory is the third qualitative method commonly used in research (Glaser & Strauss, 1967). The function of **grounded theory** is to study interactions to understand and recognize links between ideas and concepts or, in other words, to develop theory. The term *grounded* refers to the idea that the theory developed is based on or grounded in participants' reality rather than on theoretical speculation. Grounded theory is best used to study social processes and structures, hence the focus on links and interactions among ideas or categories.

Grounded theory methods often incorporate time into the study because the focus usually is on processes or change. The method itself, however, does not specify any particular timing to the data collection and analysis process. Sampling in grounded theory usually will be purposive—that is, purposely seeking participants experiencing the process or changes under study (Strauss & Corbin, 1994). Data collection in grounded theory can include interviews and careful observation of interactions and processes. As with all qualitative methods, grounded theory has a goal of avoiding placing limits or external controls on the processes being studied because the function of the method is to ground theory in natural reality.

Historical

The last general qualitative method sometimes used in research is called the **historical research method**. Its function is to answer questions about links in the past to understand the present or to plan the future. Historical research methods require the researcher to define a phenomenon in a manner that can be clearly delineated so that data sources can be identified. For example, a phenomenon that might lend itself to historical research is to understand the process of nurse practitioners' legitimization as healthcare providers. Nurse practitioner legitimization, however, is too undefined to be approached using the historical method because it is not clear what time period or data sources would be relevant. The phenomenon of credentialing of nurse practitioners as a vehicle to legitimization of the role, on the other hand, defines a focus for data sources as well as a time period because the development of credentialing occurred throughout a definable number of years. Data sources in this example would target the development and implementation of the process of credentialing nurse practitioners and how that process related to perceptions of the legitimacy of the role of nurse practitioners.

Data sources in historical research may include records, videotapes, photographs, and interviews with people involved in the phenomenon or review of published reports. As with the other qualitative methods discussed, the researcher tries to acquire as broad a sample of data sources as possible. Unlike the other methods, in the historical method, a focus of data collection includes evaluation of data sources for their reliability. For example, an editorial in the *Journal of the American Medical Association* regarding the process of nurse practitioner credentialing might reflect a bias that makes the description of the process questionable. That same editorial, however, might be a reliable data source about the professional climate in which credentialing developed. A researcher using the historical method would evaluate the data source and consider this potential bias when deciding how to use it.

We have not had a research study that has used the historical method as an example in this text. However, "Arsenic Exposure and Toxicology: A Historical Perspective" (Hughes, Beck, Chen, Lewis, & Thomas, 2011), is an example of an article that does use this method.

We have now discussed four different methods used in qualitative research, the functions of which vary. Phenomenologic methods provide in-depth data about a particular life experience and, therefore, are particularly useful in answering descriptive questions, especially when very little is known about the topic of interest. Ethnographic methods provide immersion and active participation in a particular culture or subculture, and assist in answering descriptive and linkage and connection questions. Grounded theory methods provide data about social interactions, which can be built into a theory based on reality. These methods are particularly useful in answering questions about interactions or links among social processes. Historical methods provide data about past processes to gain insight about the present and future. They answer questions about links and connections.

All the qualitative methods we have examined specifically attempt to avoid introducing external control into the study design because all are interested in gathering data that are as complex and rich as the real world. Nevertheless, all four methods entail a systematic process for sampling, data acquisition, and data analysis. Strict criteria for timing are not part of any of the methods, but time is an inherent component of the historical method, is often a part of the culture studied using ethnography, and is usually an aspect of interactional processes reported in grounded theory studies.

Throughout this section, discussing qualitative design, the word *methods* has been used more frequently than the word *design*. This is because design suggests a more formalized and standardized plan than is often present within qualitative methods. Qualitative research designs are consciously and intently unstructured and flexible to reflect the unpredictable and complex nature of phenomena as they occur in life. As we will see in the next section that discusses quantitative designs, the word *design* is more appropriate in quantitative research because quantitative methods seek to standardize as well as formalize the process of sampling, data collection, and data analysis.

QUANTITATIVE RESEARCH DESIGNS

We will once again use the three broad factors of function, time, and control to categorize quantitative designs (Fig. 9.4). The language used to describe quantitative designs can be confusing initially because terms are used in different combinations to define different methods. Rather than starting with the functions of differing designs, we start by discussing the language used to address time and control when referring to quantitative research design.

Time

Although time is a factor to study or incorporate into the fabric of a method in qualitative research, time is a specific factor that defines different research designs in quantitative research. Quantitative designs are described as either retrospective or prospective. **Retrospective designs** are those in which data are collected about past events or factors.

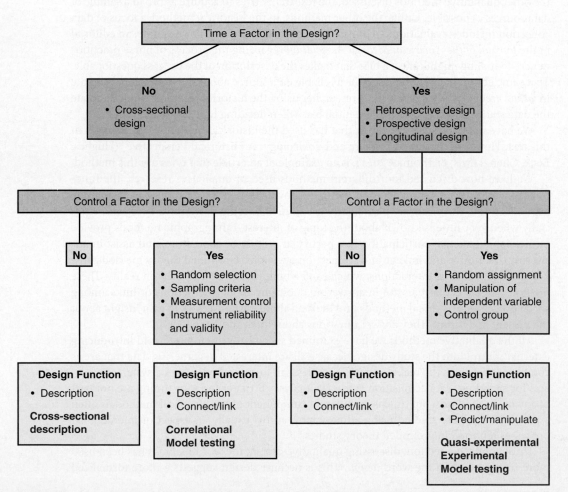

FIGURE 9.4 Three broad factors that affect research design, with associated terms and quantitative designs.

Prospective designs, like that in the research in our clinical case, are those in which data are collected about events or variables as they occur, moving forward in time. In addition to considering whether data are collected moving backward or forward in time, designs are described in terms of the time that measurement occurred. Research designs are **cross-sectional**, if they collect all data at one point in time. Research designs are called **longitudinal**, if they collect data at different time points. Therefore, a prospective study automatically is longitudinal as well. A cross-sectional study, however, does not have to be retrospective.

Consider, for example, a study of patient satisfaction with care. A retrospective and cross-sectional study would collect data from patients at some point after they visit a clinic, perhaps 1 or 2 weeks later, and ask them to recall their level of satisfaction during their visit. Data are collected at one time point looking at past experience. A study of patient satisfaction that surveys patients as they leave a clinic also would be cross-sectional because data are collected at only one time point for each subject. However, it would not be retrospective because it is not going back in time; data are being collected about variables in the present. A prospective longitudinal patient satisfaction study might collect data before a visit to a clinic, immediately after the visit, and 1 week later, looking for changes in selected variables over time. At each measurement point, the question might be "How satisfied are you right now with the clinic care?" Thus, data are not being collected about past experiences or perceptions, even when they are collected 1 week after the visit. From this example, it should be clear that it is a combination of factors that define research designs in quantitative research.

Terms used to describe the use of time in quantitative research designs include those we have discussed and another important term: *repeated measures*. **Repeated measures** mean just what the words say—a design using repeated measures repeats the same measurements at several points in time. When you see this term, it suggests that a variable or variables were measured more than just two or three times, and you can expect that the analysis of the study examines the pattern of change in the variable over time.

🛈 CORE CONCEPT 9.3 _____

The labels for quantitative research designs usually are combinations of words or terms that define the design's function, use of time, and use of approaches to provide control.

_____

Control

In addition to differences in how they consider the factor of time, quantitative research designs differ in the amount of control of extraneous factors that they attempt to impose on a study. Remember that quantitative research seeks to clearly define and measure specific variables. To do so, research designs seek to ensure that outside factors not specifically defined and measured in the study are not allowed to affect what is included in the study. Outside or extraneous factors not considered and measured within a quantitative study are sources of error. In Chapter 8, we discussed error in measurement in relation to measurement reliability and validity. We are now considering error in a broader manner, just as we examined validity of an entire study previously in the chapter. Designs in quantitative research seek to ensure the internal and external validity of the study by minimizing error. They do so by imposing different controls on the sampling, data collection, and analysis.

The areas within which research designs seek to create or to impose control include the sampling and measurement processes. Control in the sampling process can be imposed by establishing criteria for inclusion or exclusion that attempt to prevent some outside difference among subjects from confusing the findings of a study. Another method of control is the use of random sampling, by which the entire population is enumerated, and everyone has an equal chance of being asked to be in the study. A third method is random assignment because all subjects have an equal chance of being included in any particular group in the study. Thus, any differences in the subjects will likely be distributed equally within different groups that will be compared. We reviewed each of these approaches to control in Chapter 6. Quantitative research designs partly reflect and define the sampling approach that a study will take.

Control within the data collection process can be imposed by ensuring the validity and reliability of the measures or by ensuring that the measurement process itself is consistent, avoiding instrumentation threats. Control in measurement also can be imposed by creating **comparison group(s)** so that either exposure to the factors studied is manipulated in a controlled fashion or the timing of the measurement process is manipulated around a factor of interest. Study designs that include a comparison group create control by comparing subjects in two groups who differ in an independent variable of interest. Inclusion of a comparison group eliminates such threats to internal validity as history and maturation because both groups experience the same history or process of maturation. A design using a comparison group attempts to ensure that two groups are as similar as possible on most factors that could affect the dependent variable of interest and assume that they differ clearly in an independent variable. Therefore, such designs hope to isolate the influence of that independent variable on the dependent variable of interest. Study designs that include a **control group** create a greater level of control by manipulating the independent variable of interest so that the control group is not exposed to it, whereas the experimental group is. Again, a dependent variable is examined for differences to see whether the factor manipulated affects that dependent variable.

Functions of Quantitative Research Designs

Having considered the factors of time and control, we will now discuss specific quantitative designs considering these two factors as well as overall function. Quantitative research designs vary in the level of control that they impose from limited in descriptive and correlational studies to more control in quasi-experimental studies to the most control in true experimental designs.

Descriptive Designs and Correlational Studies

Descriptive designs function to portray some phenomenon of interest as accurately as possible. Correlational studies use a descriptive design to describe interrelationships among variables as accurately as possible. Researchers generally consider studies that look at correlations to be a subtype of descriptive designs and refer to them as *studies*, rather than the broader term *design*. Clearly, descriptive designs are used to answer research questions that seek to describe. **Correlational studies** are used to answer research questions that seek to link or connect. Both types focus on exerting control through the quality of the measurement—that is, by using reliable and valid measures as discussed in Chapter 8 and through sampling criteria or procedures. Descriptive and correlational studies may impose control by establishing certain criteria for inclusion or exclusion from the study. Remember, this also can be called *purposive sampling* or *use of a convenience sample*. Both types of design can impose even greater control over extraneous factors by using randomly selected samples.

Descriptive and correlational designs can be longitudinal or cross-sectional, and they can be retrospective or prospective. Decisions about how time is a factor are based on the nature of the question, the potential sample, and the measures. Some phenomena, such as growth or productivity, clearly entail a time element that would make it logical for a researcher to use a longitudinal design. However, as we discussed in Chapter 6, finding, following, and maintaining subjects over time can be difficult and costly, so some studies may use a single cross-sectional design to avoid problems of following subjects over time. Certainly, some measures can be repeated easily, whereas others cannot, because they measure stable concepts unlikely to change or because the measurement process is too intrusive to repeat often. For example, the concept of an individual's sense of coherence is a stable sense of the world and oneself within the world and, although a researcher may be interested in measuring this as a variable in a study, it would not be helpful to measure it more than once because it will remain stable. An example of an intrusive measure might be a bone marrow analysis.

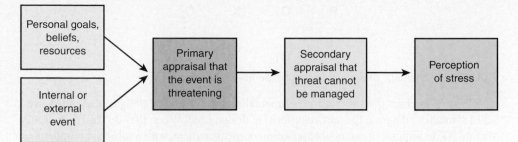

FIGURE 9.5   Schematic model of Lazarus's theory of stress.

It could be that data from weekly bone marrow tests would be ideal in evaluating a new cancer drug. However, this test is too intrusive and painful to repeat at that kind of interval.

A special type of correlational study is a design for testing a **model**. A model is the symbolic framework for a theory or part of a theory. In Chapter 2, we discussed Lazarus's theory of stress, also shown as a model in Figure 9.5. A design testing such a model identifies measures for each concept and examines how the concepts relate. A study testing Lazarus's theory would identify ways to measure the variables of personal beliefs and resources, the event, primary appraisal, secondary appraisal, and stress. Then, the study would statistically analyze relationships among the results on these measurements of the variables to see whether the relationships found were of the type and direction predicted by the model.

Often, designs for model testing are longitudinal, so some parts of the model are measured at one time point and other aspects are measured at a later time point. This allows researchers to propose causal relationships between concepts in the model. Therefore, model testing designs often attempt to answer questions that predict as well as relate.

In summary, descriptive designs function to portray a phenomenon of interest and may be retrospective, prospective, cross-sectional, or longitudinal. They also may impose varying levels of control through sampling strategies, such as purposive samples or random sampling. Correlational designs function to describe or identify interrelationships among factors of interest; they also may be retrospective, prospective, cross-sectional, or longitudinal. Because correlational designs describe relationships, you will occasionally see them called *descriptive correlational designs*. Correlational designs may use the same range of sampling strategies used in descriptive designs. Model testing designs are a special type of correlational design that usually incorporate time in some manner, either through longitudinal data collection or through use of measures that combine retrospective and concurrent data collection.

Quasi-Experimental and Experimental Research Designs

Quasi-experimental and experimental research designs function to answer questions involving prediction and the effects of manipulation. Quasi-experimental research design differs from experimental research design primarily in the amount of control imposed. Both types include control of an independent variable, but a true experimental design always includes a control group and random assignment to groups. Remember, a control group is a group of subjects who do not receive an intervention so that the control group can be compared with those who do receive the intervention (Box 9.3).

BOX 9.3
Components of Experimental Designs

- Manipulation of the independent variable
- Random assignment of subjects to groups
- A control group

$$R \quad O_1 \quad X \quad O_2$$

$$R \quad O_1 \qquad O_2$$

FIGURE 9.6 Schematic of pretest–posttest experimental design.

When researchers discuss quasi-experimental and experimental designs, they often use a set of symbols to diagram the particular form of design used. When they do this, they use the symbol "O" to indicate occasion of observation or measurement, with a subscript number designating the time point of the observation. They use the letter "X" to denote the intervention, meaning the independent variable, and they use "R" to denote that subjects were randomly assigned to groups. Figure 9.6 is an example of this type of diagram. It shows that two groups were formed using random assignment (R). Each group had measurements taken (O_1), one group received the intervention (X), and both groups had a second measurement taken (O_2). This design includes manipulation of the independent variable, random assignment, and a control group; therefore, it is experimental. Because it includes an observation both before and after the intervention, the type of design in Figure 9.6 is called a **pretest–posttest** experimental design.

Although most quasi-experimental and experimental designs are longitudinal, it is possible for an experiment to be implemented at only one time point. Figure 9.7 shows how a single time point experimental design would look. Because experimental designs always involve manipulation of an independent variable, they are never retrospective. Finally, **multifactorial** is a term sometimes associated with experimental design that refers to several independent variables being manipulated in a study. The examples we have considered have all had a single independent variable; however, some studies control and manipulate two or more independent variables.

A **quasi-experimental design** lacks either a control group or random assignment. It may not include two groups at all. Instead, it may involve a series of observations, followed by an intervention and then another series of observations (Fig. 9.8). In this case, there is manipulation of the independent variable but no control group. The threats to internal validity in this type of design include instrumentation and testing as well as selection bias and mortality. There also are quasi-experimental designs that have two groups of subjects, but the groups are nonequivalent because subjects are not randomly assigned to each group. Such a design is referred to as a *nonequivalent control group pretest–posttest quasi-experimental design*, and it entails observations of two groups, followed by one group receiving the intervention and then a second set of observations. Because both groups receive the same measurement, this quasi-experimental design is less threatened by instrumentation and testing but still is threatened by selection bias and mortality. Thus, a rather long name for a design tells us a great deal about how the research study was implemented. What if we were interested, for example, in studying the effect of positioning changes on the pain levels of hospitalized patients? If we were to find a study that randomly assigned patients to two groups and then manipulated a variable for one group but not the other, we would say that the study was most likely experimental in design. A design must include manipulation of an independent variable, a control group, and random assignment in order to be classified as experimental.

Another phrase applied to methods that we need to discuss further is repeated measures. We have already said that this phrase means that multiple measures of the same variable were taken over time. In our hypothetical study of the effect of positioning, let us assume that the researcher chose to measure a variable such as heart rate before turning the person, immediately after turning, and 5 min after turning, then 10, 15, and 25 min after turning, for a total

$$R \quad X \quad O_1$$

$$R \qquad O_1$$

FIGURE 9.7 Schematic of an experimental design with only one point of measurement.

$$O_1 \quad O_2 \quad O_3 \quad O_4 \quad X \quad O_5 \quad O_6 \quad O_7 \quad O_8$$

FIGURE 9.8 Schematic of repeated-measures quasi-experimental design.

of six measures. This is a good example of the frequency of measures you would expect if a design uses repeated measures. If a study lacked true random assignment to the intervention groups, and/or lacked a control group, the study would be labeled as quasi-experimental.

In summary, the language used to describe quantitative research designs reflects their function, such as descriptive, correlational, or experimental. Other language used to describe designs reflects how time is a component, such as retrospective, cross-sectional, or longitudinal. Finally, the language of designs reflects the level of control imposed in the study, with experimental designs imposing the greatest control over extraneous variables. We have reviewed several of the studies used throughout this book as examples of various designs. To provide familiar examples of several research designs, Table 9.4 categorizes each of the studies in this text thus far according to type of research design used.

TABLE 9.4 Categorization of Research Designs of the Articles Used Most Frequently in this Text	
CHAPTER AND REFERENCE	**RESEARCH DESIGN**
Chapters 1, 2, 4 & 5	
Cromley, T., Knatz, S., Rockwell, R. A., Neumark-Sztainer, D., Story, M., & Boutelle, K. (2012). Relationships between body satisfaction and psychological functioning and weight-related cognitions and behaviors in overweight adolescents. *Journal of Adolescent Health, 50*(6), 651–653. doi:10.1016/j.jaohealth.2011.10.252	Quantitative: Logistic regression analysis
Chapters 2 & 5	
Li, W., Rukavina, P., & Foster, C. (2013). Overweight or obese students' perceptions of caring in urban physical education programs. *Journal of Sport Behavior, 36*(2), 189.	Qualitative: Descriptive
Chapters 3 & 5	
Peck, C. N., Malhotra, K., & Kim, W. Y. (2011). Leg length discrepancy in cementless total hop arthroplasty. *Surgical Science, 2*, e183–e187. doi:10.4236/ss.2011.24040	Quantitative: Retrospective study
Chapters 4 & 5	
Ilic, D., Tepper, K., & Misso, M. (2012). Teaching evidence-based medicine literature searching skills to medical students during the clinical years: A randomized controlled trial. *Journal of the Medical Library Association, 100*(3), 190–196. doi:10.3163/1536-5050.100.3.009	Quantitative: Randomized controlled trial
Chapter 5	
Ponsford, J., Cameron, P., Fitzgerald, M., Grant, M., & Mikocka-Walus, A. (2012). Predictors of postconcussive symptoms 3 months after mild traumatic brain injury. *Neuropsychology, 26*(3), 304–313. doi:10.1037/a0027888	Quantitative: Correlational design
Chapter 7	
Ellis, N., Randall, J., & Punnett, G. (2013). The affects of a single bout of exercise on mood and self-esteem in clinically diagnosed mental health patients. *Open Journal of Medical Psychology, 2*(3), 81–85. doi:10.4236/ojmp.2013.23013	Quantitative: Correlational design
Chapter 8	
Huth, J., Peterson, J., & Lehman, J. (2013). The use of postoperative restraints in children after cleft lip or cleft palate repair: A preliminary report. *ISRN Plastic Surgery, 2013*, 1–3. http://dx.doi.org/10.5402/2013/540717	Quantitative: Comparative descriptive design
Chapter 9 (this chapter)	
Wade, D., Howell, D., Weinman, J., Hardy, R., Mythen, M., Brewin, . . . C., Raine, R. (2012). Investigating risk factors for psychological morbidity three months after intensive care: A prospective cohort study. *Critical Care, 16*(5). doi:10.1186/cc1167	Quantitative: Prospective cohort study
Chapter 10	
Grant, J. S., Vance, D. E., White, W., Keltner, N. L., & Raper, J. L. (2013). Why people living with HIV/AIDS exclude individuals from their chosen families. *Nursing: Research & Reviews, 2013*(3), 33–42	Mixed methods study
Eltahir, Y., Werners, L., Zeijlmans van Emmichoven, I., Jansen, L., Werker, P., & de Bock, G. (2013). Quality-of-life outcomes between mastectomy along and breast reconstruction: Comparison of patient-reported BREAST-Q and other health-related quality-of-life measures. *American Society of Plastic Surgeons, 132*(2), 201e–209e. doi:10.1097/PRS.0b013e31829586a7	Quantitative: Cross-sectional design

HOW CAN ONE GET THE WRONG DESIGN FOR THE RIGHT QUESTION?

Let us reflect on how the psychologist in the clinical case understood that all studies are not experimental. We have already addressed one reason for this: the research question must ask about prediction or the effects of manipulation before an experimental design will fit. For a question seeking to examine the effects of manipulation or to predict, we must have certain baseline knowledge already in place. The other reason that experimental designs are not the right design for every question involves the strengths and weaknesses of the design itself. Experimental designs are strong on control; therefore, they have the fewest threats to internal validity. That same control, however, makes experiments dissimilar from the "real" world of patient care, where variety and complexity are the rule. Therefore, the results of a study using an experimental design are generally accurate, and we can trust highly that the findings are correct. However, the findings may not be easily applied or generalized to clinical practice, where many of the factors controlled in the experiment will not be controlled.

For example, if subjects in a study on the effects of a new multiposition bed had to receive a two-dimensional CAT scan or an echocardiograph to confirm physiologic changes when the bed moved, the availability of technology would automatically reflect a certain level or location of hospital and, in most cases, a certain level of insurance coverage. Thus, uninsured patients and those from rural settings without access to tertiary care centers may likely be underrepresented or not represented in such a study. Yet, being uninsured or living in a rural setting are factors that may affect physiologic functioning and resilience. The very controls that ensured that the patients did have physiologic changes related to the multiposition bed also may limit the generalizability of the study. In reality, the controls exerted in this example probably do not greatly influence the utility of the results for more general practice; however, this example gives you an idea of why the aspects that provide control in a design also may limit the clinical usefulness of the results.

Quasi-experimental studies lose some of the internal validity of an experimental design but often gain some applicability to real life. Often, a quasi-experimental design is selected to answer a research question when the implementation of a true experimental design is not feasible. For example, researchers who want to study HIV-prevention programs with homeless women would face great difficulty in randomly assigning homeless women to different programs, because homeless people generally do not follow schedules or have circumstances that would enable them to attend programs that are not conveniently located. If the researchers tried to implement several different programs in one shelter (randomly assigning the women in the shelter to a program), it is likely that the women would share activities from the different programs, causing the programs to blur and making it impossible to isolate the effects of one compared with the other. Therefore, a researcher testing an HIV program with homeless women would likely use a quasi-experimental design, selecting homeless shelters to either receive or not receive the intervention to be tested. In contrast, if the researchers want to test HIV-prevention programs with high school students, they might more easily randomly assign subjects and create a true experiment. Nevertheless, results with high school students would not be easy to apply to the different lives and experiences of homeless women. Therefore, the very control possible with high school students would preclude the study being as useful for homeless women.

As we move to descriptive and correlational designs, control decreases even further because the researcher no longer controls the independent variable. Selection criteria or random selection, however, can still provide some control. In addition, measurement reliability and validity increase our confidence about the accuracy of the factors being studied. Because descriptive and correlational designs still impose control through sampling and measurement, the richness and diversity of real-life clinical situations is limited. Phenomenologic, ethnographic, and grounded theory designs impose the least control over the process of research and, therefore, capture the greatest detail and depth of real experiences. Yet, they can become so subjective or conceptual that the results also may be difficult to apply to real practice. Qualitative designs are not intended to develop knowledge about predictions; but, as healthcare professionals, we often seek knowledge that *will* allow us to predict.

Therefore, the answer to the question "How can one get the wrong design for the right question?" involves feasibility in terms of who or what is being studied, what measures are available, and what is already known about the problem or phenomenon. A study of the process of tobacco addiction cannot ethically manipulate the variable of exposure to tobacco, so it will, by necessity, be nonexperimental. A study of drug efficacy requires careful control of as many extraneous factors as possible, lending itself to experimental design. However, withholding drug treatment in some cases may be unethical, leading to the use of quasi-experimental design. Studies of subjective experiences, such as pain, grief, or satisfaction, require understanding best acquired through seeking the insights of those who have experienced or are experiencing the phenomenon, lending themselves to qualitative designs. Yet, a researcher may not be skilled in qualitative methods and so may choose a cross-sectional descriptive design instead.

What should be evident at this point is that study design shapes the approach taken to sampling, measurement, and data analysis. Understanding the basic language of design will allow you to understand many of the decisions made by the researcher(s) regarding the study, clarifying the approaches taken to acquiring subjects or participants and to the data collection itself. Recognizing that the terms used in quantitative design are combined differently to specify the function, control, and time factor in a design will help you to better understand the types of designs described in published research.

In addition to terms that reflect the function of and the use of control and time in a design, some designs are described as mixed methods. **Mixed methods** refer to some combination of methods in relation to function, time, or control. A study that collects retrospective data by asking parents to complete a questionnaire about family history of heart disease, their children's level of physical activity, and the parents' smoking behavior is an example of collecting data about how things were, thinking back in time. In addition, if this study then collects data of cholesterol level, blood pressure, and HbA_1C, this could be classified as a longitudinal study, because it links data from the past about activity, history, and smoking with data from the present about blood pressure, cholesterol, and HbA_1C.

Another use of the term *mixed methods* is to refer to a combination of qualitative and quantitative methods. The fictional article from Appendix B about students in a healthcare major' choices of clinical practice uses a somewhat mixed methods because it includes data collection by use of a pen-and-paper quantifiable questionnaire and a written open-ended question that was analyzed using methods associated with qualitative research. As the need for evidence-based information increases, more and more researchers are recognizing the value of both qualitative and quantitative methods to more fully answer questions of interest to healthcare professionals, which has led to increased use of a combination of qualitative and quantitative designs in single studies.

Before beginning this chapter, you were asked to consider how you might best conduct a study of the effects of college attendance on well-being. Now that we have examined various research designs and some of the advantages and disadvantages of each, let us consider some choices you would need to make if you were going to conduct such a study.

First, you could approach a study of the effects of college attendance on well-being from a qualitative perspective or a quantitative perspective. The decision would depend partly on what is already known, such as what is known about influences on well-being in college students, how healthcare programs differ from other undergraduate programs, and whether students in a healthcare major differ from other undergraduate students in some important ways that might affect well-being. If little is known about any of these factors, a qualitative study of the lived experiences of students in a healthcare major in terms of sense of well-being while in school might be the research design to use. If little is known about well-being and students in a healthcare major, a researcher might implement a grounded theory design to examine interactions that affect well-being.

A researcher also might decide to do a descriptive correlational study measuring well-being and other factors that would logically be relevant, such as general health, age, family commitments, work schedule, and grade point average, to see how they relate. If implementing a quantitative study, the researcher could decide to do measurements only at one time point and perhaps include students just entering school, those halfway through school, and those preparing to graduate. Such a study would be cross-sectional. To address problems with internal validity, the researcher would need to consider how comparable students in the three different classes were in factors that affect well-being other than college attendance.

Alternatively, a researcher might decide to do a longitudinal study, following a group of students in a healthcare major from the time they enter school to graduation. This type of study would take much time and many resources; it also would be open to such threats to internal validity as mortality, testing, and instrumentation. The question of effects of college attendance and well-being probably does not lend itself to or fit with either quasi-experimental or experimental designs, unless something already has been shown to be a factor that could be manipulated to try to change well-being.

This example demonstrates why studies addressing approximately the same question may use different research designs. As an intelligent user of research, you do not have to decide what type of design to use, but it is helpful for you to understand some considerations that go into selecting a design as well as the meaning and strengths and weaknesses of different research designs.

COMMON ERRORS IN PUBLISHED REPORTS OF RESEARCH DESIGNS

As you read published studies, there may be problems with the amount of information provided about the study design. One common problem is lack of detail about the design, leaving the reader uncertain concerning the methods used. In some cases, the only thing we are told is that a particular method or design was used. This happens more in published reports of qualitative studies than in reports of quantitative studies and may occur partly because qualitative methods were less well known or used in healthcare research in the more distant past. A written report of a study design should not simply tell the reader the label for the design; it also should describe enough of the actual process of the research study to assure the reader that the design was implemented appropriately.

For example, a study that states it uses phenomenologic methods also should tell you enough about the subjects to assure you that they were rich and appropriate sources of data and, generally, how data were collected and analyzed. A study that tells you it used an experimental design also should provide specific information about the random assignment process, creation of the control group, and manipulation of the intervention.

As with measurement in research, a study design can be complex. Nevertheless, it is the responsibility of the author(s) to communicate in writing all the essential aspects of the design so that the reader can intelligently read and understand the study. The use of a time line often helps readers to understand a study design, particularly if it is longitudinal. The other aspect that occasionally is lacking in published reports is a rationale for the choice of research design. We have discussed that a researcher has to make several decisions when selecting a design. Occasionally, the rationales for decisions, such as not including a control group, can help the reader to better understand the problems of the study and how they may affect usefulness for clinical practice.

PUBLISHED REPORTS—DID DESIGN AFFECT YOUR CONCLUSION?

The psychologist in our clinical case is seeking to understand how D.M.'s long-term mental health may be impacted as a result of his accident and hospitalization. In reading the study by Wade et al. (2012), the psychologist understands that evidence shows that there is significant correlation between ICU survivors and psychological morbidity (Wade et al., 2012). According to the study, a key factor influencing specific psychological outcomes in this population included the types of different ICU drugs given. From this perspective, the research design, a prospective cohort study, makes sense: this allowed the researchers to observe outcomes without the constraint of an experimental design, and also provided an avenue for researchers to understand what specific factors (e.g., medications given) produced which specific outcomes.

While most evidence-based studies focus on research in the form of clinical trials, this gold standard can be used only when we know enough about a topic to use a true experimental design. **Clinical trials** refer to studies that test the effectiveness of a clinical treatment, and some researchers would say that a clinical trial must be a true experiment. For many problems in clinical practice, however, there have been only a few true experimental studies, so it is not uncommon to see clinical trials defined more broadly.

Given the nature of the question and the evidence from the study, the psychologist concludes that D.M.'s long-term mental health could indeed be impacted by his stay in ICU, which gives the psychologist more insight into D.M.'s symptoms that are consistent with fear, depression, and anxiety. Having this information will help guide the psychologist in choosing the best ways to interact with D.M. to explore the factors that contributed to his current mental health, and to find ways to help D.M. optimally cope.

CRITICALLY READING THE DESCRIPTION OF THE STUDY DESIGN IN A RESEARCH REPORT FOR USE IN EVIDENCE-BASED PRACTICE

In Box 9.4, you will find questions that you can use to critically read about the design of a research study. Often the study design is part of the methods section of a research report, but since we have discussed designs in a separate chapter, we will also address questions to ask about designs as a separate component to consider when reading a report of research. The first question asks, "Did the report include a clearly identified section describing the research design?" The psychologist reading the study by Wade et al. (2012) did find a clear statement of the study design, particularly as it related to being a prospective cohort study;

BOX 9.4
How to Critically Read the Description of Study Design in a Research Report

Does the report answer the question "How were those people studied—why was the study performed that way?"

1. Did the report include a clearly identified section describing the research design?
2. Does the design make this quantitative, qualitative, or a mixed methods study?
3. Does the report address approaches taken to assure study rigor, internal validity, and/or external validity?
4. Do I think that the researcher(s) should have designed the study differently in order to answer my clinical question?

however, some research reports may fail to identify the type of design, making it necessary for you as a reader to try to classify that design based on other information in the report. If you read a report and are uncertain about the study design even after reviewing the complete method section, then it may be that the researchers failed to have a systematic plan for their study, and that would affect your trust of the total study.

The second question to ask is "Does the design make this quantitative, qualitative, or a mixed methods study?" The answer to that question allows you as a critical reader to evaluate the fit of the design to the procedures and measures used in the study. A misfit between design and actual measures would suggest that the researcher(s) may have implemented a less-than-consistent and systematic study, and would cause you to wonder about the usefulness of the results of that study for evidence based practice. For example, if a research report indicates the study design is ethnography and then indicates that data were collected using a series of written scales, we would have to wonder about the quality of the study, as this type of measurement does not fit with a qualitative design.

A third question to ask as you critically read about a study design is "Does the report address approaches taken to assure study rigor, internal validity, and/or external validity?" In order to answer this, you must be familiar with these concepts and will have to critically read the description of the implementation of the study. Finally, you will want to ask yourself "Do I think that the researcher(s) should have designed the study differently in order to answer my clinical question?" For example, the psychologist in our clinical case wants to assist D.M. in his psychosocial adjustment following hospitalization in the ICU. While reading the study about risk factors for psychological morbidity after intensive care, the psychologist recognizes that the clinical question is one about what psychological concerns (outcomes) a patient may develop after being in an ICU; therefore, the prospective cohort design used is appropriate and will give the psychologist useful evidence on which to base practice.

The psychologist realizes that without the research findings contained in the article read, the care provided may have been different and perhaps not nearly as effective in improving the patient's health. The results also suggest the importance of the healthcare provider's role in assessment of the patient's feelings. The psychologist reads the introduction, which reflects that psychosocial morbidity after ICU hospitalization is not uncommon. He begins to wonder if he has treated other patients who have also been ICU survivors, and plans in the future to ask patients, as part of a routine health history, whether they have ever been hospitalized in an ICU. Having this information may assist the psychologist in providing the best evidence-based treatment and counsel.

OUT-OF-CLASS EXERCISE

How to Set the Stage for a Study

At the end of Chapter 8, you were asked to develop some ideas for a research design in order to study the effects of college attendance on well-being. We have discussed in this chapter some possible designs that you may have considered and the need to have a better idea of what is already known before you can settle on a design. Chapter 10 discusses the background and statement of the research problem sections of research reports. It is this first part of a research report that provides the rationale for a study as well as information about previous research. Before reading Chapter 10, write one or two paragraphs that describe why a study of students in a healthcare major's well-being and the effect of attendance in college are important enough to warrant a research study. If you were going to conduct such a study, what would you need to describe at the beginning to set the stage? After you have written your case for studying the students in a healthcare major's well-being, you are ready to begin Chapter 10.

References

*Colaizzi, P. F. (1973). *Reflection and research in psychology: A phenomenological study of learning.* Dubuque, IA: Kendall/Hunt.

*Giorgi, A. (1971). Phenomenology and experimental psychology: II. In A. Giorgi, W. Fischer, & R. von Eckartsberg (Eds.), *Duquesne studies in phenomenological psychology* (*Vol. I*). Pittsburgh, PA: Duquesne University Press.

*Glaser, B. G., & Strauss, A. L. (1967). *The discovery of grounded theory: Strategies for qualitative research.* New York, NY: Aldine.

Hughes, M., Beck, B., Chen, Y., Lewis, A., & Thomas, D. (2011). Arsenic exposure and toxicology: A historical perspective. *Toxicological Sciences, 123*(2), 305–332. doi:10.1093/toxsci/kfr184

*Parse, R. R. (2001). *Qualitative inquiry: The path of sciencing.* Sudbury, MA: Jones and Bartlett Publishers and National League for Nursing Press.

*Spiegelberg, H. (1976). *The phenomenological movement* (*Vols. I and II*). The Hague: Martinus Nijhoff.

*Spradley, J. P. (1979). *The ethnographic interview.* New York, NY: Holt, Rinehart & Winston.

StatsDirect. (2013, November). *Prospective versus retrospective studies.* Retrieved from http://www.statsdirect.com/help/default.htm#basics/prospective.htm

*Strauss, A., & Corbin, J. (1994). Grounded theory methodology: An overview. In N. K. Denzin & Y. S. Lincoln (Eds.), *Handbook of qualitative research* (pp. 273–285). Thousand Oaks, CA: Sage.

*van Kaam, A. L. (1966). Application of the phenomenological method. *Existential foundations of psychology.* Pittsburgh, PA: Duquesne University Press.

Wade, D. M., Howell, D. C., Weinman, J. A., Hardy, R. J., Mythen, M. G., Brewin, C. R., . . . Raine, R. A. (2012). Investigating risk factors for psychological morbidity three months after intensive care: A prospective cohort study. *Critical Care, 16*(5). doi:10.1186/cc1167

*indicates a definitive or classic work or publication regarding this subject matter.

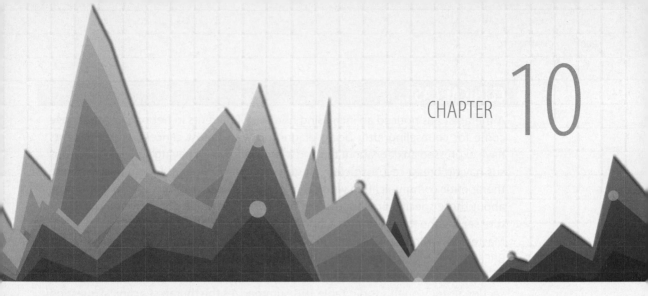

Background and the Research Problem

Why Ask That Question—What Do We Already Know?

> **LEARNING OBJECTIVE** The student will relate the background and the research problem to the research methods, results, and conclusions.

Sources of Problems for Research
Background Section of Research Reports
Literature Review Sections of Research Reports

   Directional and Nondirectional Hypotheses
   Null and Research Hypotheses

Linking the Literature Review to the Study Design
Published Reports—Has the Case Been Made for the Research Study?
Common Errors in Reports of the Background and Literature Review
Critically Reading Background and Literature Review Sections of a Research Report for Use in EBP

KEY TERMS

Conceptual framework	Research hypothesis
Deductive knowledge	Research objective
Directional hypothesis	Research purpose
Inductive knowledge	Research problem
Literature review	Research question
Nondirectional hypothesis	Secondary source
Peer review	Specific aim
Primary sources	Theoretical framework

CLINICAL CASE

A therapist has noticed an increasing number of patients in her practice that have come for counseling after being diagnosed with breast cancer. Several patients have expressed anxiety about making a choice between having a mastectomy versus having breast reconstruction surgery performed. In an effort to best facilitate therapeutic communication with these patients, the therapist wants to learn more about these specific procedures and their effects on patients. Performing a literature search, the therapist finds a study entitled, "Quality-of-Life Outcomes between Mastectomy Alone and Breast Reconstruction: Comparison of Patient-Reported BREAST-Q and Other Health-Related Quality-of-Life Matters" (Eltahir et al., 2013) (Appendix A-9). The therapist notices that the researchers decided to do a cross-sectional study on this topic. Table 10.1 summarizes the therapist's clinical question for this clinical case.

SOURCES OF PROBLEMS FOR RESEARCH

We started this book by discussing knowing and knowledge, and why research is an important source of knowledge. This led us to recognize the need to understand and intelligently use research in EBP. As we moved through discussions of the different sections of most reports of research, we ended each chapter with a "why" question: Why did the researcher come to that conclusion? Why did the researcher use those patients and those measures? Why did the researcher plan the study in that way? We are now ready to discuss the beginning of research reports, in which the most important "why" question of all is asked: Why do this study? This is the most important "why" question, because if there is no good rationale or basis for a research problem, then the rest of the study and its findings are unimportant.

One of the critical answers to "why do this study" can be found in this chapter. Studies are done to provide evidence for practice. EBP, defined as "integrating individual clinical expertise with the best available external clinical evidence from systematic research" (Sackett, Rosenberg, Gray, Haynes, & Richardson, 1996), should guide the way that all healthcare team members practice. Without evidence, best practice standards may go unheeded, important assessment information can be missed, decision making can be impaired, and

TABLE 10.1	Statement of Clinical Question from the Clinical Case
HOW DOES QUALITY OF LIFE COMPARE BETWEEN IN WOMEN WHO HAVE HAD MASTECTOMY ALONE VERSUS THOSE WHO HAVE HAD BREAST RECONSTRUCTION?	
The *Who*	137 women who had undergone mastectomy for breast cancer or prophylaxis resulting from genetic predisposition. The study population was split into two groups: those who had mastectomy alone, and those who had mastectomy with successful breast reconstruction
The *What*	Quality-of-life outcomes following mastectomy alone, or mastectomy with successful breast reconstruction
The *When*	Treatment received between 2006 and 2010
The *Where*	University Medical Center Groningen
Key search terms to find research-based evidence for practice	Breast cancer Mastectomy Quality of Life Breast reconstruction

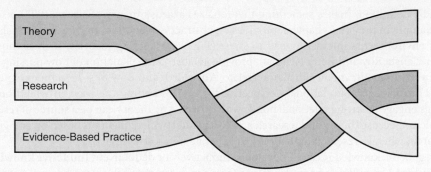

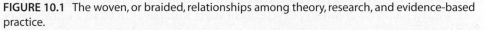

FIGURE 10.1   The woven, or braided, relationships among theory, research, and evidence-based practice.

thus, patient outcomes may decline. The reason "why" studies are conducted is to provide the critical evidence from which all healthcare providers should practice; therefore, that should be one of the primary, driving answers for "why to do this study"—to improve practice, and thus, positively influence patient outcomes.

A good **research problem** represents a knowledge gap that warrants filling and can be addressed through systematic study. Research problems are derived from several sources, but two general sources of research problems exist. They are (1) problems derived from practice and (2) problems derived from theory. Figure 10.1 illustrates how research, EBP, and theory can be viewed as one large braid because they wind together to develop knowledge.

We have focused on research questions that directly relate to EBP, and practice within the healthcare professions are the major sources for identification of gaps in knowledge that must be researched. Healthcare practice is broad and is a rich source of questions and problems for which we currently do not have answers. Examples of some of the questions that must be answered include the following:

- What techniques, approaches, and treatment options does evidence show to be most effective in addressing patient needs? (These needs may be physiological, psychosocial, developmental, spiritual, or sociocultural in nature.)
- What are the best ways to support physiologic functioning in acutely ill patients?
- How can we facilitate individual and family growth through the stress of health crises?
- How can we assist patients in making major adjustments associated with chronic illness?
- How can we facilitate and promote positive healthy living, and what constitutes a positive and healthy balanced life?
- What allows some people to adapt or cope with illness when some cannot?
- What makes some people more vulnerable to health and illness problems?
- How can we facilitate individuals and families during the transition from life to death?

These questions are broad and cannot be directly tested in a research study, but they do demonstrate the diversity of research areas that arise from professional healthcare practice. Research problems derived from practice may be based on experiences in the practice arena, may be problems derived from mandated evaluation or accrediting requirements, or may reflect social issues as they affect practice.

Theory is another source of research problems. A theory can be defined as an abstract explanation describing how different factors or phenomena relate. In Chapter 8, we discussed theoretical definitions of variables, saying that this type of definition describes a variable conceptually rather than concretely. It is the conceptual or abstract nature of the ideas that, by definition, makes something theoretical. Lazarus's theory of stress (1993), used as an example in previous chapters, provides an abstract explanation for how individuals and their environments interact to lead to stress (Fig. 9.5). Nursing theories, such as those by Sister Calista Roy and Betty Neuman, provide an abstract explanation of how nursing, persons, environment, and health all interrelate. Ainsworth and Bowlby's "Attachment Theory" (1991) provides a foundational perspective for understanding the ways in which human beings engage in strong relational bonds with others. Any theory can be a source of research problems because theory and research are closely intertwined: theory is based on and guides research, whereas research tests theory to generate new knowledge.

In general, knowledge can be developed inductively or deductively. **Inductive knowledge** is developed by pulling observations and facts generated through research together to generate theory. Inductive knowledge development starts with pieces to build a whole theory. That theory is then used to suggest further observations that might be expected, which are then used to refine the theory. **Deductive knowledge** is developed by proposing a theory regarding a phenomenon of interest. It starts with the whole and breaks down the parts of the theory, seeking observations and facts to support the abstract relationships proposed in that theory. Observations that support or refute a theory's predictions of relationships are used to revise or refine the theory, which then undergoes further testing. In healthcare, many of the observations for either inductive or deductive knowledge development arise from research studies as well as from practice, hence, the intertwining relationships among practice, research, and theory that are illustrated in Figure 10.1.

Although practice and theory are the major sources of research problems, much more is required to develop a specific narrow research problem than just identifying a broad question from either source. In the background section of a research report, we should be able to follow the trail of thinking that has led from a relatively general research problem to a specific, narrowly stated research purpose.

The first sections of most research reports are labeled "Background," "Introduction," "Problem," "Theoretical Framework," "Literature Review," or some combination of these. In all cases, these first sections of a research report should (1) provide the broad context or rationale for the problem, (2) define the problem, and (3) summarize what is already known about the problem. These three purposes are not always discrete and distinct because one purpose also may relate to another purpose. Therefore, information about what is known about a problem also may help to define it, or the context or rationale for a problem also may include what is or is not known about it. However, after reading the introductory sections of a research report, we should have a general understanding of these purposes. The purposes of context and definition are often discussed in the introduction or background section of a research report, whereas a section titled "Literature Review" often specifically describes the current state of knowledge about a problem, based upon a thorough review of the information that is already available. Our discussion will follow this division.

BACKGROUND SECTION OF RESEARCH REPORTS

To provide a context for a research problem, most study reports start with a broad and general description of a health concern derived from theory or practice. This description of the concern can be based on national health statistics; the costs of an important health problem; the goals or agenda of an organization that supports health, such as the American Medical Association (AMA); or an emerging health crisis. For example, the beginning of the report of the study "Quality-of-Life Outcomes between Mastectomy Alone and Breast Reconstruction: Comparison of Patient-Reported BREAST-Q and Other Health-Related Quality-of-Life Matters" (Eltahir et al., 2013) (Appendix A-9) states the purpose of the study conducted was to "evaluate the quality of life of women after successful breast reconstruction in comparison with those who underwent mastectomy alone" (Eltahir et al., 2013, p. 201e).

Providing the context for a specific research problem also often establishes the relevancy of the problem for healthcare. Sometimes that relevancy will be more applicable to certain disciplines based on scope of practice. In the Eltahir et al. (2013) article, the research and finding are not directly connected to one discipline within healthcare. In fact, the information found within this research study could have relevance to multiple healthcare professionals. Some research reports include a subsection at the beginning that specifically addresses the relationship between the research problem and a specific healthcare discipline, but most will not, as research can be utilized by many different members of the interdisciplinary healthcare team.

In addition to setting a broad context for a research problem that may also define the clinical relevancy of that problem, the background section of a report should narrow and refine the research problem. General problems, such as low birth weight and differences in vulnerability in rural and urban settings, are not specific enough to be easily examined using research. Even with qualitative research methods, a specific phenomenon, an aspect of a cultural group, or social interaction must be refined and delineated as the focus of the study to guide data collection and analysis.

Research problems are usually refined either through reference to the existing literature about the problem or through theoretical frameworks. Existing literature used to refine a research problem may include scholarly papers, research studies, or clinical case studies. The focus of the literature when refining the research problem is on the aspects of the problem that have been recognized, what is known about these aspects, and how they may relate. Although the background section refers to existing literature, that literature will be relatively general and address the overall research problem. Often, a background section is followed by a literature review section, in which the literature referenced is usually more focused on the particular research problem than the literature in the background section, which usually differs from the more extensive literature review because the former is relatively general and addresses the overall research problem. The literature review section often addresses the research problem after it has been refined. The background and literature review sections of a research report, then, might fit together to develop a story. The background gives us the general scene and characters, perhaps including the relationships among the characters, and it ends by presenting a specific conflict or problem among selected characters. The literature review continues the story and gives us a much more complete description of the central characters specifically relevant to that problem.

Another approach that may be used to refine a research problem, either by itself or in combination with literature, is application of a theory, theoretical framework, or conceptual framework to the research problem. A **theoretical framework** is an underlying structure that describes how abstract aspects of the research problem interrelate based on developed theories. A **conceptual framework** also is an underlying structure, but it comprises concepts and the relationships among them. We have said that a theory is an abstract explanation describing how different factors or phenomena relate. In the purest sense, these three different terms have different meanings, but understanding those meanings is not essential to intelligently using research because they all describe proposed relationships among abstract concepts.

CORE CONCEPT 10.1

Theory, theoretical frameworks, and conceptual frameworks all provide a description of the proposed relationships among abstract components that are aspects of the research problem of interest.

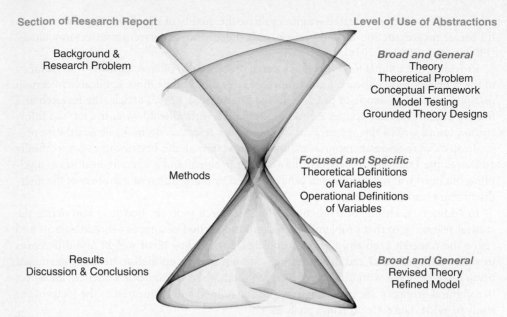

Section of Research Report

Background &
Research Problem

Methods

Results
Discussion & Conclusions

Level of Use of Abstractions

Broad and General
Theory
Theoretical Problem
Conceptual Framework
Model Testing
Grounded Theory Designs

Focused and Specific
Theoretical Definitions
of Variables
Operational Definitions
of Variables

Broad and General
Revised Theory
Refined Model

FIGURE 10.2 Relationship between sections of a research report and use of abstract language.

We must be clear that we are not talking about theoretical definitions of specific variables at this point. As shown in Figure 10.2, abstractions such as theory and theoretical definitions of variables are connected with different sections of the research report. The word *theory* does refer to something that is abstract, so theoretical definitions of variables are abstract definitions of specific variables to be studied and may derive from a specific theory or framework. However, before we can narrow in on specific variables, we must refine the research problem to a point that it can be systematically studied. As Figure 10.2 indicates by the hourglass shape, in the background section of a report, we expect that a broad and general concern, such as quality of life for patients who have undergone mastectomy with or without successful breast reconstruction, will be narrowed to a specific research purpose. The **research purpose** is a clear statement of factors that are going to be studied to shed knowledge on the research problem. These factors may also be referred to as the variables to be studied. In general, we expect the research purpose to identify the major variables. Abstract descriptions of these more narrow concepts are then included in the methods section. The discussion and conclusion sections once again use broad and more general abstractions as the results of a study are connected back to the original theory or conceptual framework.

Some research studies will note that a conceptual framework was used to develop the intervention. The use of a conceptual framework provides a rationale and support for the components of the intervention that the researchers plan to test. In most cases, the researchers do not actually test that model or framework directly; rather, it helps to identify research questions for the researchers to address in the course of the study.

In some studies, you will see terms that are referred to a *study aim* and a *research question*. These terms and several others refer to the specific focus of the research study that is being reported. Two other terms also used refer to the specific focus of a research study are *research purpose(s)* and *research objective(s)*. All of these terms mean essentially the same thing: they refer to a statement of purpose of the research and identify the variables that will be studied.

Often, the research purpose (or research question, **specific aim**, or **research objective**) also will include language that defines the type of question being asked in the research—whether the question is descriptive, relational, or predictive. For example, the research purpose for the study entitled "Psychiatric Comorbidity is Associated with increased risk of surgery in Crohn's disease" (Ananthakrishnan et al., 2013) clearly implies that the research identified an association—a connection—between these items. Titles of other research studies may use the term *distribution*, clearly indicating that we are looking for expanse in this trend. Titles that include the word *quality* implies that we are looking for distinctive characteristics to emerge as we read.

 CORE CONCEPT 10.2

The terms research purpose, research question, study, or specific aim(s) or research objective(s) all refer to the statement of the variables to be studied that are related to the broad research problem.

In summary, the background section of a research report has two major purposes: (1) to establish the context for the research problem and (2) to refine that problem to a specific research purpose. The section of the report that we are referring to as *background* may simply be the beginning of the report without any title, may be titled "Introduction," or may be titled "Background." Information that provides the broad context for the research problem may include issues from either practice or theory, and may reflect societal concerns, healthcare policy changes, or major health concerns. Refining the research problem may be accomplished using literature, theory, or both. In either case, the goal is to move from the general problem to a specific purpose or question that identifies the variables to be included in the study and often the type of question being asked.

LITERATURE REVIEW SECTIONS OF RESEARCH REPORTS

We said earlier that the use of literature to refine the research problem is not necessarily the same as the formal literature review. A **literature review** is a synthesis of the literature that describes what is known or has been studied regarding the particular research question or purpose.

Much of the literature review consists of a synthesis of existing published research, but some scholarly and theoretical work that is not actual research may also be included in the review. The literature review is more than a listing or summary of relevant research; it entails the combination of several elements or studies to provide a different or new focus on the research problem. Key points are made by summarizing the focus of a number of pertinent research studies. A recitation of all of them would be monotonous and useless. It is also within this section that researchers, such as Eltahir et al. (2013), may make reference to the fact that very little literature on the research topic exists. Box 10.1 summarizes the purposes for literature reviews.

 CORE CONCEPT 10.3

The literature review is guided by the variables that have been identified in the research purpose and aims to give the reader an overview of what is known about those variables, how those variables have been studied in the past, and with whom they have been studied.

> ## BOX 10.1
> ### Specific Purposes of the Literature Review
>
> 1. Description of what is known about the variables for the study
> 2. Description of how the variables have been studied in the past
> 3. Description of with whom the variables have been studied

The therapist in our clinical case recognizes that the authors of the Eltahir et al. (2013) article do not specifically identify their review of existing literature as a "literature review," but rather incorporate this information into the introductory section of the study, right before the "Patients and Methods" section. In this case, the purpose of the authors' research is to review existing information in order to establish that there is a gap in knowledge, which guides future research. We mentioned earlier that authors use other literature to establish and support their specific aim. However, they do not provide a formal review of the literature because that is what they have identified as the gap in knowledge that must be addressed to develop further understanding about quality-of-life outcomes for patients who have had mastectomy alone or breast reconstruction (Eltahir et al.).

To assure us that the literature review reflects the state of the science, the author must include current or recent studies. Usually, we would expect that most of the literature cited in a literature review has been published within 3 years (optimally) of the date of the study or the publication of the report, and no greater than 5 years from the date of study or report publication. However, sometimes little research has been conducted on selected variables, there has been a gap in time since the problem was addressed, or some important or classic studies may have been done more than 3 to 5 years ago. In these cases, we may appropriately see literature cited that was published more than 3 to 5 years ago. We care about how current the literature cited is because we want to know that the researcher is building on the most current knowledge related to the problem of interest.

Another way of ensuring that a study, either proposed or reported, is based on current knowledge is its use of primary sources. **Primary sources** are the sources of information as originally written. To be accurate and current, it is important that the researcher has read and synthesized the actual research reports or scholarly papers that are relevant to the study. A **secondary source** is someone else's description or interpretation of a primary source. For example, Grant et al. (2013) (Appendix A-10) state that Serovich et al. (2010) found that the concept of family as a unique relationship was one reason that HIV-positive men who have sex with men (MSM) place value on their family of origin. This example reflects a primary source because Grant et al. must have read Serovich et al.'s study and reported on what they read. However, suppose that another researcher named "Smith" wanted to study reasons that this population value their family of origin, had read Grant et al.'s research report, and then stated in the literature "Serovich et al. (2010) found that the concept of family as a unique relationship was one reason that HIV-positive men who have sex with men (MSM) place value on their family of origin" (Grant et al., 2013) (Appendix A-10). In this case, Smith would be citing a secondary source: Smith has not read the Serovich et al. study, but only Grant et al.'s description of it. We know this because Smith tells us the names of the authors who reported the original study, then references different authors, in this case, Grant et al., as the source of the information.

One problem with secondary sources is the potential for inadvertent error or distortion of the findings of a study. Think about the childhood game of telephone, in which six or seven children sit in a circle, and one child starts a message around the circle by whispering it into the ear of the child next to him or her. That child then whispers the message that he or she heard into the next child's ear. As we all know, by the time the message gets around the circle, it is likely to have changed significantly from what was originally stated. The same problem can occur with reports of research or other scholarly work. The greater the number of times that the work is interpreted beyond the original, the greater the possibility that the actual results will be distorted or changed.

The second reason that we expect a researcher to use primary sources is because the researcher must carefully choose quality sources to support his or her current research study. If we depend on Grant et al.'s sentence about Serovich et al.'s study, we are also depending on Grant et al.'s judgment about the quality of that study related to the reason that HIV-positive men who have sex with men place value on their family of origin.

In addition to the use of current and primary sources, the healthcare team member in the clinical case should expect to see literature that has been published in refereed or peer-reviewed journals. We mentioned in Chapter 1 that the quality of information acquired on the World Wide Web must be carefully evaluated because anyone can create a Web site and claim to be an authority on a subject. Similarly, there is variety in the quality of published literature. A standard that ensures a published report has been carefully scrutinized for quality is the use of peer review. **Peer review** means that the manuscript for the published report has been read and critiqued by two or more peers before being accepted for publication. *Refereed* is another term that means that there was critical review of manuscripts before being accepted for publication. Manuscripts that are peer reviewed are intentionally sent to individuals who have expertise in the manuscript's topic. Therefore, the reviewers' comments are likely to reflect current and well-established knowledge. Not all sources of reports on research are peer reviewed or refereed. You can find out whether a particular publication is refereed by checking the author's guidelines for a journal—often available on a Web site, and always in the journal itself.

All of the studies used as examples in this chapter are from peer-reviewed journals. However, not all of the citations listed when doing a search using search programs such as CINAHL will be from peer-reviewed publications. As an intelligent discerner of evidence used for clinical practice, you should consider not only the content of the study, but also the type of publication. When you read research published in refereed journals, you know that the published report has been reviewed by several individuals who have expertise in the research area, giving you some assurance about the quality of the study before you read it.

Part of what assures us of the quality of a literature review and, therefore, the knowledge on which the study was based, is that the literature cited was from refereed publications. Therefore, the therapist in our clinical case will read background literature contained within studies, as well as systematic reviews, expecting that recent literature, from primary sources and peer-reviewed journals, will provide information about what is known about quality of life for patients who have had mastectomy alone or breast reconstruction.

A literature review should provide focused information about the specific variable(s) to be examined in a study. The review should provide some understanding of what is known about the variables, how they have been studied in the past, and with whom they have been studied. This should logically support the design and methods for the research study reported. Returning to our earlier analogy, by the time the literature review is completed, the major plot and subplots for the story should be clear. For those plots to make sense, we must understand the characters and their past "relationships" or stories.

After the literature review, some research reports include detailed research questions or hypotheses, if those elements are applicable to the study. In particular, we do not expect such information in a study using a qualitative approach because the emphasis should be on understanding the whole of an experience or a phenomenon, rather than breaking it down and studying its discrete parts. We also do not expect detailed research questions or hypotheses from quantitative studies whose purpose is general description. However, studies that test theory and predictions from theory or attempt to test the effect of manipulation usually have focused detailed research questions or hypotheses.

We said earlier that a research problem is broad and general, while a research purpose is narrowly stated, may also be called a research question, and will specify the factor(s) or variable(s) to be examined. These are considered to be "detailed" research questions. Another way to think about these questions is as subquestions to the narrow and specific question or purpose of the study. For example, in the Discussion section of the article by Eltahir et al. (2013), the researchers state that their study could not account for all variations of perception of quality of life over time. Factors such as nipple reconstruction, nipple tattooing, or secondary corrective surgery were identified as other factors that may influence perception of quality of life, and therefore, each of these represents more detail that could be included in future research that seeks to understand qualify of life experienced by patients who undergo breast reconstruction.

Information like this can break down the larger research purpose into more detailed and specific questions. The questions include not only the specific variables of interest in the study but also the specific relationship to be tested and the time frame for that testing. As an intelligent reader and user of research in EBP, you should understand that it is important to know that most reports of research studies start with a general problem, move to a more refined research purpose or question, and then, if appropriate, develop specific measurable questions or hypotheses, as illustrated in Figure 10.3. The research problem, purpose, and question are descriptions of the knowledge sought by the study that differ in their depth and specificity, but content from one may overlap with another at times. They also may differ in the actual terms used, such as the research purpose being called a specific aim or the research questions being written as objectives. However, a research report should include at least two, and often three, levels of depth and specificity of statements about the knowledge being sought in the study. These levels are differentiated by the specificity of the statements, with the problem being general, the purpose stating the variables for the study, and the questions or hypotheses stating specific measurable predictions or relationships.

In Chapters 2 and 5, we defined a hypothesis as a prediction regarding the relationships or effects of selected factors on other factors. We now know that the factors in a study are called *variables*. A research question and a **research hypothesis** are often opposite sides of the same coin, because they both state predictions about relationships among variables. A **research question** puts the predictions in the form of a question, whereas a hypothesis puts the predictions in the form of a statement. There are two types of research hypotheses and questions: directional and nondirectional.

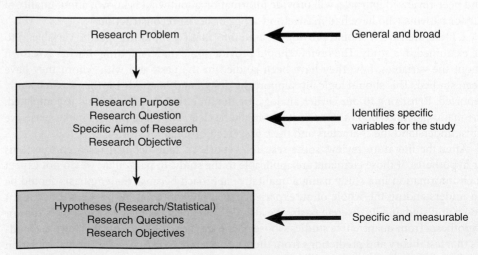

FIGURE 10.3 Levels of development of the statements of the knowledge sought by the study.

Directional and Nondirectional Hypotheses

A hypothesis may predict whether there will be a relationship between two variables, or it may state the nature of the relationship between them. When we speak about the nature of a relationship, we are referring to whether the relationship is positive or negative; another word for this is the *direction* of the relationship. We talked about negative and positive relationships in Chapter 5, when we discussed correlations. A positive relationship exists between two variables if one increases as the other increases and vice versa. A negative relationship exists if one variable increases as the other variable decreases. Figure 10.4 illustrates a positive relationship between number of freckles and sun exposure, and a negative relationship between hours of work and ability to concentrate. A **directional hypothesis** predicts that two variables will be related and as well predicts the direction of that relationship. It will predict, for example, that as the score for one variable increases, the score for a second variable will increase. A **nondirectional hypothesis** predicts that two variables will be related but does not predict the direction of that relationship.

Research questions can also be directional and nondirectional. If a researcher asks, "Is there a relationship between sun exposure and number of freckles?" this would be a nondirectional question. If a researcher asks, "Do the number of freckles increase as the amount of sun exposure increases?" this would be a directional research question. Whether a hypothesis or research question is directional or not depends on the current level of knowledge about the variables of interest or the extent to which theory has been developed about the variables. A well-developed theory proposes not only relationships among factors but also the direction of those relationships. Therefore, a study using such a theory would be more likely to have directional hypotheses.

If we look at the Grant et al. (2013) study (Appendix A-10), we find that the authors had one specific question. In fact, their specific question is the title of the study itself: "Why people living with HIV/AIDS exclude individuals from their chosen families?" This question was nondirectional, simply asking the reasons that individuals living with HIV/AIDS may exclude family members, rather than predicting that these individuals are more likely to exclude parents than siblings from their lives. An example of a directional research question might have been "Do people living with HIV/AIDS more frequently exclude parents from their lives than they exclude siblings?" This question includes a proposed direction for the effect of the intervention—that is, the intervention is proposed to reflect that parents are excluded more often than siblings are excluded from the lives of people living with HIV/AIDS.

Null and Research Hypotheses

In addition to hypotheses being directional or nondirectional, there are two forms for hypotheses: the null and research forms. We described research and null hypotheses in Chapter 5. The research hypothesis predicts relationships or differences in variables, whereas the null

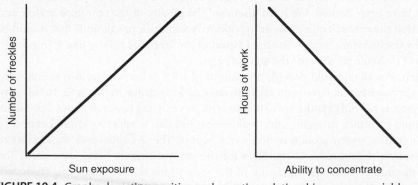

FIGURE 10.4 Graphs depicting positive and negative relationships among variables.

hypothesis states that there will be no relationship or differences among variables. Remember that the null hypothesis is developed for statistical purposes and represents the assumption made in inferential statistics that most relationships or differences that may be found in any particular sample might have occurred by chance alone. Only when a difference or relationship among variables found in a sample is so large that it would only occur by chance in fewer than 5% of samples can the null hypothesis or statistical hypothesis be rejected. Usually, when a study has a null hypothesis, an alternate hypothesis also is stated, and that alternate hypothesis will predict both a relationship and a direction to that relationship. The idea of a "null" form is not applied to research questions, only to predictions in the form of statements.

To illustrate the concept of null hypothesis, let us think about a study examining pregnancy behaviors to predict pregnancy outcomes using statistical hypotheses. Suppose that the purpose of the study was "to describe and compare the patterns of health-related behaviors, including smoking, alcohol use, use of prenatal care, exercise, and nutrition among women in rural and urban settings, and to test the relationship among these behaviors and the outcomes of low birth weight and premature birth." Two sets of possible hypotheses could be stated: First set of possible hypotheses comprises the following:

H_0: There will be no differences in the pattern of tobacco use among pregnant women from urban and rural settings.

H_1: Women from rural settings will use tobacco more when pregnant than will women from urban settings.

Second set of possible hypotheses comprises the following:

H_0: Timing and regularity of use of prenatal care will not be related to birthweight among rural and urban samples.

H_1: Earlier and more regular use of prenatal care will decrease the incidence of low-birth-weight infants in both the rural and urban samples.

The symbol "H_0" represents the null hypothesis, and "H_1" represents the alternate hypothesis. You can see that the null hypothesis is a neutral or negative prediction, written primarily to support the assumptions of inferential statistics. A study that is using research hypotheses without null hypotheses also may use the symbol of an uppercase "H," but they will be numbered consecutively as H_1, H_2, H_3, and so on. A researcher should only include hypotheses at the beginning of a study if there is some basis for the predictions from either previous research or theory, and the literature review should include the information from theory or research that supports the hypotheses.

LINKING THE LITERATURE REVIEW TO THE STUDY DESIGN

When we first discussed the literature review, we said that it should give us an overview of what is known about the study variables, how they have been previously studied, and with whom they have been studied. We have discussed the quality of the literature review and mentioned that the research questions or hypotheses are specific predictions that should be supported by the literature review. The final aspect of the literature review that is important is the support it should provide for the study design.

The literature review should provide a synthesis of what is known but also should synthesize the approaches that have been taken to develop knowledge in this area. In this way, a literature review not only synthesizes but also critiques existing research about a problem. A true critique identifies strengths and weaknesses, and this is what we should expect to see in the literature review section of a research report. The strengths and weaknesses of previous research should serve as the basis for the study currently being described. The researcher should tell us at the beginning of the report how the results of this study will fit within the overall structure of knowledge about the problem. For example, Grant et al.

(2013) (Appendix A-10) identify in the review of literature that most studies demonstrate that "because of the isolation, rejection, and stigmatization that are usually associated with HIV/AIDS, some people living with HIV (PLWH) become distant from their traditional families" (p. 35). They go on to state that, "PLWH manage to create chosen families that include those they consider family. Proximity, support, love, and acceptance, and biological ties appear to be important in defining the chosen families of PLWH. HIV disclosure appeared to . . . [be] . . . a gradual process and more PLWH disclosed . . . [their condition] . . . to those who provided emotional support and socialized with them" (p. 35).

This information supports a mixed method design because it identifies that human feelings (which are associated with qualitative methodology) influences choice (which can be quantified) of individuals that PLWH consider as their family. The authors also state that there is a need to understand the "ways that these social processes influence HIV vulnerability" (Grant et al., 2013, p. 35) which indicates how the findings from their study could fit with and increase existing knowledge.

A literature review may specifically address problems in study design from previous research or limitations of past samples. The literature review also may synthesize and critique the existing literature without directly addressing design and sampling issues. However, in either case, one of the purposes of the literature review is to identify the rationale for the design used in the study. Like a well-written story, each section or chapter should build a foundation for the next section or chapter. Choices of research design should be based on approaches taken in the past, with the goal of improving on or expanding on previous knowledge.

In summary, the background and literature review sections of a research report set the stage for the remainder of the study. The background gives the broad context for the research problem and an overview of factors relevant to that problem. This overview may present an abstract set of concepts and their relationships to one another called a *theory, conceptual framework,* or *theoretical framework.* The background usually ends with a statement of a research purpose or questions that specify the variables to be studied. The literature review starts with the purpose and describes the current state of the science in relation to the study variables. To do so, the literature review must be current and use mostly primary sources from peer-reviewed journals. The literature review should include what is known about the variables, and how and with whom they have been studied. It establishes the basis for the design of the study and may end in specific research questions or hypotheses.

PUBLISHED REPORTS—HAS THE CASE BEEN MADE FOR THE RESEARCH STUDY?

We began this study wondering about quality-of-life outcomes for patients who have had mastectomy alone and breast reconstruction (Eltahir et al., 2013). If we examine the literature review found in the Eltahir et al. (2013) article, we find that some studies in the past have focused on this issue. The authors' critique of existing literature reflects that one study showed no significant different in quality-of-life outcomes between women who underwent mastectomy alone, versus lumpectomy, versus breast reconstruction; another study identified that rigorous patient-reported outcomes data should be the focus of future research, and a systematic review (Winters et al., in Eltahir et al., 2013) identified that most studies on this topic were weakly designed, with marked limitations, and likely biased (Eltahir et al., 2013). The information about findings and limitations of previous studies set the stage for the researchers' review, using clearly identified inclusion and exclusion criteria in order to organize and categorize their findings.

After reading the introduction of the Eltahir et al.'s (2013) article, the therapist in our clinical case has more information to use in understanding the findings from the review, understanding the general problem that the study is attempting to address, and understanding the specific aim of the review. The therapist notes that this research shows that patients do benefit from breast reconstruction, and that more importantly, patient education is an important key to empowering patients to make autonomous, informed decisions about their individualized treatment plan (Eltahir et al., 2013). The therapist understands that empowerment can greatly reduce patient anxiety. Therefore, she is confident in this evidence-based information that will guide her dialog with patients, which will include encouragement for patients to seek full information from their medical professional about all available individualized treatment options before making a decision.

At the end of Chapter 9, you were asked to make a case for why a study of the well-being of students in healthcare major should be implemented. After reading this chapter, you should have a clearer idea about how you might have developed that rationale and why it can be an important part of a research report. The background and literature review set the stage for the rest of the research report by giving us a general setting for the study in terms of the problem; the specific purpose of the study, including the study variables; and an understanding of how this study will fit with current theory and research-based knowledge.

COMMON ERRORS IN REPORTS OF THE BACKGROUND AND LITERATURE REVIEW

One of the first errors that may occur in the background and literature review sections of a research report is a failure to develop a consistent link among the research problem, the research purpose, and any specific hypotheses or questions. The fictional article that describes the study of nursing students' choices of practice after graduation (Appendix B) gives a good example of a background that does not directly link the problem, purpose, and research questions. The introduction to that report discusses the general problem of the nursing shortage and the need for workforce planning. It then states that in addition to the sheer number of students, we must consider choice of practice in workforce planning, indicating that specific sites for practice will have greater needs for nurses in the future. International differences are mentioned, but there is no further mention of international aspects through the rest of the report. The next section, titled "Background," continues with the thread that students who will choose the most severe shortage sites should be targeted for recruitment to schools of nursing and concludes with a research purpose to "examine the relationships among nursing students' demographic characteristics and their choices for practice following graduation." At this point, the connections become weak. After the research purpose, the author lists three specific questions, the first of which addresses specific demographic variables (age, gender, race, and marital status), but the second and third introduce new variables, students' well-being and students' experiences that relate to their choices of practice, that have not been mentioned at any point in the preceding section. This is like an author of fiction placing an entirely new character into the middle of a story without connecting that character to anything or anyone in the previous part of the story.

The example in the fictional article is somewhat extreme, and what makes it an even poorer example is that no literature review is included. Consequently, we have no idea of what research has been done with students and choice of practice, what methods were used to conduct the research, or what types of students were studied. Published research reports vary in the consistency and links that they draw among the research problem, the purpose, and specific measurable questions. If, as an intelligent reader of research, you finish the background and literature review section and still do not know what is going to be studied and why, one explanation may be that connections among the problem, the purpose, and the research questions have not been clearly or consistently identified in this section of the report.

A second problem that can occur is a failure to provide the information needed to fulfill the important purposes for these sections. For example, a literature review may provide a thoughtful synthesis of what is known about the variables of interest in the study but may fail to connect it to the purpose of the study being reported. This can leave us uncertain concerning the basis for the researcher's selection of research design and approach to measurement or how the study will fit with current knowledge.

Another problem that can occur is a failure to adequately reference statements. If the author of a research report makes a statement about the variables of interest that reflects knowledge that is not common and does not provide a reference, then we are left wondering how much we can trust the statement. We must wonder whether the statement is simply the opinion of the researcher, some stray fact that was found on the Internet, or a well-documented research-based piece of knowledge. Occasionally, the number of references imbedded in a sentence, in a literature review, can almost be distracting from the meaning of the sentence, but those references assure us that the information is well founded and accurate.

The last potential problems with background and literature review sections of research reports are those we have discussed: the use of secondary sources and out-of-date references. The point of these beginning sections is to give us a clear and accurate picture of the state of knowledge about the research problem and to develop a coherent set of connections between that knowledge and the specific research purpose and questions. Secondary sources and references that are all more than 3 to 5 years older than the date of publication of the study do not give us much confidence that the study will fit well with current levels of knowledge.

CRITICALLY READING BACKGROUND AND LITERATURE REVIEW SECTIONS OF A RESEARCH REPORT FOR USE IN EBP

There are seven questions that you can ask yourself as you read the background and literature review sections of research reports, and these are listed in Box 10.2. We will take these one by one and examine each more closely. First, and most obvious, is "Does the report include a clearly identified background and/or literature review section?" Several of the reports that we have read in previous chapters do not clearly identify the background or literature review; they simply start with a statement of a problem or concern and then describe literature relevant to that problem, eventually concluding with a research question or purpose. The lack of specific headings may or may not interfere with your understanding about why a study was implemented. You will have to judge whether this is a problem.

BOX 10.2
How to Critically Read the Background Section of a Research Report?

Does the report answer the question "Why ask that question—what do we know?"

1. Does the report include a clearly identified background and/or literature review section?
2. Do I think the background discusses aspects of my clinical question?
3. Does the literature help me understand why the research question is important to nursing?
4. Is the majority of the literature cited current (less than 3 to 5 years old) or very important to understanding the research question?
5. If a nursing or other theory was presented, does it connect to my clinical question?
6. Is the specific research question/problem/hypothesis connected logically to the literature and/or theory presented in the background section?
7. Is the specific research question/problem/hypothesis relevant or related to my clinical question?

A second question is "Do I think the background discusses aspects of my clinical question?" The therapist in our clinical case selected this article to gain a better understanding of quality of life in patients who underwent mastectomy alone versus breast reconstruction (Eltahir et al., 2013). A third question that is related is "Does the literature help me understand why the research question is important to my specific healthcare profession, and/or my particular patient?" One aspect that we would expect to find in the literature review, sometimes explicitly and at other times implicitly, is identification of the relevance of the research question to the healthcare team member's healthcare profession, and/or the healthcare team member's patient.

The next question to ask yourself is "Is the majority of the literature cited current (less than 3 to 5 years old) or very important to understanding the research question?" Some reports may include literature that is dated and neither seems relevant nor addresses the stated problem for the research. Keep in mind that there will be times that the researchers need to refer to historical research studies, yet if the majority of the literature is excessively dated or irrelevant to the stated research problem, you will want to question whether that article has relevant enough information to be considered the best evidence available.

The fifth question, "If theory was presented, does it connect to my clinical question?" also addresses congruency and logical building of content in a background and literature review. If you read any research report and find in it a description of a theory that is not later connected to the purpose or question addressed in the research, you should wonder why it was included at all. As we stated earlier, theory can be a very important source of research problems, and often a background section describes a theoretical framework or conceptual model to support the approach taken to a clinical problem. But if that theoretical framework or conceptual model does not seem to be relevant to your clinical question and is not used in a specific manner to establish the research study, then it is superfluous and detracts from the reader's understanding of a study.

The sixth and seventh questions are related: "Is the specific research question/problem/hypothesis connected logically to the literature and/or theory presented in the background section?" and "Is the specific research question/problem/hypothesis relevant or related to my clinical question?" Thus, these questions critically examine the specific research purpose or question or hypotheses, and ask whether these flowed from the background and literature review, providing a specific focus for the research study that addresses the clinical question of interest. Remember the analogy of these sections resembling a story. If this story concludes with an unrelated ending, we clearly recognize that it is not a very good story. Similarly, if the specific research question, problem, or hypothesis is not connected to the background and literature review "story" that has preceded it, the quality of those sections have to be questioned. Moreover, if the specific research question, problem, or hypothesis does not seem relevant to the clinical question of interest, then reading and understanding the rest of the report will not be particularly useful.

OUT-OF-CLASS EXERCISE

Pulling It All Together

We have now completed the second section of this book. We have looked at the entire research report, starting with the conclusions and moving forward to the background and literature review. As we discussed the sections, we also focused on selected aspects of the research process. The last two chapters return to the traditional approach to discussing research: starting at the beginning of a study or report and moving to the end. We discuss how the research process is related to the published research report. We also examine the history of research and how EBP and quality improvement relate to the research process. To prepare you for these chapters and to help you pull together the different sections of a research report, write an abstract that describes a research problem addressed by the in-class exercise. Decide on one question that you think could have been answered by that study. Then, in approximately 250 words (one page, double spaced), write an abstract that includes (1) background, (2) objective or purpose, (3) methods, (4) results, and (5) conclusions. If you have had the opportunity, you may be able to use real results generated in your class. If not, make up the results. The point of the exercise is to write a concise description of a research study using the specific language of research. Go back and read some of the abstracts of the research reports that we have used in this book or find some published research of interest to you to serve as examples of what your abstract should look like. Remember that abstracts are organized differently in different journals, but for this exercise, try to use the five headings listed in this paragraph.

If you did not have an in-class study, you may want to take the fictional article from Appendix B and think of another research question that might be addressed, given the variables in that study, or at least rewrite the abstract for the study using the headings listed in the previous paragraph. After you have completed this exercise, you are ready to move on to Chapter 11.

References

*Ainsworth, M. D. S., & Bowlby, J. (1991). An ethological approach to personality development. *American Psychologist*, 46, 331–341.

Ananthakrishnan, A. N., Gainer, V. S., Perez, R. G., Cai, T., Cheng, S. C., Savova, G., . . . Liao, K. P. (2013). Psychiatric co-morbidity is associated with increased risk of surgery in Crohn's disease. *Alimentary pharmacology & therapeutics*, 37(4), 445–454.

Eltahir, Y., Werners, L., Dreise, M. M., van Emmichoven, I. A., Jansen, L., Werker, P. M., & de Bock, G. H. (2013). Quality-of-life outcomes between mastectomy along and breast reconstruction: Comparison of patient reported BREAST-Q and other health-related quality-of-life measures. *Plastic and Reconstructive Surgery*, 132(2), 201e–209e. doi:10.1097/PRS.0b013e31829586a7

Grant, J., Vance, D., White, W., Keltner, N., & Raper, J. (2013). Why people living with HIV/AIDS exclude individuals from their chosen families. *Nursing: Research & Reviews*, 2013(3), 33–42.

*Sackett, D. L., Rosenberg, W. M. C., Gray, J. A. M., Haynes, R. B., & Richardson, W. S. (1996). Evidence based medicine: What it is and what it isn't. *British Medical Journal*, 312(7023), 71–72.

*indicates a definitive or classic work or publication regarding this subject matter.

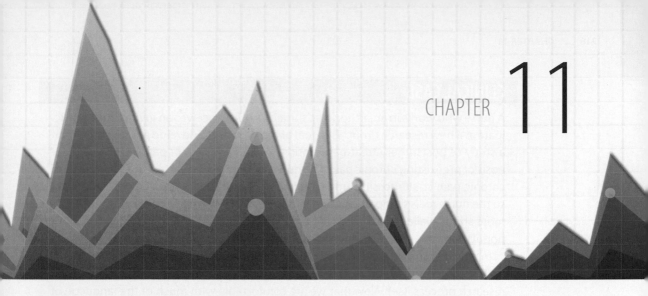

CHAPTER 11

The Research Process

How Is the Research Process Related to a Published Research Report?

LEARNING OBJECTIVE The student will relate the process of research to the sections of published research reports and to the healthcare decision making processes.

The Research Process

Define and Describe the Knowledge Gap or Problem
Develop a Plan to Gather Information
Implement the Study
Analyze and Interpret the Results
Disseminate the Findings

Research Process Contrasted to the Research Report
Factors that Affect the Research Process
Generating Knowledge Through Research Can Be Fun!
Published Reports—What Do You Conclude Now?
Conclusion

KEY TERMS

Aggregated data
Assumptions
Codebook

Dissemination
Pilot study

CLINICAL CASE

A nurse who works in an orthopedic surgeon's office receives an invitation to participate in a new research group. The goal of the group is to develop and to implement
a study of postsurgery treatment options to address pain in patients with a diagnosis of preexisting chronic pain. The nurse recognizes that an existing diagnosis of
chronic pain could possibly impact a patient's perception of pain postoperatively,
so the nurse feels that participation in this research group would allow him to learn
more about available postsurgical treatments that could be of benefit to his patient
population.

In previous chapters, we learned about the different sections of a research report
and discussed the process of doing research, but we have not yet focused on the
research process itself. Now that we are comfortable with much of the language of
research and with some fundamental elements of the aspects of the research process that are reflected in a research report, it is time to look at the research process
as a whole. This chapter describes the research process from beginning to end, links
that process to the research report, and discusses the relationship between the research process and healthcare decision making processes.

THE RESEARCH PROCESS

In Chapter 2, we briefly described the five steps of the research process:

1. Define and describe the knowledge gap or problem.
2. Develop a detailed plan to gather information to address the problem or gap in
   knowledge.
3. Implement the study.
4. Analyze and interpret the results of the study.
5. Disseminate the findings of the study.

A process is, by definition, fluid and flexible. Processes include a series of steps, or activities, which must be taken in order to achieve results. Sometimes, certain steps within a
process are necessary before one can successfully move to the next step. In other cases, the
steps do not always follow one another in a step-by-step manner. Sometimes, these steps
occur simultaneously, and at other times, the results of a step in the process leads cyclically
to returning to a preceding step.

CORE CONCEPT 11.1

The steps of the research process are not always linear: they may overlap or be
revisited during the research process.

A refined research purpose is necessary before beginning to develop a detailed research
plan, but it is possible that as a plan is developed, the research purpose may be revisited
and refined further. Similarly, a research plan is needed before a study is implemented,
but it is possible that as the study is implemented, the plan will be revised. In fact, in most

qualitative methods, the methods are expected to change as the study progresses. Although this chapter discusses the steps of the research process in order, the actual process may be more fluid and flexible in action.

Define and Describe the Knowledge Gap or Problem

The nurse in our clinical case finds that by attending the first meeting of the group; this is the start of the first step in the research process. The lead researcher begins by describing a question that has been developed based on the previous work with patients with chronic pain who have undergone surgical hip replacement. The researcher has noticed that in many cases, these patients have reported an increase in the severity of their chronic pain after undergoing hip replacement surgery. One member of the research group wonders what factors contribute to patients' perception of chronic pain before and after surgery. Another member states their belief that opioid pain medication should automatically be increased after surgery, since it stands to reason that pain perception increases in the postoperative state. Other members of the group state that they believe that patients overestimate the severity of their pain, and that no adjustment in opioid medication should be prescribed postsurgery. Then, another member of the group suggests that a surgeon's willingness to fully assess the patient's chronic pain status is an important factor in determining what postsurgical treatments may be needed. The nurse in our clinical case suggests that coexisting diagnoses, such as depression, may influence the patient's perception of severity of chronic pain.

It is obvious to the nurse that at this point in the group's process, there is no agreement about the knowledge gap that must be addressed. Each individual's input about the factors influencing perception of chronic pain, and use of opioid medications for this condition before and after hip replacement surgery, is different, and is based on their own personal professional experience. Creating a flowchart of all the ideas that have been discussed is suggested. Once a group sees all its ideas in a flowchart, it begins to identify some of the areas that it must explore further. For example, the group identifies that it must find out what is known about the use of opioids for chronic pain after hip replacement surgery. The uses of opioids for chronic pain, and the status of having undergone hip replacement surgery, are recognized as two separate, yet connected, concepts. The group agrees that it will focus on the use of opioids for chronic pain after hip replacement surgery, but will consider how the use of opioids for chronic pain prior to hip replacement surgery may also be a factor in continued use postoperatively. They also agree that they need to know more about patient perceptions of chronic pain in the preoperative and postoperative stages. The members of the group divide the list of various ideas they have discussed and agree to conduct a literature review focusing on a particular subset of ideas, returning in 2 weeks to share what they have found. The process described in this hypothetical situation illustrates aspects of the first step in the research process.

The information required for this first step will be acquired from existing theory and research to identify what is known about the problem and the relevant factors related to the problem. This step also requires thoughtful analysis because rarely does theory or past research easily blend into an obvious research purpose. At this point in the research process, often what is needed is an explosion of ideas and information, all of which then must be thoughtfully analyzed and synthesized to develop a refined purpose. The brainstorming session that our nurse experienced may be the first of several sessions in which many ideas are explored, validation and information about those ideas are sought and digested, and new ideas are generated. This step can be both exciting and frustrating: exciting because of the amount to be discovered about a problem of interest and frustrating because of the amount to digest and integrate to develop a refined research purpose.

For example, our hypothetical research group may find a great deal of information about opioid use for treatment of chronic pain. They also may find a good amount of information about how patients perceive (general) pain. However, they discover that little has been done in comparing and contrasting perceptions of chronic pain preoperatively and postoperatively, nor in studying the use of opioids for chronic pain after a procedure as specific as hip replacement surgery. Perhaps, the focus primarily has been on treating general postoperative pain. The group does find theory about the concept of postoperative opioid use. They also found several studies that conclude by recognizing the importance of control of chronic pain. Yet, they find few current research studies that link postoperative opioid use to chronic pain after hip replacement surgery, or that measure the use of opioids for chronic pain preoperatively versus postoperatively. Despite this lack of literature, the nurse believes, from personal professional experience, that there is a connection that may influence how patients experience chronic pain postoperatively versus preoperatively that in turn, influences the amount of opioids that may be necessary to effectively treat the pain.

All of these findings leave the group with even more information than they compiled when they brainstormed and with no immediately obvious connections between all the possible factors that it might consider. This is what was meant by an "explosion of information": as ideas are analyzed in this step of the research process, they sometimes explode into multiple new ideas to explore.

Despite the potential explosion of information, notice that our hypothetical group has now acquired a foundation of knowledge about what is known, has been theoretically considered, or has been studied in the past. Developing that foundation of knowledge is the goal of the first step of the research process. That foundation of existing knowledge should include existing research, practice experience, and any appropriate and relevant theory. The challenge then becomes synthesizing the existing knowledge; critically examining practice experience, theory, and past research; and identifying a research purpose that includes specific factors or variables to be studied. Notice also that the foundation of knowledge located strongly supports the relevancy of the problem that this group has identified for healthcare practice.

In addition to establishing a foundation of knowledge about the research problem, another part of this first step entails identifying assumptions that are embedded in the approach to the problem and the purposes being considered. **Assumptions** are ideas that are taken for granted or viewed as truth without conscious or explicit testing. Assumptions can be difficult to identify, because they are ideas that we "just know" or "all understand" and are usually unspoken. However, assumptions can sometimes impact how a research problem is viewed so that the approach to knowledge development is limited in some way. Identifying the assumptions embedded in a study can be helpful because we may realize that the assumptions must be researched and confirmed before we can move forward in knowledge development. In the hypothetical study that we are discussing, there is an assumption that patients with existing chronic pain who undergo hip replacement surgery will postoperatively experience continuation of, and possibly an increase in, chronic pain.

As the research problem is refined into a specific purpose, the types of questions that will be addressed and the approach likely to be taken are often beginning to be identified. We previously discussed how research questions that address prediction or examine the effects of manipulation of a variable require a relatively large amount of background or foundational knowledge. It becomes increasingly clear to our hypothetical research group that not enough research or theory exists about comparison and contrast of perception of chronic pain, nor use of opioids for chronic pain before and after hip replacement surgery, to make predictions or to plan to manipulate any factor. Because the researchers cannot find studies and theory that convince them to predict that a certain variable will have a desired outcome, they realize that they must consider questions about perceptions of chronic pain preoperatively and postoperatively, and relationships between variables influencing opioid use before and after hip replacement surgery.

The group also begins to consider whether a qualitative, quantitative, or mixed methods approach is most logical as it begins to refine the general problem of understanding opioid use for chronic pain before and after hip replacement surgery. Some of the group argues that because so little has been studied regarding this relationship, the first study should be phenomenological so that the researchers can understand how the patient perceive chronic pain before and after surgery. Others believe that theories about relationships about the use of opioids for generalized chronic pain, as well as past research about opioid use for postsurgical pain, provide a set of relevant factors that can be measured and tested to see how they affect opioid use for chronic pain before and after hip replacement surgery. These members think that a correlational study is what is needed.

It is not uncommon that during the first step of the research process, several potential research studies are identified that are relevant to the problem. Refining a problem clarifies the nature of the gaps in knowledge as well as the factors relevant to the problem. In many cases, the problems of interest to healthcare are too complex to address in a single study. Let us assume for now that after several meetings, substantial discussion, and review of theory and the literature, the hypothetical group in our clinical case agrees on a tentative purpose: to identify and examine factors that affect patient perception of chronic pain before and after hip replacement surgery, and opioid use for treatment and management of this chronic pain preoperatively and postoperatively. These factors become the variables of our study. This purpose will probably need further refining, which will occur as the group moves into the second step of the research process. In this next step, the group takes the purpose it has identified, and develops a specific research plan that includes the research design and methods of measurement and sampling.

Develop a Plan to Gather Information

As the purpose for a study is refined, ideas about gathering information about the problem being studied also begin to generate. As researchers review past research studies regarding the problem, they consider not only the findings from that research but also the methods and samples used. This helps to clarify gaps in knowledge, and identifies measures and approaches that previously have been successful in addressing the problem. For example, our hypothetical research group has found that most studies of opioid use for chronic pain have been conducted with adults who suffer from generalized chronic pain rather than (more specifically) with adults with chronic pain who have had a surgical procedure for hip replacement. They also found that many of the studies have focused on a single episodic analysis of perceptions of chronic pain as the focus of study. Because this group is interested in long-term management of chronic pain after hip replacement surgery, it knows that it needs a different research method, since looking at an isolated episodic analysis will not provide the information they need.

The second step of the research process is complex, and involves many considerations and decisions. This step includes deciding on the general approach to be taken to the study and a specific research design; identifying and developing plans for the study sample or participants; and planning the measurement process, including specific techniques, measures, and timing. Finally, at the end of this step, an IRB proposal must be written and submitted in preparation for implementation of the study.

The group in our clinical case eventually decides that a mixed methods approach makes the most sense, beginning with a phenomenological study of patients' perceptions of chronic pain. It plans to follow this with a descriptive correlational study about how the factors they have identified from research and practice affect opioid use for chronic pain before and after surgery. This becomes the purpose of their research: to understand patients' perception of chronic pain, and to investigate the role of opioid use for chronic pain before and after hip replacement surgery.

The refined purpose described reflects several decisions that have been made by the research group. It has decided that a phenomenological approach is appropriate because it will help the researchers understand the perception of chronic pain that patients who undergo a surgical experience for hip replacement, both preoperatively and postoperatively. The group has ruled out doing a true longitudinal study, as this requires more time and resources than a cross-sectional correlational study. The group has also settled on two outcomes—understanding perception of chronic pain, and the role of opioid use in treating this condition in patients before and after hip replacement surgery.

Thus, the second step of the research process requires critical thinking and decision making. Researchers must consider what is known, what has been shown to work, and what is feasible. The last consideration includes issues of time, cost, established measures or approaches, and other resources, such as space or access to samples. We will discuss these further when we discuss factors that affect research.

Decisions about the best possible methods for implementing the chosen study designs must also be made during this part of the research process. In the case of the phenomenological phase of the hypothetical study, researchers must make decisions about methods of data collection, such as interviews, observations, or use of journaling, as well as the timing for the data collection. Similarly, to implement the descriptive correlational phase of the study, researchers will have to make decisions about measures, such as chart audits, and the use of a questionnaire (or other instrument) or a structured interview. The issues of rigor, validity, and reliability that we discussed in Chapters 8 and 9 are central to making these decisions about methods and measurement.

Another important part of the second step is deciding on the sample for the study and approaches to the process of sampling, as discussed in Chapter 6. Although the group plans to measure opioid use for chronic pain before and after hip replacement surgery, it recognizes that the length of time into each patient's postoperative phase may affect their individual results. The phenomenological phase of the study will benefit from researchers' talking with several patients who have experienced chronic pain before and after hip replacement surgery. After discussion, the research group decides to limit the study to persons who experienced chronic pain for 2 years or more before having hip replacement surgery, and are not more than 2 years past hip replacement surgery. This decision is based on the experience of the researcher, our nurse in the clinical case, and several other group members who suggest that patients experience pain, and treatments for pain, differently at varying times within their lifespan.

In addition to deciding who will participate in the study, the group in our clinical case must consider how comfortable patients will be when talking about their personal experiences with pain, opioid use, and hip replacement surgery when they know there is a study in progress. This would be an example of the Hawthorne effect described in Chapter 9. Patients might be concerned about repercussions on their care if they express any negative feelings. These issues could lead to a threat to internal validity from testing and to researcher effects threatening external validity. The research group decides to use individuals who are not associated with the patients' healthcare providers in any way as data collectors and to put extra effort into ensuring anonymity of participants and subjects to address this concern.

The hypothetical group in our clinical case will make other specific decisions as it moves through the second step, and the details of these decisions could probably fill several chapters. Overall, this process is based on a further exploration of the past research to identify research designs and methods that have been used, measures that are available and sampling considerations. This research literature, along with the realities of the specific setting for the research, the knowledge and experience of the researchers, and resources such as time and money, all will be considered in developing a detailed plan to gather information about the research purpose. Box 11.1 summarizes these and other considerations affecting the development of the research plan.

> **BOX 11.1**
> **Considerations Affecting the Development of the Detailed Research Plan**
>
> - Methods and samples used in previous research
> - Potential setting(s) for the study
> - Experience and knowledge of the researcher(s)
> - Resources available, such as time and money
> - Subject safety and rights
> - Rigor, reliability, and validity

Once a detailed plan is developed, the last part of this second step is to ensure the protection of human subjects and to acquire the resources needed for the study. We discussed informed consent and the role of IRBs in Chapter 7. IRB approval will require a written proposal describing the study background, purpose, literature review, design, and measures, and how the rights of subjects will be assured. Depending where a study will be conducted, IRB approval from multiple locations may be required. Developing this type of IRB proposal not only helps a researcher or research group to tighten the details of their plan of study but also takes time and must be considered when planning a time line for a research study. In addition, many studies cannot be implemented without acquiring some outside resources to support the time and materials needed. Depending on the complexity of the proposed study and the resources inherent in the study site, researchers often must write and submit proposals for funding before they can implement it. This process can take weeks to months. However, both the review of IRB proposals and the funding proposals provide outside input into the plans for a research study and often significantly improve those plans before the study is implemented.

Implement the Study

The third step in the research process is to implement the study. This is when the advance planning and decisions can pay off and when unexpected issues can arise. One of the biggest responsibilities of the researcher during implementation is to maintain meticulous documentation of the sampling and data collection process. This documentation allows the researcher to later clearly identify any points in the study at which plans were changed and the rationale for decisions made during the implementation process. Areas that may need to be addressed and documented during this step include data about numbers and characteristics of those who were approached to be in the study but declined or later dropped out, any revisions in sampling criteria, any changes in the timing or the measurement process, and any anecdotal or incidental data that becomes relevant during the study implementation.

In Chapters 6 and 8, we discussed things that can go wrong with sampling and measurement, and how important it is to consider those aspects when deciding on the usefulness of research for practice. The careful documentation kept by researchers during the study implementation is the basis for reporting information that will allow us to evaluate the sampling and measurement process. In addition, incidents or occurrences that are unexpected may have a big effect on the meaning of results of a study. For example, suppose that patients who had one particular surgeon declined to be in our hypothetical study. Or, suppose that as the study is implemented, patients start approaching the research staff and ask to participate before they have been recruited. Either of these observations suggests that there may be some underlying factor at work during the process of study implementation. In the first case, that factor may be a surgeon eliminate, who has told patients not to participate, because the surgeon is unhappy about the study, thus eliminating data about relationships with a provider who is controlling. In the second case, the underlying factor might be that patients have a strong need to talk about their experiences with chronic pain before and after hip replacement surgery, which this study is meeting. This unmet need may be important to consider when gaining understanding about patients' experiences with chronic pain. One could speculate about the meaning of either observation, but what is important is to document the observation for future consideration as the results of the study are analyzed.

During the study implementation, the steps of the research process may be particularly fluid, moving back and forth between this step and the previous step of planning or to the next step of analysis and interpretation. As we discussed in Chapter 8, in the implementation step, qualitative methods depend on a spiraling process of data collection followed by data analysis and interpretation that informs the next round of data collection. Sometimes, during the study implementation, the plans for sampling prove to be unrealistic, perhaps because criteria are too strict or because the desired subjects for the study are not willing to participate. The researchers will then have to revise their sampling plan to implement the study. Or perhaps data collectors note that all subjects are confused and have difficulty answering some part of a questionnaire. The researchers will have to use this information to decide whether to change their measures in the middle of their study or to continue with a measure that may have problems with reliability. These are just a few examples of the many kinds of problems that can be encountered during the study implementation. The process requires time, care, consistency, and ongoing monitoring.

Analyze and Interpret the Results

The fourth step of the research process involves the analysis and interpretation of study results. As we indicated, this step may be interwoven with the step of implementation in a qualitative study. In contrast, most of the data analysis in a quantitative study is usually reserved until the entire data collection process is complete. This difference reflects the differences in philosophy behind the two types of approaches. A qualitative method uses data as it is generated to build additional data, with the goal of arriving at information that is dense and thick to inform our understanding of a phenomenon. Quantitative methods strive to control and isolate phenomena to understand each discrete element. Therefore, quantitative methods defer analysis of most of the data until the collection process is complete to avoid contaminating the data collection process with ideas generated from the analysis. The exception to this is in analysis of sample characteristics. A purposive sample or a matched sample, as discussed in Chapter 6, requires the analysis of subject characteristics during the study implementation to effectively implement the sampling plan.

Data analysis, whether carried out in a qualitative or quantitative study, requires the same level of meticulous care and documentation that is needed during the implementation step of the research process. In qualitative research, this is accomplished through the audit trail and notations within the software programs that are often used during data analysis. In quantitative research, decisions about data analysis are often documented in a codebook. In research, a **codebook** is a record of the categorization, labeling, and manipulation of data about variables in a quantitative study. It includes information about how each of the variables in the study was measured; how the data from the study were reviewed and transferred into computer files; and all decisions made regarding the management of problems, such as incomplete responses or confusing responses. Like an audit trail, a codebook provides a detailed description of how the data from a study were managed.

Qualitative data are often collected in an interview, so the first thing that must be done is to transcribe the data into a word-processing program. This can be a very time-consuming process that the researcher must plan for when designing the study. Once transcribed, the data can be either loaded into a qualitative analysis program or printed and analyzed on hard copy. In either case, data management often includes careful reading and listening to interviews that have been transcribed to ensure that the transcription is accurate and complete. Similarly, quantitative data have to be entered into computer software programs to be analyzed. This can be done in several ways, including direct entry of numbers from quantitative measurement into a data file or use of an optical scanner that reads and records numbers of a data collection measure into a data file. In either case, once it is in a data file, the data must be carefully examined for accuracy. Human error in keying numbers into a file or computer error in scanning answer sheets can significantly affect and even invalidate study results.

The researcher can proceed with the analysis and interpretation of the results once data have been put into a form that allows that process. As discussed in Chapters 4 and 5, data analysis is complex and challenging. It also is an exciting time in the research process, because the researchers begin to find out what their study says about the research problem that started this whole process. In addition to information about data management, codebooks in quantitative data analysis often include information about decisions regarding analysis approaches and the mathematical manipulation of the data. For example, a researcher can decide to use a mean score of items from a measure of a variable in the analysis or to use a score that is just the sum of all the items. Alternatively, a researcher may decide to study all subjects as one large group in which members have differences on a variable of interest or to divide subjects into two groups that clearly differ on that variable. All of these types of decisions are usually documented in the codebook so that as the research progresses, the researcher can recall those decisions and the rationale behind them. Thus, both the audit trail and the codebook reflect documentation of data management and analysis, which are important aspects of the fourth step of the research process.

Interpretation is the last part of this step. Interpretation of the results of a study entails pulling the whole process together into a meaningful whole. The theory and research literature that served as a foundation for the study, the decisions made in the planning step of the process, and the decisions and observations that were made during the implementation step all must be considered and tied into the results of a study. At this point, the expertise of the researchers and their personal knowledge and experience are also used in interpreting results. For example, suppose that during the implementation of the hypothetical study introduced earlier in this chapter, patients started hearing about the study and asking staff to be included. The research team will have to decide why this occurred and how it affected the data collected. The research team in our clinical case may decide that this interest in participating in the study reflected a strong need on the patients' part to express their feelings about chronic pain that they have experienced. Or, they may project that the interest in participating in the study provides a forum for patients who want to express their displeasure with how their chronic pain has been managed by their healthcare provider after hip replacement surgery. These are different interpretations and would have different meanings for the results of the study. It is important to remember that these subjective interpretations do not necessarily represent the reality of the findings; a different study would need to be done to accurately understand the true meaning of the actions of the patients who asked to be included in the study.

Disseminate the Findings

The last step of the research process brings us back to where we started in this book—to the research report. **Dissemination** of research findings refers to the spreading of knowledge and is an essential step in the research process because knowledge development is wasted unless it becomes known so that it can be used. The dissemination of research findings may be accomplished in several ways. Findings may be disseminated through a report of the research to the agency or organization that funded or hosted the study. This type of dissemination is targeted at the specific groups that were closely involved in the study. Often, the results of a research study also are reported back to participants in that study. In addition, findings from a study may be verbally reported in the form of presentations to agencies or funding groups, or at scholarly and professional meetings. Findings from research are reported in published journals in print and online formats, and are sometimes disseminated to the public through the lay press, television, or other medium. Each of these types of approaches to dissemination of findings targets different groups of potential users of the research, with the report to those closely involved in the study clearly reaching a much smaller group than a published article in a major professional journal.

Because research dissemination targets different groups, the depth and detail of the dissemination vary. However, in all cases, the goal of dissemination is to accurately share the knowledge gained from the research so that it is useful and meaningful to the targeted recipients of that knowledge. For example, a summary of a research study that is being sent out in a regional newsletter will probably focus on a brief description of the problem, the sample, and one or two key findings. A presentation of a paper reporting the findings of a study at a professional meeting will usually be limited to 15 or 20 min, allowing inclusion of more detail than a newsletter column but less than what would be included in a published report in a research journal. A published report in a practice-focused journal will probably include fewer specifics about the research process than a report appearing in a research journal. However, in all cases, the researcher must be sure that the findings of a study are clearly and accurately stated.

The other consideration that is important for all types of dissemination is ensuring the anonymity of subjects or participants in a study. This requires that data primarily are reported in the aggregate and that there is careful scrutiny of that data. **Aggregated data** mean that the results from the study are reported for the entire sample rather than for individual members in the group. Usually, when data are aggregated, no specific result from the study can be attributed to any participant in the study. However, with a small sample, it is possible that even with aggregated data and elimination of any traditional identifiers, the anonymity of individual subjects might be lost.

For example, suppose that the hypothetical study we are discussing in this chapter acquired a sample of 50 subjects. One characteristic of subjects that will be reported is race, and perhaps only three subjects in the study were from a certain culture. Further, suppose that there was one finding stating a difference in patients' perceptions of staff by race, with Hispanic patients reporting much more negative experiences with outcomes associated with opioid use for chronic pain following hip replacement surgery. The staff on the surgical unit could read those results and likely know immediately which patients reported negative experiences because they have so few Hispanic patients, thus eliminating the anonymity of those patients. In this type of circumstance, it is possible that a result may have to be withheld from dissemination to protect the rights of the subjects in the study. Given that the reason the results may breech anonymity is because the numbers of Hispanic patients was so small and, therefore, that the results may have happened by chance alone and must be confirmed with a larger sample, the withholding of such a result does not jeopardize knowledge development.

It should be noted that even at this last step in the research process, a researcher might revisit an earlier step. Sometimes only when writing up the findings of a study does a researcher discover the need to consider and report a specific descriptive result or conduct a particular statistical test. Sometimes after sharing findings from a study with others, suggestions are made for additional analysis that may shed further light on the research problem. Of course, the findings from a study often raise new questions or suggest new research problems, taking us back to the first step.

It should be clear from this description of the research process that it is complex, exacting, and challenging (Box 11.2). The dissemination product of that research often does not provide a full picture of all the thought and work that went into a research study. Throughout this book, we have discussed common errors that can occur in a research report. However, any report of research deserves to be read with respect because of the effort and risk taken by the researcher to implement the research process and then make public the results of his or her efforts. Few research studies are perfect, and research reports certainly vary in their

BOX 11.2
Characteristics of the Research Process

- Systematic
- Exacting
- Complex
- Challenging

completeness and usefulness to practice. However, reports of research reflect a substantial time commitment of one or more individuals to address a gap in knowledge through the use of the complex and often strenuous process of research. The next section looks more closely at how and why publications of research do not always fully reflect the research process.

RESEARCH PROCESS CONTRASTED TO THE RESEARCH REPORT

In Chapter 2, we discussed the relationship between the research process and the sections of a research report. This relationship is illustrated in Figure 11.1. Now that we have discussed the research process in more detail, a fuller comparison of the process to the research report is possible.

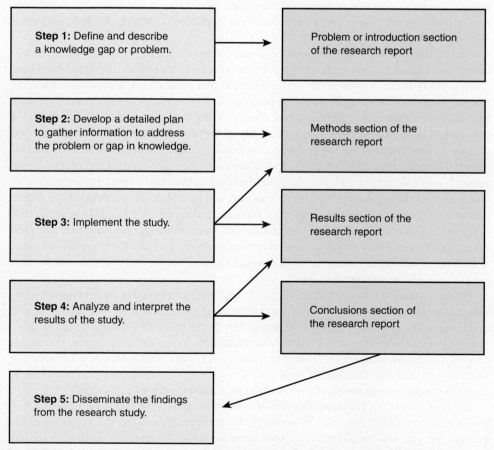

FIGURE 11.1 The relationship between the research process and the sections of a research report.

The first step of the research process of describing and defining the knowledge gap or problem is summarized in the background and literature review sections of a research report. These sections give us the context for a research problem, and tell us about relevant theory and research regarding aspects of the problem. The information included in the report is a synopsis of the much more extensive information that was gathered and synthesized during the first step in the research process. The research purpose and specific questions or hypotheses that conclude the first sections of a report reflect the final refinement of the research problem into specific variables and a specific type of research question.

The second step of the research process is reflected in the methods section of a research report. The methods section tells us the study design, sampling plan, methods of measurement, and procedures. Again, all of the previous research, practicalities, and experience that enter into the decisions about settings for a study, the sample, and the measurement are distilled into a few paragraphs describing the final decisions that were reached about the study plan.

The third step of study implementation is usually reflected in the results section of a research report because it is there that we learn who participated in the study. We may also see part of the implementation of the study reflected in the methods section if what occurred during the implementation process changed the sampling or measurement approaches taken. In either case, the information included in a report rarely reflects all of the details of a study's implementation.

The fourth step of analysis and interpretation of the results of a study is reflected in both the results and conclusions sections of a research report. Of all the steps of the research process, probably this one is most fully described in the report. However, even with this step, a great deal more goes into the process than is reflected in the results and conclusion sections of most reports.

Finally, the fifth step in the research process is the research report itself. However, developing and publishing a research study report also requires more effort than may be obvious when looking at the final product. The publication of a research study depends on several factors. These include the fit between the purpose of the study and the emphasis of journals that publish research, the relevance and quality of the research study, and the ability of the researcher to express clearly and succinctly all the pertinent elements that are needed to fully understand and use the research. The first two factors primarily affect the user of research because they affect what research is available through journals and online. Some research journals publish all types of research in each issue; others develop themes for different issues, limiting the types of studies that they will publish at any particular time. Other journals reflect specialties, such as obstetric nursing, and are only interested in research that is relevant to that specialty. Some journals do not want to publish research that is highly theoretical because they target readers who want practical and practice-focused information. To disseminate the study findings, a researcher first has to find journals that fit with the purpose of the completed study.

We mentioned in Chapter 10 that research reports from refereed or peer-reviewed journals are considered more credible, and are more respected, because they have been reviewed and critiqued by experts in the area of the research. Some research is not published because problems with the quality of the research are identified during the review process that decreases the meaningfulness or validity of the study's results. This does not mean that the research was bad, but simply that some flaw or aspect of the study creates enough doubt about the findings or meaning of the results to preclude warranting publication.

Another factor that affects publication of research studies is the ability of the researcher to express in writing adequate information to accurately describe the entire research process. As you will recall, many of the common errors in research reports discussed throughout this book were errors of omission or lack of complete information. We have now seen how much more thought and work goes into the research process than can go into a research report. The challenge for a researcher, and for the reviewers and editors who contribute to the final publication, is to describe clearly and completely all the aspects of the research process that were relevant to the particular study. The goal is to provide the readers with enough information to allow them to fully understand the study and to make intelligent decisions about the usefulness and meaning of the research for practice. One way that this is accomplished is by using the language of research to limit the need to fully explain each study aspect. Yet, that very language of research may interfere with using research in practice because the practitioner may not be familiar with or understand that language.

FACTORS THAT AFFECT THE RESEARCH PROCESS

In the previous section, we discussed factors that affect the publication of research studies. What about factors those affect whether a research study is implemented? Potential barriers to the implementation of research include lack of knowledge; lack of resources, such as money, time, or both; and lack of methods or measures.

Occasionally, research is not implemented because those who see a problem do not have the knowledge or skill to carry out the research process. For example, a healthcare team member in practice may see an important problem, but be unable to find others who have a similar interest with the skills to implement the research. The healthcare team member also might not be experienced enough to know that the problem they have identified could qualify as a research study. Similarly, a community or a group of patients may see a problem that is not recognized as important by providers or by those who are prepared to implement research.

Research requires time and effort, and is not without expense. Some research is not implemented because there are no resources to support the particular study. Expenses in research range from routine small costs, such as copying expenses and paper, to potentially huge costs for sophisticated measures, such as ultrasounds or specialized laboratory testing. Costs are associated with the researcher's time and the time of others, such as data collectors or workers who enter data. Costs are associated with providing space and equipment needed for some research. As well, costs may be directly associated with subjects in the study, such as incentive payments, or reimbursement for travel or lodging.

Financial support for research can come from numerous sources, including individuals; local, regional, or national foundations or organizations; or the government. In almost every case, to receive financial support for a study, a researcher must prepare a proposal describing the study and identifying how the study will help to meet the goals of the funding source. Herein lies another limit or potential barrier to some research.

Sources of financial support for research usually have goals or initiatives that relate to the purpose of the group providing the support. Occasionally, these goals are specific, such as those of the National Alzheimer's Association, which are to support research into the mechanisms and treatment of Alzheimer's disease. Sometimes these goals are broad, such as the goal of the National Institute for Nursing Research (NINR) to support knowledge development in nursing. However, even the NINR, with its broad goal, has research priorities and target areas for research, such as studies with vulnerable populations, which may influence the success of a particular study in receiving funding. The Web site of a professional organization, such as the American Medical Association (2014), usually publishes its research priorities. When developing a proposal for a research study, decisions about the study purpose, sample, or methods may be based, at least in part, on the goals and priorities of the potential funding source.

In addition to direct financial support for research, sources of indirect support also may affect the types of research implemented. In the medical profession large healthcare organizations and universities who offer degree programs in medicine often employ individuals with the expectation that they will implement research as part of their role. These organizations pay for part of the time a researcher spends on research because the results of research fit with the mission of the organization. A nurse researcher in a large metropolitan medical center, for example, may not need to find financial support for his or her time but may need to limit the types of research implemented to problems directly relevant to delivery of tertiary healthcare.

Another factor that affects the implementation of research is the availability of safe and tested methods and measures to study what we are interested in studying. For example, we may be interested in predictors of pancreatic cancer, because it is so lethal but have no effective way to identify the dependent variable of interest—pancreatic cancer—until an individual is so ill that it is no longer feasible to implement measurement of selected biologic or psychosocial parameters. Or a researcher may be interested in a concept, such as empathy, but finds that no instruments have been developed that can be used to measure empathy. Sometimes, it is unethical to implement a study using what might be the best design validity because of the need to protect the rights of human subjects, as discussed in Chapter 7.

One approach that researchers can take to address some of the limits related to measures and methods is to implement a pilot study. A **pilot study** is a small research study that develops and demonstrates the effectiveness of selected measures and methods. Occasionally, this type of study is used to demonstrate the potential importance of a selected factor to a research problem. At other times, it is used to demonstrate the reliability or validity of selected measures in a unique situation or sample. A pilot study also may be used to demonstrate the ability of the researcher(s) to implement a study. Because knowledge development regarding any particular gap in knowledge is a process that takes time and usually requires multiple studies, pilot studies can be an important first step in building a research program.

GENERATING KNOWLEDGE THROUGH RESEARCH CAN BE FUN!

We started this book by stating that the goal was not to make you a researcher but to give you the knowledge and tools needed to understand and use research intelligently within the context of evidence based practice. However, we do not want to end this chapter, or this book, with an emphasis on how complex and arduous the research process can be or the many potential barriers there can be to both implementing and publishing research. The research process is a wonderful and exciting challenge. It is like a giant interactive puzzle because as each piece is solved and fit into place, the rest of the pieces change and must be addressed in their new form, given what has already been completed. Fitting each piece into the puzzle can be extremely satisfying, and finishing small sections of the puzzle through completion of a research study can be rewarding.

Part of the reason the research process is fun because it is a continuous learning experience for those involved. When one is trying to develop new knowledge, the challenges of planning and implementing a valid and meaningful study always require problem-solving and creative solutions, so the opportunity to learn and create can be immense. More and more, we are recognizing that most research is best approached by using an interdisciplinary team which includes members from different backgrounds and professional disciplines. This allows the knowledge regarding a research problem to be wide ranging and enhances the potential for a high-quality product.

We started this chapter with the nurse joining a newly formed group seeking to address a research problem. We talked about the process employed by this group and how that process relates to the research report. As we discussed the research process, you may have noticed some similarities between it and decision making processes that healthcare team members use when working with patients. For one thing, both are processes, and both have been broken down into steps. In the broadest sense, these processes are similar because they are used to solve problems. Both a research problem and a patient care problem (whether the patient is an individual, family, or community) can be viewed as a complicated puzzle, where often only some of the pieces are available at any time point.

Both types of problems are initially addressed through gathering information. In the healthcare decision making processes, this gathering of information is referred to as assessment, and in the research process, it is referred to as describing and refining the knowledge gap or problem. However, in both cases, we are collecting information to guide us in understanding the problem and formulating a plan.

The second, third, and fourth steps within these processes may initially appear similar, although they differ in some major ways. Although the second step of the healthcare decision making processes is planning for care and/or treatment based upon the given evidence, and the second step of the research process is developing a detailed plan, the two processes differ because they have fundamentally different purposes. The purpose of healthcare decision making processes is to provide informed, scientifically based care and/or treatment for human responses to potential or actual health problems – thus, we now better understand this process, which is "**evidence-based practice**." The purpose of the research process is to develop or validate knowledge. The goal of EBP is taking action, based upon understanding the best information available coupled with the patient's autonomous choices, to promote the established outcome of improved health. The goal of the research process is to acquire new knowledge, and the outcomes for that new knowledge cannot be known until the knowledge is established. Therefore, the second and third steps of EBP address planning and implementing care and/or treatment, whereas the second and third steps of the research process address planning and implementing acquisition of new information. As a result, the fourth steps of these two processes have different focuses because evaluation of EBP is concerned with outcomes, whereas data analysis and interpretation associated with the research process are concerned with understanding. Table 11.1 summarizes the similarities and differences between the two processes.

Although there are some similarities and differences in the processes of EBP and research, it is essential that there be a strong relationship between the two. The research process should provide knowledge that is the basis for making evidence-based decisions. This is why this entire book focuses on understanding, discerning, and intelligently using research in practice. In addition, EBP will often be the source of problems that need to be addressed using the research process. As we plan, implement, and evaluate EBPs, we often find new problems or face questions about the best ways to achieve our outcome of improved health, which generates the need for new or more updated research.

TABLE 11.1	**Comparison of the Research Process and the Healthcare Decision Making Processes**	
	RESEARCH PROCESS	HEALTHCARE DECISION MAKING PROCESSES (EVIDENCE-BASED PRACTICE)
Similarities	A process with steps	A process with steps
	A form of problem solving	A form of problem solving
	Complex "puzzle"	Complex "puzzle"
Differences	Purpose is to develop knowledge	Purpose is to provide scientifically based care
	Plans and implements knowledge acquisition	Plans and implements delivery of care
	Analysis and interpretation concerned with knowing	Evaluation concerned with outcomes

CORE CONCEPT 11.2

While different in purpose, EBP shares several steps with the research process.

Apply

PUBLISHED REPORTS—WHAT DO YOU CONCLUDE NOW?

We have used numerous research study reports in this book as examples of how research can be used and related to clinical practice. In several cases, the studies examined a research problem from the two different approaches of qualitative and quantitative methods. None of the studies that we examined could be called perfect, and to expect them to be so is unreasonable, but each made a meaningful contribution to our knowledge about patients and patient care. No one study, however, gave us the full answer to our clinical questions and often had clear limitations in trying to apply the findings to our nurse's clinical case. This is often a frustration for healthcare team members in practice. With a better understanding of the research process, it should be clearer now why usually no single study fully answers a clinical question. Clinical questions are usually too complex, and too many variables and factors must be considered and examined for any one study to provide a complete answer. However, as research studies about a particular clinical problem accumulate, we should see answers begin to unfold. This is the essence of EBP, which explicitly recognizes the need for a discernment of knowledge regarding a problem to ensure the best and safest delivery of healthcare. Excellence in delivery of evidence-based care is one of the qualities recognized and valued by many healthcare accrediting organizations such as The Joint Commission (TJC, 2014) and the Healthcare Facilities Accreditation Program (HFAP, 2014).

Therefore, what do you conclude now about the needs of the school nurse from Chapter 1, who is facing complex planning for the 17-year-old adolescent patient who is struggling with physiologic and psychological issues related to her weight? What do you conclude about how the orthopedic surgeon from Chapter 3 who is seeing C.T. following a left total hip arthroplasty (THA), and how the surgeon should proceed, recognizing that the patient has back pain and is concerned about leg length differences? You should now be able to accomplish the following tasks and answer five questions as you read the research we have reviewed. As you look at these questions, realize how much you have learned and how much you now know regarding research.

- You can read and understand the background and literature review of a report to find out "Why was the research question asked—what do we already know?"
- You can read the design and methods sections of a research report to find out "How were those people studied—why was the study performed that way?"
- You can read the sampling section of the research report to find out "To what types of patients do these research conclusions apply?"
- You can read the results and conclusions sections of the report to find out "Why the authors reached their conclusions—what did they actually find?"
- Finally, you can use the answers from the above four questions to decide "What is the answer to the question—what did the study conclude?"

You also now know that finding the "answer" to your question will only be the beginning, and that it may give you new knowledge and insight into patient care but may also leave you asking even more questions.

CONCLUSION

The authors hope that as you read research, and practice according to the best evidence available, you will develop a professional appreciation for EBP. Although every healthcare team member is not expected to plan and implement research, there are several roles for all of us within the research process, such as participation in planning a study or in subject recruitment and data collection, and there is professional accountability and expectation that we all practice according to the best evidence. If you have come away from this book with an understanding of how to better read and discern research for use in EBP, then you are well on your way to providing even more competent, comprehensive patient care through this process. Just as the use of research is EBP is a process of constant movement towards better provision of exceptional patient care, so is the journey of lifelong learning to consistently incorporate current best practices into your everyday practice as a healthcare professional. We hope that the information contained in this book will be a most useful part of *your* journey.

References

American Medical Association. (2014, January). *Other Research Opportunities*. Retrieved from http://www.ama-assn.org/ama/pub/about-ama/ama-foundation/our-programs/medical-education/other-research-opportunities.page?

HFAP. (2014, January). *Healthcare Facilities Accreditation Program*. Retrieved from http://www.hfap.org

TJC. (2014, January). *The Joint Commission*. Retrieved from http://www.jointcommission.org

*indicates a definitive or classic work or publication regarding this subject matter.

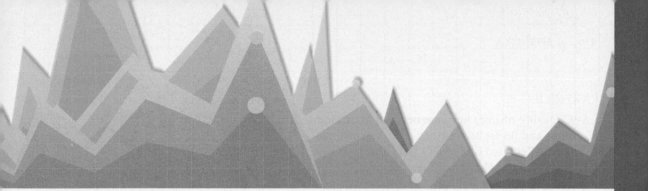

Appendix A

Research Articles

The ten articles contained in this appendix are referred to and discussed in various chapters throughout the text. While articles may be mentioned in several chapters, they normally correspond to topics specific to one or two chapters.

The following table will help link the articles to the chapters in which they are discussed:

ARTICLE	AUTHORS/DATE	CORRESPONDING CHAPTERS
A-1. Relationships Between Body Satisfaction and Psychological Functioning and Weight-Related Cognitions and Behaviors in Overweight Adolescents	Cromley et al./2012	1, 2, 4, 5
A-2. Overweight or Obese Students' Perceptions of Caring in Urban Physical Education Programs	Li et al./2013	2, 4, 5, 6
A-3. Leg Length Discrepancy in Cementless Total Hip Arthroplasty	Peck et al./2011	3, 5
A-4. Teaching Evidence-Based Medicine Literature Searching Skills to Medical Students During the Clinical Years: A Randomized Controlled Trial	Ilic et al./2012	4, 5, 6
A-5. Predictors of Postconcussive Symptoms 3 Months After Mild Traumatic Brain Injury	Ponsford et al./2012	5, 6
A-6. The Affects of a Single Bout of Exercise on Mood and Self-Esteem in Clinically Diagnosed Mental Health Patients	Ellis et al./2013	7
A-7. The Use of Postoperative Restraints in Children after Cleft lip or Cleft Palate Repair: A Preliminary Report.	Huth et al.	8
A-8. Investigating Risk Factors for Psychological Morbidity Three Months After Intensive Care: A Prospective Cohort Study	Wade et al.	9

(*Continued*)

ARTICLE	AUTHORS/DATE	CORRESPONDING CHAPTERS
A-9. Quality-of-Life Outcomes between Mastectomy Alone and Breast Reconstruction: Comparison of Patient-Reported BREAST-Q and Other Health-Related Quality-of-Life Measures	Eltahir et al.	10
A-10. Why People Living with HIV/AIDS Exclude Individuals From Their Chosen Families	Grant et al.	10

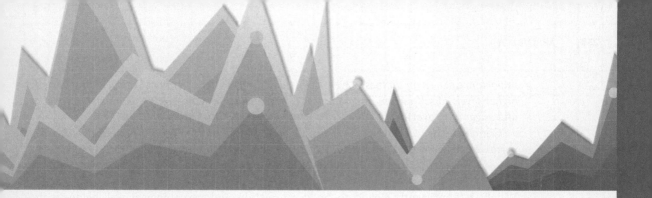

Appendix A-1

Adolescent health brief

Relationships Between Body Satisfaction and Psychological Functioning and Weight-Related Cognitions and Behaviors in Overweight Adolescents

Taya Cromley, Ph.D.[a], Stephanie Knatz, M.A.[b,c], Roxanne Rockwell, M.A.[b,c], Dianne Neumark-Sztainer, Ph.D., M.P.H., R.D.[d,e], Mary Story, Ph.D., R.D.[d,e], and Kerri Boutelle, Ph.D.[b,c,e,f]

Article history: Received April 13, 2011; Accepted October 27, 2011

Keywords: Overweight adolescents; Body satisfaction; Weight control behaviors; Adolescent psychological functioning

Abstract

Purpose: *To examine how differences in body satisfaction may influence weight control behaviors, eating, weight and shape concerns, and psychological well-being among overweight adolescents.*

Methods: *A group of 103 overweight adolescents completed a survey assessing body satisfaction, weight control behaviors, eating-related thoughts and behaviors, importance placed on thinness, self-esteem, anger, and symptoms of depression and anxiety between 2004 and 2006. Logistic regression analyses compared overweight adolescents with high and low body satisfaction.*

Results: *Higher body satisfaction was associated with a lower likelihood of engaging in unhealthy weight control behaviors, less frequent fears of losing control over eating, and less*

[a] Department of Psychology, University of California, Los Angeles, California
[b] Department of Pediatrics, University of California, San Diego, La Jolla, California
[c] Department of Psychiatry, University of California, San Diego, La Jolla, California
[d] Department of Pediatrics, Adolescent Health, University of Minnesota, Minneapolis, Minnesota
[e] Division of Epidemiology and Community Health, School of Public Health, University of Minnesota, Minneapolis, Minnesota
[f] Rady Children's Hospital, San Diego, California

1054-139X/$ - see front matter © 2012 Society for Adolescent Health and Medicine. All rights reserved. doi:10.1016/j.jadohealth.2011.10.252

importance placed on thinness. Overweight adolescents with higher body satisfaction reported higher levels of self-esteem and were less likely to endorse symptoms of depression, anxiety, and anger than overweight adolescents with lower body satisfaction.

Conclusions: *Adolescents with higher body satisfaction may be protected against the negative behavioral and psychological factors associated with overweight.*

Weight is consistently linked to body satisfaction and psychological well-being, with overweight youth expressing lower body satisfaction and poorer psychological functioning [1]. Few studies have evaluated differences in behavior and psychological functioning in overweight youth with high body satisfaction. If a positive relationship between body satisfaction and behavioral and psychological well-being exists among overweight adolescents, then improved body satisfaction could be a key component of interventions for overweight youth, particularly cognitive-behavioral interventions that target negative thoughts about the self to ultimately promote engagement in positive health behaviors.

Although studies suggest that lower levels of body satisfaction may be a risk factor for more health-compromising behaviors and fewer health-promoting behaviors [2], body satisfaction may also serve as a protective factor with regard to weight and behavior. A longitudinal study examining the relationship between body satisfaction and weight found that overweight girls with higher body satisfaction gained less weight at 5-year follow-up than overweight girls with lower body satisfaction [3].

The aim of this study was to examine differences in self-reported body satisfaction among overweight adolescents in relation to weight control behaviors, eating in secret, fear of losing control while eating, importance placed on thinness, and psychological well-being (depression, anxiety, anger, and self-esteem). It was hypothesized that overweight youth with higher body satisfaction would engage in fewer unhealthy weight control behaviors (UWCB) and eating disordered behaviors and would report better psychological functioning than overweight youth with lower body satisfaction.

Methods

Study design and participants. Data were collected as part of Successful Adolescent Losers, a descriptive study of overweight adolescents who lost weight and those who did not [4]. Participants were recruited using public marketing strategies (e.g., flyers) from the Minneapolis/St. Paul area between 2004 and 2006. Study procedures were approved by the Institutional Review Board at the University of Minnesota. Only adolescents classified as overweight or obese (body mass index ≥85th percentile for gender and age) were included in the analyses (Table A1.1).

Measures. The following measures were part of the 73-item Successful Adolescent Losers survey, a self-report instrument that assesses behavioral and psychological factors potentially associated with weight in adolescence [4].

Weight control behaviors. Participants were asked about their use of 32 strategies to reduce or maintain weight, adapted from Project EAT [5]. A factor analysis identified four domains of weight control behaviors: healthy weight control behaviors UWCB, "other" dietary changes, and behavior change strategies [4]. Healthy weight control behaviors were dichotomized into ≥6 versus ≤5 using the distribution median. UWCB, behavior change strategies, and "other" dietary changes were dichotomized into any versus none.

Eating-related behaviors and cognitions. Frequency of eating in secret and fear of losing control while eating (both in the past month) were measured by using items from the Eating Disorder Examination Questionnaire [6]. Using the distribution median, these variables were dichotomized into ≥5 days versus ≤4 days. Importance of being thin was assessed with a 4-point Likert scale ranging from "not at all important" to "very important."

TABLE A1.1	Demographics of sample of overweight adolescents and mean (SD) scale scores for continuous dependent variables			
	TOTAL SAMPLE (N = 103)	HIGH BS (N = 50)	LOW BS (N = 53)	P
Gender				.06
Female	67 (65.0%)	28 (56.0%)	39 (73.6%)	
Male	36 (35.0%)	22 (44.0%)	14 (26.4%)	
Mean age	15.2 (range: 12–20; SD = 2.15)	15.6 (SD = 2.2)	14.9 (SD = 2.1)	.11
Ethnicity				.16
White	61 (59.2%)	31 (62.0%)	30 (56.6%)	
Multiethnic	16 (15.5%)	5 (10.0%)	11 (20.8%)	
African American	15 (14.6%)	7 (14.0%)	8 (15.1%)	
American Indian	6 (5.8%)	4 (8.0%)	2 (3.8%)	
Asian	2 (1.9%)	0	2 (3.8%)	
Other	3 (2.9%)	3 (6.0%)	0	
Mean weight loss (lbs)	7.1 (range 0-65; SD = 11.6)	6.7 (SD = 10.1)	7.5 (SD = 12.9)	.71
Mean BMI	31.5 (range 21.7-45.1; SD = 5.1)	30.8 (SD = 4.1)	32.2 (SD = 5.8)	.18
Mean scale scores: eating behaviors and cognitions				
Secretive eating	3.4 (6.4)	2.1 (4.6)	4.5 (7.9)	
Importance of thinness	3.0 (.92)	2.7 (.89)	3.3 (.86)	
Fear of losing control	5.1 (8.2)	2.6 (5.0)	7.5 (9.9)	
Mean scale scores: psychological functioning				
Depression	13.1 (11.5)	9.2 (7.2)	16.8 (13.5)	
Anxiety	16.4 (4.4)	14.4 (3.6)	18.4 (4.2)	
Anger	20.2 (6.4)	18.2 (5.0)	22.1 (7.1)	

BS = body satisfaction; SD = standard deviation.

Psychological functioning. Depression was measured using the Center for Epidemiological Studies Depression Scale for Children [7]. Anger and anxiety were measured using the Spielberger State-Trait Personality Inventory [8]. Self-esteem was measured using the Rosenberg Self-Esteem Scale [9].

Body satisfaction. Body satisfaction was assessed with a modified version of the Body Shape Satisfaction Scale [10]. Participants rated their satisfaction with 10 body features (weight, shape, waist, etc.), with lower scores indicating less body satisfaction (range: 10–60). Responses were dichotomized using a median split (high >32.1; low <32.0).

Weight status. Height and weight was measured using standardized equipment and procedures. Cutoff points for gender- and age-specific BMI percentile values were based on growth charts from the Centers for Disease Control and Prevention.

Data analysis. Statistical analyses were conducted using SPSS (version 15.0). There were no significant differences between the "high" (n = 50) and "low" (n = 53) body satisfaction groups on demographics or weight loss (see Table A1.1). Logistic regression analyses compared high and low body satisfaction in relation to dependent variables. Models controlling for gender and BMI were ran separately, but results were not significantly different from the unadjusted model, which is presented here.

Results. Overweight adolescents with higher body satisfaction were less likely to engage in UWCB than adolescents with lower body satisfaction, but differences were not found for other weight control behaviors. Adolescents with higher body satisfaction were also less likely to report fear of losing control over eating and less importance placed on thinness. No differences were found for eating in secret. Finally, overweight adolescents with higher body satisfaction endorsed fewer symptoms of depression, anxiety, and anger, and higher self-esteem (Table A1.2).

TABLE A1.2	Logistic associations between adolescent body satisfaction (high/low) weight control behaviors, eating, weight and shape concerns, and psychological functioning among overweight adolescents (N = 103)			
		BODY SATISFACTION		
	B	SE	OR	95% CI
Weight control behaviors				
HWCB	−.01	.41	.99	[.44, 2.22]
UWCB	−.89	.41	.41*	[.18, .93]
BCS	−.61	.40	.54	[.25, 1.19]
ODC	.82	.74	2.27	[.54, 9.63]
Eating, weight, and shape concerns				
Eating in secret	−.46	.42	.63	[.28, 1.44]
Fear of losing control over eating	−1.02	.41	.36**	[.16, .81]
Importance placed on thinness	−.74	.24	.48**	[.30, .77]
Psychological functioning				
Depression	−.07	.02	.93**	[.89, .97]
Self-esteem	.20	.05	1.22**	[1.11, 1.34]
Anxiety	−.27	.07	.76**	[.67, .87]
Anger	−.11	.04	.90**	[.84, .97]

Beta, standard error, odds ratio, and 95% confidence intervals presented. OR = odds ratio; CI = confidence interval; HWCB = healthy weight control behaviors; UWCB = unhealthy weight control behaviors; BCS = behavior change strategies; ODC = other dietary changes.
*$p \leq .05$.
**$p \leq .01$.

Discussion. Overall, lower body satisfaction in overweight adolescents is associated with less positive behavioral and emotional functioning. Consistent with previous literature [2], adolescents with lower body satisfaction were more likely to engage in UWCB, such as fasting, skipping meals, vomiting, or using laxatives, diuretics, or diet pills. Adolescents with higher body satisfaction reported lower levels of depression, anxiety, and anger, higher levels of self-esteem, and less concern about thinness and fear of losing control over food. These results suggest that overweight adolescents who feel better about their bodies may be more resilient, with potentially less risk for developing or exhibiting psychological comorbidities associated with overweight [1].

Strengths of this study include the inclusion of questions on weight-related behaviors and psychological functioning in an overweight sample. Limitations of the study include the small sample and large age range of participants, use of self-report, the cross-sectional nature of the study, and the abbreviated nature of the psychological measures.

Findings from this study suggest that body satisfaction may protect against negative behavioral and psychological comorbidities associated with overweight. Cognitive behavioral interventions with overweight adolescents should focus on enhancing body satisfaction while providing motivation and skills to engage in more effective weight-control behaviors. Targeting cognitions related to body satisfaction in treatment with overweight adolescents may need to be done in conjunction with, or before, attempting to engage clients in behaviorally-oriented interventions geared toward prevention of unhealthy weight control strategies.

Acknowledgment
The study was supported by University of Minnesota Children's Vikings Grant.

References
1. Paxton SJ, Neumark-Sztainer D, Hannan PJ, Eisenberg ME. Body dissatisfaction prospectively predicts depressive mood and low self-esteem in adolescent girls and boys. *J Clin Child Adolesc Psychol* 2006;35:539–49.

2. Neumark-Sztainer D, Paxton SJ, Hannan PJ, et al. Does body satisfaction matter? Five-year longitudinal associations between body satisfaction and health behaviors in adolescent females and males. *J Adolesc Health* 2006;39:244–51.

3. Van den Berg P, Neumark-Sztainer D. Fat 'n happy 5 years later: Is it bad for overweight girls to like their bodies? *J Adolesc Health* 2007;41:415–7.

4. Boutelle KN, Libbey H, Neumark-Sztainer D, Story M. Weight control strategies of overweight adolescents who successfully lost weight. *J Am Diet Assoc* 2009;109:2029–35.

5. Haines J, Neumark-Sztainer D, Eisenberg ME, Hannan PJ. Weight teasing and disordered eating behaviors in adolescents: Longitudinal findings from project EAT (eating among teens). *Pediatrics* 2006;117:209–15.

6. Luce KH, Crowther JH. The reliability of the eating disorder examination-self-report questionnaire version (EDE-Q). *Int J Eat Disord* 1999;25:349–51.

7. Faulstich ME, Carey MP, Ruggiero L, et al. Assessment of depression in childhood and adolescence: An evaluation of the center for epidemiological studies depression scale for children (CES-DC). *Am J Psychiatry* 1986;143:1024–7.

8. Spielberger C, Reheiser E. Measuring anxiety, anger, depression, and curiosity as emotional states and personality traits with the STAI, STAXI, and STPI. In: Hilsenroth MJ, Segal DL, eds. *Comprehensive Handbook of Psychological Assessment*, Vol 2. Hoboken, NJ: John Wiley & Sons, Inc, 2003:p. 70–85.

9. Rosenberg M. *Society and the Adolescent Self-Image*. Princeton, NJ: Princeton University Press, 1965.

10. Pingitore R, Spring B, Garfield D. Gender differences in body satisfaction. *Obes Res* 1997;5:402–9.

Appendix A-2

Overweight or Obese Students' Perceptions of Caring in Urban Physical Education Programs

Weidong Li, Ph.D.
The Ohio State University

Paul B. Rukavina
Adelphi University

Chelsea Foster
The Ohio State University

The purpose of the study was to explore overweight or obese students 'perceptions of caring in urban physical education (PE) programs. Forty-seven overweight or obese students were recruited and participated in a semi-structured interview. Inductive analysis and constant comparison were used to analyze the data. The findings indicated that overweight students perceived being cared-for when their peers were supportive, and when teachers made instructional adaptations, built interpersonal rapport, and created a positive, motivational climate in PE. It is suggested that to create a caring climate, teachers need to allow overweight or obese students to work at their ability level, provide quality instruction and feedback and make developmentally appropriate instructional adaptations, foster a positive, motivational learning climate, create a connection between teacher and student (interpersonal rapport), and create a learning community with positive peer interactions. Creating an inclusive environment that enhances their sense of caring and belonging, has a great potential to increase overweight or obese students' engagement in PE.

Due to weight stigmatization (Cramer & Steinwert, 1998; Puhl & Brownell, 2001; Tiggemann & Wilson-Barrett, 1998), overweight or obese students are often teased and commonly excluded from participating in physical activity (PA) (Faith, Leone, Ayers, Heo, & Pietrobelli, 2002; Pierce & Wardle, 1997; Storch et al., 2007) and physical education (PE) (Bauer, Yang, & Austin, 2004; Fox & Edmunds, 2000; Li & Rukavina, 2012; Trout & Graber, 2009). Because of potential psychological and emotional damage for overweight or obese students as a result of weight-related teasing (e.g., Eisenberg, Neumark-Sztainer, & Story, 2003; Puhl & Brownell, 2003) and serious health implications as a result of living a physically inactive lifestyle, it has become increasingly critical that PE teachers create a safe, caring and inclusive learning climate to enhance overweight or obese students' engagement and learning in PE, thus developing and sustaining a healthy, physically active lifestyle.

A perceived caring learning climate has great potential to affect overweight or obese students' engagement and learning in PE for two reasons: 1) overweight or obese students are socially isolated and commonly excluded from participation in PE (Bauer et al., 2004; Fox & Edmunds, 2000; Li & Rukavina, 2012; Trout & Graber, 2009). 2) Research has demonstrated that caring teaching behaviors are strongly linked to positive attitudes and motivation to learn among general student population in general education (Battistich, Solomon, Watson, & Schaps, 1997; Wentzel, 1997; Wentzel & Asher, 1995) and PE (e.g., Cothran & Ennis, 1999,2000; Larson, 2006). According to Noddings (1984, 1992), the ethic of caring is created through making a connection between the 'one-caring' and the 'cared-for'. This interactive, relational process is composed of engrossment, action and reciprocity. Engrossment refers to the one's desire to understand the person's, who is cared-for, physical and personal situation. For example, the teacher who cares for an overweight or obese child learns about their individual characteristics, such as home life, health habits, or interests. Caring is then communicated through the carer's actions. Noddings (1984) defines actions as any behaviors or communications that are geared toward the welfare, protection and enhancement of the one being cared for. And finally, caring can only exist when the one being cared for reciprocates or responds to the actions or presence of the 'one caring'. For example, if a teacher gave an overweight or obese student a compliment on their basketball jump shot, the student would reciprocate by practicing harder or following the teacher's instructions.

In general education, the interpersonal interactions between teachers and students are considered as being at the core of the teaching-learning processes (e.g., Bruner, 1996; Noddings, 1992, 2002). A number of studies have investigated the relationship between students' perceptions of caring and their attitudes and motivation. The findings have demonstrated that students' perceptions of being cared for are strongly connected to students' evaluation of their teachers and their perceptions of cognitive and affective learning (Teven & McCroskey, 1997), their attitudes toward school (e.g., Battistich, Solomon, Watson, & Schaps, 1997), and student motivation to learn (Wentzel, 1997; Wentzel & Asher, 1995).

Researchers in the field of PE have also conducted research on students' perceptions of caring (e.g., Cothran & Ennis, 1999, 2000; Ennis et al., 1997; Larson, 2006). Consistent with the findings from general education, the findings in school PE have indicated that teaching caring behaviors were strongly related to students' attitude toward PE and their engagement in PE (e.g., Cothran & Ennis, 1999, 2000; Cothran, Hodges Kulinna, & Garrahy, 2003; Ennis et al., 1997; Larson, 2006). Students participated more in PE when they perceived that teachers were willing to work with them, showed an authentic attentiveness for their well-being, and fostered a safe and supportive learning environment that focused on personal growth and cooperation.

Larson (2006) has argued that the uniqueness of PE contexts can offer opportunities for caring teaching behaviors to emerge that can be dissimilar to those in general education. Larson investigated perceptions of caring teaching among 518 United States elementary and secondary students using critical incident forms to elicit descriptions of caring teaching. The findings revealed 11 clusters of caring teaching behaviors: 1) Showed me how to do a skill; 2) honored my request to choose an activity; 3) gave me a compliment; 4) confronted my behavior; 5) inquired about my health; 6) attended to me when I was injured; 7) allowed me to re-do my test; 8) motivated me; 9) played/participated with me during class; 10) persuaded me; 11) showed concern for my future health. These 11 clusters were further sorted into three subcategories: Recognize me; help me learn; and trust/respect me, and a primary category of pay attention to me. Even though certain caring teaching behaviors are PE context specific, the central concept of caring is the same regardless of the context.

The previous studies, however, have mainly focused on perceptions of caring among the general student population. Little is known about overweight or obese students' perceptions of caring. In PE, it is expected that teachers provide differentiated instruction for all students, including overweight and obese students (National Association for Sports and Physical Education: NASPE, 2001). For example, PE teachers may simplify the skills for overweight or obese students to work on or allocate more time and attention to them. PE teachers may also give advice to overweight or obese students on losing weight. It is unclear how these instructional modifications based on overweight or obese students' skills and abilities would be perceived. Due to the internalization of weight stigma and sensitivity of obesity in PA, it is possible that overweight or obese students may interpret these teaching practices as negative. In addition, the previous literature has investigated perceptions of caring behaviors in relation to teachers. However, no research has been conducted to examine perceptions of caring behaviors exhibited by their peers. To effectively and successfully include overweight or obese students in PE, there is an urgent need to understand their perceptions of caring from their teachers and peers. Therefore, the purpose of the present study was to qualitatively describe perceptions of caring among 47 overweight or obese students in urban PE programs. The information gathered from the present study can better inform practitioners and teachers of strategies for effective inclusion.

Method. A descriptive qualitative research design was employed to explore the perceptions of caring among overweight and obese adolescents in an urban city school district in the South-em USA. The present study was part of a larger one, which investigated overweight or obese adolescents' experience in PE (Li & Rukavina, 2012; Li, Rukavina, & Wright, 2012).

Setting. The setting in which the data were collected was a Southern urban city school district in the United States, which delivers education to more than 119,000 students in grades K-12. There are many challenges that the district faces: Approximately 87% are African Americans, 71% of the students receive free or reduced lunch, and 61% of the students graduate with a high school degree. Moreover, 19.7% of high school students in this school district were overweight and additionally 16.2% were obese (Eaton et al., 2008).

Participants. The study was delimited to overweight and obese students, which made recruitment difficult due to the sensitivity of the topic. This is consistent with other studies that have investigated issues related to childhood overweight and obesity (e.g., O'Keefe & Coat, 2009; Trout & Graber, 2009). Selection bias or bias from recruiting from a particular sub-population in the city school district was minimized by using a variety of methods, such as recruitment through the schools, summer camps (organized through a community recreation center), distributing flyers to weight loss clinics, and participant word of mouth. All participants were enrolled in school PE classes (six high schools, three middle schools, and one k-6 elementary school) during the study or in the previous year.

Forty-seven students who had a body mass index (BMI) greater than the 85th percentage (19 males and 28 females; 14 European Americans and 33 African Americans) participated in the study. Their ages ranged from 11 to 19 year olds {$M = 14.86$, $SD = 1.97$). At first, students were visually identified as being overweight or obese by the first two investigators or their PE teachers. We then measured their height and weight to calculate BMI adjusted for gender and age. The adolescents' BMI ranged from 25 to 62.2 (Overweight = BMI of 25-29.9; Obese = BMI of 30 or greater). The participants were self-selecting volunteers. Both child assent and parental consent were obtained. Demographic variables included age, gender, grade, and ethnicity. Adolescent participants and their family were provided $50 for participation in the study.

Recruitment. Recruitment was a lengthy and rigorous process. At first, we recruited from the city schools to identify a pool of adolescents and their parents. The PE teacher handed consent forms to the students and if they and their parents were interested. Due to the sensitivity of the topic, much care was taken with interpersonal communication with the participants and their families. A heterogeneous and adequate sample size was ensured through several methods. Consent forms were handed out at multiple schools, flyers were handed out at summer camps organized through a local community center and weight loss clinics, and we asked the adolescents to tell their friends about the study (i.e., word of mouth). Recruitment was also completed with flyers. The flyers included information similar to what was written in the consent form, but were more general. Specific details were provided to parties that contacted the researchers. Child assent and parental consent were obtained if they were interested. At the clinics, the supervising physician handed out the flyers to the families in the waiting room. If the family was interested in the study, the researchers would explain the consent form and answer any questions they may have. For the participants that were recruited from the schools, multiple approvals were obtained, which included the PE teacher, school principal and school district. For recruitment from the weight loss clinics and summer camps, administrative approval was obtained. All participants' and their guardians' consent were obtained prior to the start of the study as required from the University IRB.

Data Collection. Data were collected about perceptions of caring using interviews from overweight or obese adolescents. Knowledge about sensitive topics, such as talking about one's weight and how teachers care, are best achieved with interviews because of the flexibility in conversations and means of achieving a personal connection (Edmunds, 2005). A conversational style face-to-face interview was guided by two initial questions: 1) What are the situations where you feel being cared-for by your PE teachers? 2) What are these situations where you feel being cared-for by your peers? Based upon participant's responses, their comments were followed by prompts to gain further information or clarification. These questions were a part of larger interview that addressed their experience in PE and weight-related teasing and coping. The overall interview for the larger study lasted about 40 minutes on average. The first two researchers conducted the interviews privately at the first author's university office, participant's home, or school or weight loss clinics offices. Both researchers had training in qualitative research and experience conducting interviews. The participants were provided choices and they selected the place where they felt most comfortable being interviewed and fit their schedule and family commitments.

Prior to the beginning of the interview, the interview was framed through establishing a personal connection with participants to put them at ease (Kvale, 1996), discussing the study and explaining the importance of having overweight students' voices heard. Participants were assured at any time they could stop and take a break or drop from the study without any penalty if they felt uncomfortable during the interview. After all the interviews were transcribed and coded, six students volunteered to participate in a focus group for an interpretative member check. All participants provided permissions to audio-tape their interview.

Data Coding and Analysis. Each participant was assigned an ID number for identification to facilitate analysis and reporting of the data. Audio tapes were transcribed verbatim, and inductive content analysis and constant comparison were used to analyze the data (Denzin & Lincoln, 1994). The first phase of the analysis involved the first two authors reading the interviews multiple times to ensure familiarity with the data. Following the first phase, both researchers deliberated and identified the most consistent concepts emerged from the data and developed an initial coding template upon a 100% agreement. Seven participants' interviews were then independently double-coded by both researchers and the inter-rater reliability was assessed using the formula: number of agreements/ (number of agreements + number of disagreement). A reliability coefficient of 0.93 was obtained. The disagreements were discussed and changes were made until both researchers reached a 100% agreement. For the remaining interviews, each investigator independently coded the data. The major concepts that arose most frequently were then identified and formed into upper level themes by the first author. A peer debriefing session was held with the second author and changes were made to the identified themes until reaching a 100% agreement. Finally, the interpretation of the themes and the relationships among the themes were identified. Data from the focus group were incorporated as the narratives were written. A final reshaping of the themes was completed after the focus group.

Data Trustworthiness. Multiple procedures and strategies were used to establish trustworthiness of the data (Creswell, 2003). First, we recruited as diverse a sample as possible of overweight or obese students so that the themes would represent the diverse population inherent in the urban city school. Second, peer debriefing was completed with a colleague who was adept and experienced in qualitative research. The peer de-briefer provided insights in regard to data collection procedures, formation of conceptual linkages, overall representation of the data, alternate interpretations, and focus group interview procedures. Third, transcripts were mailed to all participants for review using the addresses provided during the interview. They were asked to read, check for accuracy and mail them back with the self-addressed stamped envelope. Only ten of the transcripts were received. The rest of transcripts were returned due to incomplete address information or family relocations without any forwarding address. Of the received transcripts, participants only made typographical and grammatical errors. Fourth, an interpretative member check was performed with a focus group interview. Six adolescent participants were recruited and participated voluntarily in the focus group with consent from their parents. All of the themes and the relationships among them were presented to the participants to check for the accuracy of the interpretations. We also further explored issues that emerged from the themes. Finally, a search of negative cases was completed to refute the themes or provide an alternative viewpoint throughout the entire data analysis process.

Findings. Themes are illustrated through overweight or obese adolescents' voices taken from the individual and focus group interviews. Four major themes emerged from the data, which included teachers' instructional adaptations, a positive, motivational climate (e.g., choices, made it fun, not put them "on the spot"), built interpersonal rapport (e.g., gave advice, did things with them), and supportive peers.

Teachers' Instructional Adaptations. Instructional adaptations are an important component of pedagogical content knowledge (PCK) (Shulman, 1987). A key feature of instructional adaptations to diverse learners is how teachers can transform content knowledge to their diverse backgrounds and varied abilities and skill levels (Shulman, 1987). For the present study, three different types of instructional adaptations were mentioned by the overweight students: task support, refinements, and task simplification. Even though these instructional adaptations were made specifically to accommodate overweight or obese students' physical limitations and capabilities as a result of their body size and shape, overweight or obese adolescents in the present study felt being cared-for by these teaching behaviors. First, overweight students commented on how they felt cared-for when the PE teacher would provide support for the task, such as spotting them with a difficult exercise. One overweight student commented,

> When the PE teacher tell you to do something and you can't do it, they will try to help you with it, like if you are trying to do a toe touch, I mean not a toe touch but a hand stand or something they will go up there and hold your feet, and then let go and you will still be up there and they will help you with something like that.

Overweight or obese students also reported that they felt cared-for when their PE teachers provided specific feedback to refine the tasks. PE teachers would show overweight or obese students how to do the skill correctly or provide specific feedback on the skill execution, (e.g., dancing, soccer, and basketball). For example, one overweight student commented, "When I was playing kickball a few weeks ago, I tried to catch the ball and missed it, just by a little bit. Coach was like, next time, stand in front of it. Don't be scared of it." Overweight students felt good when they were successful and learned it. Another overweight student perceived the teacher's comment as caring when the teacher listened to him after the teacher provided him feedback. The student commented,

> PE teacher help me understand things that I don't understand and things that he showed us how to do, he will go back over and show me how to do it and his way, and I show him I do it in the way that I know how. He accepts it as that.

Other overweight students felt cared-for when teachers simplified the task if they were tired or could not finish what everybody else was assigned, such as running laps or doing other fitness activities. One student reported,

> Yeah, they care about us a lot because they tell us, they try to help us get better and don't slack or whatever. And sometimes, if they know we can't do it, like if we're too overweight, like most people if they know we can't do it, they will just tell us, we have to do ten of everything. They just tell some people that they know can't do it to just do five or four.

Other times, the overweight student appreciated when the teacher allowed them to sit on the side, such as when they became too tired. One overweight student commented,

> When I just got finished running up and down the bleachers and I didn't feel like playing basketball, so he let me sit out that day because he see I couldn't catch my breath. We were outside playing baseball. When I got in the sun, I got real bad headaches. So he let me go sit in the shade, up under the tree, and watch them play.

Knowing that overweight students tire more easily than the other students and adapting the task for them was important to them. They felt connected to them especially when they knew the teacher understood what it was like to be overweight. One student commented,

> I mean, the physical education teacher, she was kind of heavy, and she won't make it so hard that the bigger people they get tired quicker than the smaller people or the people who have problems doing stuff, she won't make it too hard for them or she'll say that you go to keep going, keep pushing yourself, so you can be the best you can be.

A Positive Motivational Climate. Many overweight or obese students felt being cared-for when PE teachers created a positive motivational learning climate. There exist two different types of motivational learning climates in an achievement motivation context: An ego involved versus a task involved learning climates (e.g., Ames & Ames, 1984; Ames & Archer, 1988; Meece, BlUmenfeld, & Hoyle, 1988). An ego involved learning climate focuses on social comparisons. Whereas a task involved learning climate is one where teachers focus on cooperative learning, effort, and personal improvement rather than social comparison and performing the best with minimal effort. An ego-involved motivational learning climate is positively associated with an ego goal orientation. Whereas a task involved motivational learning climate is positively related to a task goal orientation. For students who adopt a task goal orientation, they are likely to exhibit adaptive motivational and behavioral responses in physical education (e.g., Li & Lee, 2004 for a review; Xiang, McBride, Bruene, & Liu, 2007). In the present study, students talked about how they felt cared-for when they had choices to run the number of laps they wanted to run or if they were in the weight room. One overweight student commented,

> She [PE teacher] let you go where you want to stand and choose how you want to do it . . . she said you do it as a group so you don't stand out . . . . . she won't say that these people get these amounts of weight and these people get these weights. She let you pick your own weight.

Thus, when teachers designed fun activities where students got to feel they worked at their ability level and their ability was not being spotlighted or compared to other students, they felt cared-for.

Overweight students commented that they felt cared-for when the teacher focused on improvement in challenging, developmentally appropriate activities and were very supportive as they put in effort. Encouragement was very important to the overweight students. They felt cared-for and supported when the teachers encouraged them to do better. For example, one student who was overweight commented, "She [PE teacher] will not give up on me like if I couldn't do. She tell me keep on trying, trying until I get it right." Another overweight student reported,

> When I was doing the running thing, um, he [PE teacher] would always encourage me: 'Yeah come on you can, you can do it you can keep going just a little bit farther'. He's always encouraged me and all the other kids . . .

Sometimes overweight students knew they were not putting in a lot of effort and liked it or felt cared-for when the teacher reinforced their expectations. They commented, "Yeah, they care about us a lot because they tell us, they try to help us get better and don't slack or whatever." And then, after they put in the effort, the overweight students felt cared-for when teachers would give them a compliment or recognized the effort they put forth. One overweight student commented, " . . . at the end of the PE, they'll be like 'you did good today, you really did good.' Stuff like that." These PE teachers expected overweight or obese students to improve, and then encouraged and complimented them when they tried to achieve them. The overweight students really appreciated the "motivation" provided by the teacher, which in turn, helped them succeed at their own level.

Built Interpersonal Rapport. Building interpersonal rapport was another dimension of caring that emerged from the data. Open communication with students, especially with ones that are disenfranchised, is an effective strategy to establish a connection and further to get to the root cause of what is troubling them. In these situations, the teacher communicates through nonverbal and verbal communication that the student "matters", which most of the time is not expected teacher behavior or typically experienced by the students. In the present study, overweight or obese students felt being cared-for when PE teachers paid attention and made personal connections with them. One student said he liked when the teacher told him stories.

> Well, I've always been good with my teachers pretty much, like the one coach he was really funny like .... he'd always tell these funny stories and I'd go to him after class and like if I couldn't remember a part of the story I'd ask him to tell me . . .

Other overweight students felt cared-for when the teachers responded by being nice and making them feel special. For example, when students did good and kept quiet in class, teachers responded with rewards, such as letting them play basketball or providing special treats. Or they really liked it when teachers participated in activities. Overweight students felt cared-for or special when the teachers selected them and allowed them to be on their team.

In other situations, personal connections were made when the teachers talked to overweight or obese students about improving in a sport or improving their current health (e.g., losing weight). These personal connections are often specifically related to the overweight or obese students' unique characteristics. For example, one overweight student reported, "my PE teachers and coaches help me out a lot. They'll tell me about my weight, or sometimes they'll tell me I need to be playing football and stuff like that." Overweight students felt cared-for when teachers gave them information about their performance or weight status, offered to help them, and gave them opportunities or information on how they could improve.

PE involves movement and physical interaction with equipment and other people, so often there are injuries or mishaps. Sometimes teachers would warn students of safety issues like running on bleachers, such as make sure you "catch yourself". Other times, if an accident would happen, students were injured or happened to stumble, their PE teachers would come over to see if they were okay. For example, one overweight student commented,

If I stumble, they [PE teachers] usually come and see if I need ice or anything, make sure I can still walk, they look at it, make sure there is no damage done. And then they ask me 'am I okay', and I say yeah and they be 'Are you sure?' I would be like 'yeah', so I guess they have very caring personality, making sure that I'm ok if I stumble.

Another overweight student said if the injury was bigger, it was nice that the teacher would suggest that they go to see the nurse. Often overweight students had negative interactions with their peers due to weight stigma. When overweight students got teased by their peers and felt hurt, teachers came over and say things to cheer her up even though the teachers did not say anything to the teasers. Overweight students felt cared-for when they gave them advice on how to cope with teasing. One overweight student commented,

Yeah, they tell me, 'Don't worry about what other people say about you because, what they said about you, is the same thing as they say about other people too. So don't worry about what they say just keep it to yourself and keep rolling but if you feel like it's hurting you too bad then come tell somebody that you really know, and we will get on them about it' . . .

The teachers gave strategies to the overweight students and reinforced to them that they would be there for them if it got really bad, such as when teasing incidents evolved into physical altercations. This happens when overweight students do not have the coping mechanisms to deal with the teasing. How the teacher reacts and handles the fights made a big difference in how the overweight students handle the content in PE. One overweight student commented,

They [PE teachers] always stuck up for me oh certain things so if I were getting to fighting or something like that or whatever they would always stick up for me, I mean they would never let things get too out of hand things like that so I mean I just made me feel comfortable sticking with the physical fitness.

Supportive Peers.   Peer acceptance and friends' support are critical to the development of an individual's social and emotional functioning (La Greca & Bearman, 2000). Overweight or obese students felt being cared-for if they received support and encouragement during activities in PE or even outside school from their peers or friends. These supportive behaviors varied in many different forms, ranging from helping overweight students learn the subject matter in PE, providing emotional and social support, to encouraging them to keep trying. Some overweight students felt being cared-for when their friends helped them to learn motor skills or lose weight by working out with them. For example, one overweight student reported, "I was having problems with basketball, and then a couple days after school he invited me to come down and play with his friends and he showed me a couple good tricks on how to play." Another overweight student reported, "Like, on my weight, they'd like me to do better, and sometimes we'll go to the bottom of the gym and we'll be lifting weights, and I'll be losing weight and stuff." Another overweight student also commented, "When we have to run and stuff, they will be like 'come on you can do it'. They also tried to run with me so I don't stop."

Overweight students also felt be cared-for when their friends did not pick on them, buffered them from the teasers, played sports and did exercise together with them, or selected them on teams and backed up on their weakness or let them have time to shine if they are better at something. For example, one overweight student reported,

I have like one good, good friend, if she hear people talking about me she will say 'don't talk about her, you don't know anything about her, that's mean' and she would be like 'don't worry about them, they don't know no better' and she would just say something like that to make me feel good, and I love her, she's my best friend. Because she always help me like, help me with everything like showing me how to do it, and she would be like 'I could help you' and my other friends they would laugh you know how girls do, talk behind your back and then when you go confront them it's a whole other story. So I just have one good friend.

Overweight students felt being cared when peers were concerned about their well-beings by providing comfort when they got hurt, felt sad about their peers cheating in a game, or had a death in their family. For example, one overweight student commented,

> I was sitting there sad and kind of all to myself and they all came over there and was like it's going to be ok and they tried to do things to make me get mind off of my grandmother's death, which did help a lot.

In other situations, overweight students felt being cared-for when peers encouraged them to keep trying or demonstrate confidence in them to do the activities. Sometimes, their peers even slowed themselves down for overweight students to catch up with them. For example, one overweight student commented,

> When we are like doing our exercises or whatever, like say if I'm tired, and I don't do them right, sometimes they try to give us extra numbers on them, but sometimes they tell me 'You can do it,' and 'Just keep on trying you can do it.' if we were doing pushups, I just lay there if I'm tired, and they tell me I can do it and don't quit and keep doing it and then I just start doing it.

Another overweight student reported how his peers slowed down so that he could catch up with them.

> When I am running, and I get tired, they say keep on going and when I can't catch anybody, they say that um, 'we'll slow down for you,' because um, they can run fast and I can't run that fast, they say 'we'll slow down so you can run and catch us'.

Discussions and Implications. The purpose of the present study was to examine overweight or obese students' perceptions of caring in PE. Four themes emerged from our data: teachers' instructional adaptations, a positive, motivational learning climate, built interpersonal rapport, and supportive peers. According to Noddings (1984, 1992), the ethic of caring is created through making a connection between the 'one-caring' and the 'cared-for'. This interactive, relational process consists of three components: Engrossment, action and reciprocity. As illustrated from our themes, the ethics of caring was enacted between overweight or obese students and their teachers and peers in PE. Peers and PE teachers engrossed or considered overweight or obese students' personal physical situation (e.g., history of teasing, body shape and size), and conveyed regard and desire for overweight or obese students' well-being (e.g., Noddings, 1984) through their actions. These actions included teachers' making instructional adaptations, creating of a positive motivational learning climate, and building an interpersonal rapport, and peers' providing instructional assistance, feedback, and encouragement. Overweight or obese students perceived that their PE teachers' and peers' actions were to improve their well-being. As a result, overweight or obese students responded to their teachers' and peers' actions in many different positive ways, such as showing appreciation, being positive, and being more engaged. These findings are consistent with studies in general PE where students are more engaged when they perceive teacher caring (e.g., Cothran & Ennis, 1999, 2000; Cothran, Hodges Kulinna, & Garrahy, 2003; Ennis et al., 1997- Larson, 2006).

The quality of teacher-student interactions (i.e., instructional adaptations, feedback, social interactions, learning climates) has a great impact on students' engagement and learning in PE (Ayvazo & Ward, 2011; Carlson, 1995; Li & Lee, 2004; Silverman & Subramaniam, 1999). The findings showed that overweight or obese students reported that they felt being cared-for by their teachers when PE teachers made instructional adaptations to their abilities and skills, such as refinements (feedback), task supports and simplifications. Due to their body weight, overweight or obese students generally have difficulty performing the same instructional tasks as their peers, such as fitness activities and playing sports. To effectively and successfully include overweight or obese students in PE, teachers need to strategically design appropriate instructional tasks and make corresponding adaptations to the original stated tasks based on the responses from these students. By doing so, overweight or obese students would felt being cared-for and thus be more willing to engage in PE. Due to the sensitivity of obesity, PE teachers very often worry that content adaptations may make overweight or obese students feel embarrassed by "spotlighting" them. The data from the present study showed that these teaching behaviors made overweight or obese students feel good and be more motivated to learn.

Previous research on achievement motivation has demonstrated that when PE teachers foster a learning climate focusing on learning mastery and personal improvements (For a review, see Li & Lee, 2004), empower students with choices and autonomy (e.g., Hellison & Walsh, 2002), and make PE fun and enjoyable (e.g., Chen & Ennis, 2004; Li, Lee, & Solmon, 2005,2008), students are likely to display more adaptive motivational and behavioral responses. The findings of the present study showed that overweight or obese students felt being cared-for (engrossment and action) and therefore reciprocated, or were motivated to be engaged in PE when teachers foster a positive, motivational learning climate. Effective motivational strategies for successful inclusion of overweight or obese students include, empowering students with leadership opportunities and choices, listening to students' voices, providing autonomy support, teaching personal and social responsibility, focusing on personal improvement and effort, and setting realistic individualized goals.

Lowman (1984) has defined teaching excellence along two dimensions: good interpersonal rapport and effective teaching skills. Good interpersonal rapport is a key to teaching excellence because it involves mutual appreciation, trust and a sense that teachers and students understand and share each other's concerns (Lowman, 1984). There is a plethora of anecdotal evidence, supporting the key role that good interpersonal rapport plays in effective teaching in PE. The findings of the present study have showed that overweight or obese felt being cared-for and were more motivated to be engaged in PE when teachers had good interpersonal rapport with them. Practical strategies for building good interpersonal rapport with overweight or obese students include being nice, listening to their voices, appreciating and working with the differences with them, paying attention to them when they feel sad, stumble, or get injuries, being on their sides when they need support, and giving advice on living a healthy lifestyle. There is a lack of valid and reliable measurement of assessing. interpersonal rapport in PE and little research has been conducted to examine how interpersonal rapport contribute to effective teaching. This is an important area of research worthy of future endeavor.

The previous studies have mainly focused on teachers' caring behaviors (Larson, 2006; Lee & Ravizza, 2008) and not student-peer interactions that lead to caring. Peer acceptance and friends' support play a critical role in the development of an individual's social and emotional functioning (e.g., La Greca & Bearman, 2000). The present study extended the literature on perceptions of caring by examining the caring behaviors from peers and friends in PE. Our data showed that overweight or obese students felt being cared-for when their peers and friends helped them learn the skills, encouraged them to keep trying, and supported them emotionally and socially, etc. This was especially evident in situations where overweight or obese students could be teased or where their body shape and size puts them at a disadvantage and they need to work harder than other students. The supportive behaviors from peers and friends have become an important motivator for overweight or obese students to continually be engaged in PE.

The findings of the present study and the previous literature in PE (Larson, 2006; Lee & Ravizza, 2008) and general education (e.g., Hayes, Ryan, & Zseller, 1994; McCros-key, 1992) have also demonstrated that the essence of the concept of caring is context free. However, the specific caring behaviors are influenced by a particular context and student population. Many caring behaviors reported by overweight or obese students in the present study were context-specific responses to their unique characteristics and experience in PE. For example, teachers in the present study provided advice on how to cope with weight-related teasing and let overweight or obese students sit out of the activities when they could not catch their breath. Peer friends in the present study worked out together with overweight or obese students to help them lose weight. These context specific caring behaviors provide critical insights for PE teachers to develop and implement strategies to successfully and effectively include overweight or obese student in PE.

Recently, Newton et al. (2007) developed a measurement of caring in physical activity settings: The Caring Climate Scale (CCS). The CCS is a 13-item questionnaire with a five point Likert scale. It assesses the degree to which an individual perceives a participant learning environment as being inviting, safe, supportive, valuable, and respectful. Even though the preliminary study showed that the CCS measurement was valid and reliable (Newton et al., 2007), caring was conceptually defined as a single-dimensional construct. The findings from the previous studies (Larson, 2006; Lee & Ravizza, 2008) and the present study have suggested that the concept of caring is a multiple-dimensional rather than single-dimensional construct. It consists of three dimensions, including instructions, interpersonal rapport, and the type of learning environments from both teachers and peers. Currently, there is a lack of a valid and reliable measurement of perceptions of caring in PE from a multi-dimensional perspective. Information from both students and expert teachers on how they set up inclusive learning environments and care about students could provide excellent information to design this instrument. This is an important area worthy of future research to move forward the literature on caring in PE.

There were some limitations in the present study. The data were collected in an urban school district located in the Southern United States. The findings of the present study may be not transferable to southern suburban or rural areas or other areas of the country due to social-cultural and economic differences. Another limitation is that a single one-time interview research design was used (except for those who participated in the focus group). Interviews were used because of several constraining factors, including lacking access to participants, difficulty in scheduling multiple interviews due to parents' work schedule and school schedules, dangerous nature of inner city neighborhoods, and the emotionally charged nature of obesity and weight-related teasing. Future research should include data from other resources for triangulations.

Our findings have significant teaching implications. It is suggested that to create a caring climate, teachers need to allow overweight or obese students to work at their ability level, provide quality instruction and feedback and make developmentally appropriate instructional adaptations, foster a positive, motivational learning climate, create a connection between teacher and student (interpersonal rapport), and create a learning community with positive peer interactions. Creating an inclusive environment that enhances their sense of caring and belonging, has a great potential to increase overweight or obese students' engagement in PE.

References

Ames, C., & Ames, R. (Eds.). (1989). *Research on motivation in education: Goals and cognition (Vol. 3)*. San Diego: Academic Press.

Ames, C., & Archer, J. (1988). Achievement goals in the classroom: Students' learning strategies and motivation processes. *Journal of Educational Psychology, 80*, 260–267.

Ayvazo, S. & Ward, P. (2011). Pedagogical content knowledge of experienced teachers in physical education: Functional analysis of adaptations. *Research Quarterly for Exercise and Sport, 82*, 675–684.

Battistich, V., Solomon, D., Watson, M., & Schaps, E. (1997). Caring school communities. *Educational Psychologist, 32*, 137–151.

Bauer, K. W., Yang, Y. W., & Austin, S. B. (2004). "How can we stay healthy when you're throwing all of this in front of us?" Findings from focus groups and interviews in middle schools on environmental influences on nutrition and physical activity. *Health Education and Behavior, 31*, 34–46.

Bruner, J. (1996). *Cultural education*. Cambridge, MA: Harvard University Press.

Carlson, T. B. (1995). We hate gym: Student alienation from physical education. *Journal of Teaching in Physical Education, 14*, 467–477.

Chen, A., & Ennis, C. D. (2004). Goals, interests, and learning in physical education. *The Journal of Educational Research, 97*, 329–339.

Cothran, D. J., & Ennis, C. D. (1999). Alone in a crowd: Meeting students' needs for relevance and connection in urban high school physical education. *Journal of Teaching in Physical Education, 18*, 234–247.

Cothran, D. J. & Ennis, C. D. (2000). Building bridges to student engagement: Communicating respect and care for students in urban high schools. *Journal of Research & Development in Education, 33*, 106–117.

Cothran, D. J., Hodges Kulinna, P., & Garrahy, D. A. (2003). "This is kind of giving a secret away.": Students' perspectives on effective class management. *Teaching and Teacher Education, 19*, 435–444.

Cramer, P., & Steinwert, T. (1998). Thin is good, fat is bad: How early does it begin? *Journal of Applied Developmental Psychology, 19*, 429–451.

Creswell, J. W. (2003). *Research design: Qualitative, quantitative, and mixed methods approaches* (2nd ed.). Thousand Oaks, CA: Sage Publications, Inc.

Denzin, N. & Lincoln, Y. (1994). *Handbook of qualitative research*. Thousand Oak, CA: Sage Publications.

Eaton, D. K., Kann, L., Kinchen, S., Shanklin, S., Ross, J., Hawkins, J., . . . Wechsler, H. (2008). Youth Risk Behavior Surveillance—United States, 2007. *Morbidity & Mortality Weekly Report, 57(ss-4)*, 1–131.

Edmunds, L. D. (2005). Parents' perceptions of health professionals' responses when seeking help for their overweight children. *Family Practice, 22*, 287–292.

Eisenberg, M. E., Neumark-Sztainer, D., & Story, M. (2003). Associations of weight-based teasing and emotional well-being among adolescents. *Archives of Pediatric and Adolescent Medicine, 157*, 733–738.

Ennis, C. D., Cothran, D. J., Stockin, K. D., Owens, L. M., Loftus, S. J., Swanson, L, & Hopsicker, P. (1997). Implementing a curriculum in a context of fear and disengagement. *Journal of Teaching in Physical Education, 17*, 58–72.

Faith, M. S., Leone, M. A., Ayers, T. S., Heo, M., & Pietrobelli, A. (2002). Weight criticism during physical activity, coping skills, and reported physical activity in children. *Pediatrics, 110*, e23.

Fox, K. R., & Edmunds, L. D. (2000). Understanding the world of the "fat kid": Schools help provide a better experience? *Reclaiming Child Youth: Journal of Emotion Behavior Problems, 9*, 177–181.

Hayes, C., Ryan, A., & Zseller, E. (1994). The middle school child's perceptions of caring teachers. *American Journal of Education, 103*, 1–19.

Hellison, D., & Walsh, D. (2002). Responsibility-based youth programs evaluation: Investigating the investigations. *Quest, 54*, 292–307.

Kvale, S. (1996). *Interviews: An introduction to qualitative research interviewing*. Thousand Oaks, CA: Sage Publications.

La Greca, A. & Bearman, K. (2000). Commentary: Children with pediatric conditions: Can peers' impressions be managed? And what about their friends? *Journal of Pediatric Psychology, 25*, 147–149.

Larson, A. (2006). Student perception of caring teaching in physical education. *Sport, Education, and Society, 11*, 337–352.

Lee, O. & Ravizza, D. (2008). Physical education pre-service teachers' conceptions of caring. *Education, 128* (3), 460–472.

Li, W., & Lee, A. M. (2004). A review of conceptions of ability and related motivational constructs in achievement motivation. *Quest, 56*, 439–461.

Li, W., Lee, A. M. & Solmon, M. A. (2005). Relationships among dispositional ability conceptions, intrinsic motivation, perceived competence, experience, persistence, and performance. *Journal of Teaching in Physical Education, 24*, 51–65.

Li, W., Lee, A. M., & Solmon, M. A. (2008). Effects of dispositional ability conceptions, manipulated learning environments, and intrinsic motivation on persistence and performance: An interaction approach. *Research Quarterly for Exercise and Sport, 79*, 51–61.

Li. W. & Rukavina, P. (2012). The nature, occurring contexts, and psychological implications of weight-related teasing in urban physical education programs. *Research Quarterly for Exercise and Sport, 83*, 308–317.

Li, W., Rukavina, P., & Wright, P. (2012). Coping against weight-related teasing among adolescents perceived to be overweight or obese in urban physical education. *Journal of Teaching in Physical Education, 31*, 182–199.

Lowman, J. (1984). *Mastering the techniques of teaching*. San Francisco, CA: Jossey-Bass.

McCroskey, J.C. (1992). *An introduction to communication in the classroom*. Edina, MN: Burgess International.

Meece, J. L., Blumenfeld, P. B., & Hoyle, R. H. (1988). Students' goal orientations and cognitive engagement in classroom activities. *Journal of Educational Psychology, 80*, 514–523.

National Association for Sport and Physical Education (NASPE) (2001). *National standards for beginning physical education teachers*. Reston, VA: National Association for Sport and Physical Education.

Newton, M., Fry, M., Watson, D., Gano-Overway, L., Kim, M., Magyar, M., & Guivemau, M. (2007). Psychometric properties of the caring climate scale in a physical activity setting. *Revista de Psicologia del Deporte, 16*, 67–84.

Noddings, N. (1984). *Caring: A feminine approach to ethics and moral education*. Los Angeles, CA: University of California Press.

Noddings, N. (1992). *The challenge to care in schools: An alternative approach to education*. New York, NY: Teachers College Press.

Noddings, N. (2002). *Educating moral people: A caring alternative to character education*. New York, NY: Teachers College Press.

O'Keefe, M., & Coat, S. (2009). Consulting parents on childhood obesity and implications for medical student learning. *Journal of Pediatrics and Child Health, 45*, 573–576.

Pierce, J. W., & Wardle, J. (1997). Cause and effect beliefs and self-esteem of overweight children. *Journal of Child Psychology and Psychiatry and Allied Disciplines, 38*, 645–650.

Puhl, R., & Brownell, K. D. (2001). Bias, discrimination, and obesity. *Obesity Research, 9*, 788–805.

Puhl, R., & Brownell, K. D. (2003). Ways of coping with obesity stigma: Review and conceptual analysis. *Eating Behaviors, 4*, 53–78.

Shulman, L. S. (1987). Knowledge and teaching: Foundations of the new reform. *Harvard Educational Review, 57*, 1–22.

Silverman, S., & Subramaniam, P. R. (1999). Student attitude toward physical education and physical activity: A review of measurement issues and outcomes. *Journal of Teaching in Physical Education, 19*, 97–125.

Storch, E. A., Milsom, V. A., DeBraganza, N., Lewin, A. B., Geffken, G. R., & Silverstein, J. H. (2007). Peer victimization, psychosocial adjustment, and physical activity in overweight and at-risk-for-overweight youth. *Journal of Pediatric Psychology, 32*, 80–89.

Teven, J. J., & McCroskey, J. C. (1997). The relationship of perceived teacher caring with student learning and teacher evaluation. *Communication Education, 46*, 1–9.

Tiggemann, M., & Wilson-Barrett, E. (1998). Children's figure ratings: Relationship to self-esteem and negative stereotyping. *International Journal of Eating Disorder, 23*, 83–88.

Trout, J., & Graber, K. C. (2009). Perceptions of overweight students concerning their experience in physical education. *Journal of Teaching in Physical Education, 28*, 272–292.

Wentzel, K. (1997). Student motivation in middle school: The role of perceived pedagogical caring. *Journal of Educational Psychology, 89*, 411–419.

Wentzel, K. & Asher, S. (1995). The academic lives of neglected, rejected, popular, and controversial children. *Child Development, 66*, 754–763.

Xiang, P., McBride, R. E., Bruene, A., & Liu, Y. (2007). Achievement goal orientation patterns and fifth graders' motivation in physical education running programs. *Pediatric Exercise Science, 19*, 179–191.

Author's Note

This project is part of a larger one, funded by American Association of Health, Physical Education, Recreation, and Dance—Research Consortium Grant Programs.

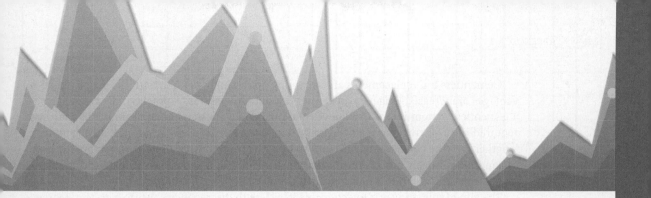

Appendix A-3

Leg Length Discrepancy in Cementless Total Hip Arthroplasty

Christopher N. Peck, Karan Malhotra, Winston Y. Kim
Department of Trauma and Orthopaedics, Salford Royal Hospital NHS Foundation Trust, Manchester, Britain

Received August 17, 2010; revised April 8, 2011; accepted April 18, 2011

Surgical Science, 2011, 2, 183–187
doi:10.4236/ss.2011.24040 Published Online June 2011 (http://www.SciRP.org/journal/ss)

Abstract

The use of cementless total hip arthroplasty (THA) is on the increase. In order to achieve rotational and axial stability larger implants may be required than originally templated for. This could potentially result in a larger leg length inequality. Our objective was to determine whether there is greater inequality in leg length post-operatively in cementless THA as compared to cemented implants. 136 consecutive patients undergoing elective THA between June 2007 and May 2008 were included. Post-operative digital radiographs were examined to determine leg length. Twenty seven patients (20%) underwent a cemented procedure and 109 (80%) a cementless procedure. In the cemented group the mean leg length discrepancy was 7.3 mm (range 19 mm short to 21 mm long). In the cementless group the mean measured leg length discrepancy was 6.3 mm (range 18 mm short to 23 mm long). There was no significant difference between the two groups (P = 0.443). This study shows that with accurate pre-operative templating, both cemented and cementless procedures produce comparable and acceptable leg length discrepancies.

Keywords: *Hip, Arthroplasty, Cementless, Leg Length*

1. Introduction. Total hip arthroplasty is a very successful operation in the management of end stage hip osteoarthritis with over 64,000 primary procedures being performed in the UK last year [9]. Leg length discrepancy (LLD) is a well documented complication of total hip replacement. It has been shown to correlate strongly with patient dissatisfaction [5,8,11,17] and is a leading cause of litigation [4]. Reports in the literature show a change in leg length following THA from 21 mm short to 35 mm long [5,7,15]. Studies have shown that a discrepancy greater than 10 mm can result in a limp, back pain, sciatica, stiffness, hip dislocation, the need for a shoe raise and early failure [7,13,15,17]. These problems are particularly problematic in the younger population where the impact on quality of life may be more marked.

Cementless hip replacements are becoming increasingly popular with the perceived advantages of increased longevity and easier revision procedures. A potential disadvantage of a cementless system is that to achieve rotational and axial stability larger implants may be required intra-operatively than originally templated for. This may result in inadvertent leg lengthening. The converse may occur if stability is achieved with a smaller implant. The use of a modular implant system means that the surgeon can make adjustments to the final leg length if necessary but this may affect the overall stability of the joint.

The aim of this study was to determine if leg length discrepancy exists to a greater degree in cementless THA compared with cemented hip replacements.

2. Patients and Methods. This retrospective study was performed at a single institution, a large University Teaching Hospital in the North-West of England. All surgeries were carried out by one of five lower limb arthroplasty consultants. The inclusion criteria were all patients undergoing a primary elective total hip arthroplasty (THA) between June 2007 and May 2008. Patients were excluded if the contralat-eral hip had already been replaced.

Preoperative templating was done using an overlay technique on hard film copies of digital radiographs. The size of the acetabular cup was templated first and its centre of rotation marked. Using this, the size of the femoral stem was determined and the proposed neck cut that would best reproduce the normal neck-shaft angle and offset. All procedures were carried out under either a general or spinal anaesthetic and were performed with the patient in the lateral position through a posterior approach. Leg length was assessed intra-operatively by comparing the relative position of the knees through the drapes and the soft tissue tension during trial reduction. The cemented femoral implants used were the collarless polished taper (CPT) (Zimmer, Swindon, UK) and the Exeter stem (Stryker, Howmedica Osteonics, Berkshire, UK). The cementless femoral implants used were the Zimmer M/L Taper Hip Prosthesis with standard and extended offsets and modular heads and the CLS Zimmer cementless stem (Zimmer, Swindon, UK).

All post-operative radiographs were in the digital format on the Patient Archive and Communication System (PACS, General Electric) and measurements were made using the systems integrated measurement tools. An-tero-posterior digital radiographs of the pelvis, centred on the pubic symphysis with the hips internally rotated 15° were taken on the first post-operative day, prior to mobilisation. Limb length inequality was calculated using the method described by Woolson *et al.* [16] and subsequently by a number of other authors [5,8,11,12,15]. This is measured as the perpendicular distance from the inter-teardrop line to the most prominent point on the lesser trochanter of the femur. The distance on the post-operative side was compared to the contralateral limb which was assumed to be equal to the initial length of the operated limb before development of joint disease. Magnification was adjusted for by using a standard estimation of 20% magnification consistent with the literature [3,10,14,15]. All measurements were made on the initial post-operative radiographs and were made to the nearest millimetre by a single observer not involved in the surgical procedures. Each measurement was taken twice, at the same sitting, and an average value used to reduce intra-observer errors.

All data was analysed using Excel for Windows (Microsoft). Continuous parametric data were analysed using the two sample T-test and nonparametric data were analysed using the chi squared test ($p < 0.05$ was considered as significant).

3. Results. Between June 2007 and May 2008 166 patients underwent a primary total hip arthroplasty (THA). Thirty patients had a pre-existing contralateral hip replacement and so were excluded. Of the 136 patients in the study 27 (20%) underwent a cemented THA and 109 (80%) a cementless procedure. Fifty eight (43%) patients were male and 78 (57%)

were female. The mean age of patients was 66.7 years in the cemented group and 66.4 in the ce-mentless (Table A3.1).

Post-operatively in the cemented group seven patients (26%) had some degree of radiographic shortening, 19 (74%) had some degree of lengthening and one patient (4%) had equal leg lengths. In the cementless group 32 patients (29%) had some degree of radiographic shortening, 67 (61%) had some degree of lengthening and 10 patients (9%) had equal leg lengths. There was no significant difference between these proportions (P = 0.949).

When corrected for an estimated magnification of 20% the mean radiographic limb length inequality regardless of direction was 7.3 mm in the cemented group and 6.3 mm in the cementless group (P = 0.496). In the cemented group two patients (7%) had shortening greater than 10 mm (mean 16.5 mm) and four patients (15%) had lengthening greater than 10 mm (mean 17.3 mm). In the cementless group five patients (5%) had shortening greater than 10 mm (mean 14.0 mm) and 17 patients (16%) had lengthening greater than 10mm (mean 14.0 mm). There was no significant difference between these groups (P = 0.331 for shortening, P = 0.140 for lengthening). These results are summarised in Table A3.1.

4. Discussion. To be successful, hip replacement surgery needs to accurately reconstruct the patient's own anatomy and bio-mechanics. This includes reproducing the centre of rotation of the hip joint, the offset and leg length. This requires the appropriate selection and orientation of implants and if not done appropriately will lead to post operative complications and patient dissatisfaction.

Leg length discrepancy can have a significant impact on patient satisfaction and is one of the leading causes of the litigation following THA in America [4,7]. Leg lengthening is much less tolerated than leg shortening, with lengthening over 10 mm being very poorly tolerated by the patient [16]. Lengthening of the operated limb can lead to joint stiffness, sciatic nerve palsy, low back pain, early failure of the prosthesis and the need for revision surgery [7,13,15,17]. Shortening can impair hip abduction and increase the risk of dislocation [13].

In a study of 75 patients Konyves et al. [5] showed that the post-operative Oxford Hip Score was significantly worse in patients with leg lengthening compared to those with equal leg lengths. Most other studies confirm that a discrepancy in leg length has a direct adverse effect on clinical and functional outcome [8,11,17]. In contrast, White et al. [15] showed no statistically significant difference in the Harris Hip Score and SF 36 Health Survey in patients with radiological leg lengthening or shortening. However, their outcome scores were measured at six months after surgery so long-term problems were not assessed. Furthermore it has been suggested that the Harris Hip Score may not fully take into account the patients' subjective experience of pain [17]. The position of the acetabular component

TABLE A3.1	Patient demographics and post-operative radiographic leg length discrepancy (LLD) in cemented and cementless THA. (SD Standard Deviation).		
	CEMENTED THA	CEMENTLESS THA	SIGNIFICANCE
Number of Patients	27 (20%)	109 (80%)	
Mean Age (Range)	66.7 years (30 - 87)	66.4 years (37 - 88)	p = 0.930
Males (M)/Females (F)	M = 15 (56%) F = 12 (44%)	M = 43 (39%) F = 66 (61%)	
Overall mean LLD (SD)	7.3 mm (6.0)	6.3 mm (4.9 mm)	p = 0.496
Mean (SD) Shortened LLD [Range]	6.8 mm (7.2) [1 to 19 mm]	6.8 mm (4.0) [1 to 18 mm]	p = 0.956
Mean (SD) Lengthened LLD [Range]	8.0 mm (5.5) [1 to 21 mm]	7.0 mm (5.0) [1 to 23 mm]	p = 0.475

has a much smaller impact on leg length, it has been shown that only 2% of patients with a leg length discrepancy were attributed to the position of the acetabular component [5].

True and apparent leg length should be measured pre-operatively in all patients to guide the surgeon as to how the joint should be reconstructed [7]. Intra-operatively, with the patient in the lateral position, leg length can be judged by comparing the relative knee and ankle position and by assessment of soft tissue tension. However, this is not always accurate as any small change in the position of the patient can lead to a big change in apparent leg length and be misleading [11,16]. An additional part of the preoperative plan is hip templating which is routinely used to guide the surgeon towards the size and placement of implants, the neck length, offset, level of the femoral osteotomy and the restoration of limb length required. This can be done by the traditional overlay method or by using a computer package for digital radiographs. These methods have been shown to have variable correlation with the actual implants used [2,14] and so may be deceptive to the surgeon leading to difficulty in achieving equal leg lengths.

Despite evidence of better short to medium term results for cemented implants there is an increasing tendency towards cementless fixation with the perceived advantages of increased longevity and easier revision procedures. In 2008 33% of implants were cementless compared to 21% in 2004 and this trend looks set to continue [9]. With cementless hip replacements rotational and axial stability is achieved intra-operatively by a press fit technique. We felt that in many cases a larger implant was required to accomplish this than was originally tem-plated for with the possibility of inadvertently causing leg length discrepancy. The majority of cementless components increase in offset with increasing component size and therefore lengthen the limb. Modular implant systems may allow the surgeon to make adjustments to the final leg length if necessary but this may affect the overall stability of the joint. Final adjustments would be impossible with a mono-block system. In a laboratory study Barink *et al.* [1] assessed how well two different cementless hip systems matched the final rasp position. Using synthetic and cadaveric femurs the average rasp-stem mismatch was within 2 mm in three different planes, the mismatch being larger in the cadaveric femurs. The authors felt that this mismatch was of low clinical relevance. However, any mismatch may be misleading when performing a trial reduction to determine the final implant size. As far as we are aware this study has not been repeated with other cementless stems leaving any mismatch with these systems unknown.

There are very few clinical or radiological studies in the literature evaluating leg length discrepancy in ce-mentless hip replacements. In a radiographic analysis Leonard *et al.* [6] compared cemented and cementless hip replacements for offset and limb length. They showed that cementless procedures resulted in a greater degree of leg lengthening with a mean of 5.6 mm compared to 3.8 mm in the cemented group, this was statistically significant. Our results show an overall mean leg length discrepancy of 7.3 mm in the cemented group and 6.3 mm in the cementless group which is consistent with other published series [5,7,15]. In contrast to Leonard *et al.* [6] we found no significant difference in ra-diographic leg length discrepancy between cementless and cemented implants. This may simply be due to the spread of our results shown by the high standard deviations, possibly due to the five different surgeons per forming the hip replacements. However, no measure of spread was provided in Leonard's paper.

We acknowledge the limitations of the present study which should be considered when interpreting the results. The surgeries were carried out by five different consultants in lower limb reconstruction each with their own variations on templating and intraoperative methods to equalise leg lengths. No account was taken of the pre-existing limb length which can have a direct impact on the post operative limb length. Additionally, no assessment was made of disease in the contralateral hip which may also have a bearing on a surgeons desired final leg length of the operated hip. Due to the retrospective nature of the study we were unable to compare the size of the prosthesis used with the size of prosthesis templated for. This would have given us a better understanding as to whether the size of final implants may have changed leg length.

The general limitations of using radiographs to make our measurements include the variation in positioning of the pelvis with respect to the x-ray film and variations in relative magnification due to distance from the film. However, as these factors affect both hips and we are comparing the difference between the two it is reasonable to use plain radiographs to assess leg length. Our methods of measuring leg length discrepancy have been used in numerous other studies [5,8,11,12,15] and are considered to be accurate and reliable. To calculate the magnification the radiographic diameter of the prosthetic femoral head can be compared to the actual diameter of the prosthesis. This data was not available in the current study so a standard magnification factor of 20% was used to adjust the actual measurements taken from the radiographs. However, this is the standard magnification used in most templating systems and consistent with other studies [3,10,14,15].

5. Conclusions. In conclusion, total hip arthroplasty is a safe, effective and reproducible treatment for end stage degenerative hip disease. The current trend is towards the use of ce-mentless implants particularly in the younger patient. Our study shows that there is no significant difference in leg length discrepancy between cementless and cemented implants. This suggests that with accurate pre-operative templating both cemented and cementless procedures produce comparable and acceptable leg length discrepancies.

6. Conflict of Interest Statement. No benefits in any form have been received or will be received from a commercial party related directly or indirectly to the subject of this article.

7. References

1. M. Barink, H. Meuers, M. Spruit, C. F. Fankhauser and N. Verdonschot, "How Close Does an Uncemented Hip Stem Match the Final Rasp Position?," *Acta Orthopaedica Belgica*, Vol. 70, No. 6, 2004, pp. 534–539.
2. L. W. Carter, D. O. Stovall and T. R. Young, "Determination of Accuracy of Preoperative Templating of Non-cemented Femoral Prostheses," *The Journal of Arthroplasty*, Vol. 10, No. 4, 1995, pp.507–513. doi:10.1016/S0883-5403(05)80153-6
3. K. S. Conn, M. T. Clarke and J. P. Hallett, "A Simple Guide to Determine the Magnification of Radiographs and to Improve the Accuracy of Preoperative Templating," *Journal of Bone and Joint Surgery*, Vol. 84-B, No. 2, 2002, pp. 269–272. doi:10.1302/0301-620X.84B2.12599
4. A. A. Hofmann and M. C. Skrzynski, "Leg Length Inequality and Nerve Palsy in Total Hip Arthroplasty: A Lawyer Awaits," *Orthopaedics*, Vol. 23, No. 9, 2000, pp. 943–944.
5. A. Konyves and G. C. Bannister, "The Importance of Leg Length Discrepancy after Total Hip Arthroplasty," *Journal of Bone and Joint Surgery*, Vol. 87-B, No. 2, 2005, pp. 155–157.
6. M. Leonard, P. Magill, P. Kiely and G. Khayyat, "Radiographic Comparison of Cemented and Uncemented Total Hip Arthroplasty and Hip Resurfacing," *European Journal of Orthopaedic Surgery and Traumatology*, Vol. 17, No. 6, 2007, pp. 583–586. doi:10.1007/s00590-007-0228-y
7. W. J. Maloney and J. A. Keeney, "Leg Length Discrepancy after Total Hip Arthroplasty," *The Journal of Arthroplasty*, Vol. 19, No. 4, 2004, pp. 108–110. doi:10.1016/j.arth.2004.02.018
8. S. B. Murphy and T. M. Ecker, "Evaluation of a New Leg Length Measurement Algorithm in Hip Arthroplasty," *Clinical Orthopaedics and Related Research*, Vol. 463, 2007, pp. 85–89.
9. National Joint Registry 6th Annual Report, 2009. http://www.njrcentre.org.uk/njrcentre/linkclick.aspx?fileticket=euukur4jpyc%3d&tabid=86&mid=523
10. M. J. Oddy, M. J. Jones, C. J. Pendergrass, J. R. Pilling and J. A. Wimhurst, "*Assessment of Reproducibility and Accuracy in Templating Hybrid Total Hip Arthroplasty Using Digital Radiographs*," *Journal of Bone and Joint Surgery*, Vol. 88, No. 5, 2006, pp. 581–585.
11. C. S. Ranawat, R. R. Rao, J. A. Rodriguez and H. S. Bhende, "Correction of Limb-Length Inequality During Total Hip Arthroplasty," *The Journal of Arthroplasty*, Vol. 16, No. 6, 2001, pp. 715–721. doi:10.1054/arth.2001.24442

12. N. Sugano, T. Nishii, H. Miki, H. Yoshikawa, Y. Sato, and S. Tamura, "Mid-Term Results of Cementless Total Hip Replacement Using a Ceramic on Ceramic Bearing with and Without Computer Navigation," *Journal of Bone and Joint Surgery*, Vol. 89, No. 4, 2007, pp. 455–460.

13. K. T. Suh, S. J. Cheon and D. W. Kim, "Comparison of Preoperative Templating with Post-Operative Assessment in Cementless Total Hip Arthroplasty," *Acta Orthopaedica Scandinavica*, Vol. 75, No. 1, 2004, pp. 40–44. doi:10.1080/00016470410001708070

14. A. Unnanuntana, D. Wagner and S. B. Goodman, "The Accuracy of Preoperative Templating in Cementless Total Hip Arthroplasty," *The Journal of Arthroplasty*, Vol. 24, No. 2, 2009, pp. 180–186. doi:10.1016/j.arth.2007.10.032

15. T. O. White and T. W. Dougall, "Arthroplasty of the Hip Leg Length Is Not Important," *Journal of Bone and Joint Surgery*, Vol. 84-B, No. 3, 2002, pp. 335–338. doi:10.1302/0301-620X.84B3.12460

16. S. T. Woolson, J. M. Hartford and A. Sawyer, "Results of a Method of Leg-Length Equalization for Patients Undergoing Primary Total Hip Replacement," *The Journal of Arthroplasty*, Vol. 14, No. 2, 1999, pp. 159–164. doi:10.1016/S0883-5403(99)90119-5

17. V. Wylde, S. L. Whitehouse, A. H. Taylor, G. C. Bannister and A. W. Blom, "Prevalence and Functional Impact of Patient-Perceived Leg Length Discrepancy after Hip Replacement," *International Orthopaedics*, Vol. 33, No. 4, 2009, pp. 905–909. doi:10.1007/s00264-008-0563-6

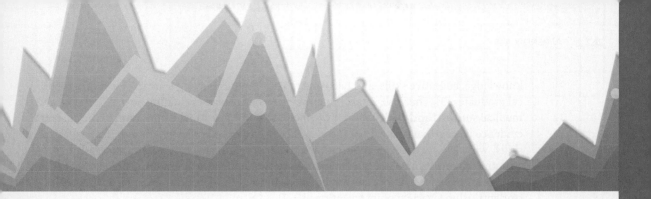

Appendix A-4

Teaching Evidence-Based Medicine Literature Searching Skills to Medical Students During the Clinical Years: A Randomized Controlled Trial

Dragan Ilic, PhD; Katrina Tepper, BSc (Hons); Marie Misso, PhD

See end of article for authors' affiliations.
DOI: http://dx.doi.org/10.3163/1536-5050.100.3.009

Objectives: *Constructing an answerable question and effectively searching the medical literature are key steps in practicing evidence-based medicine (EBM). This study aimed to identify the effectiveness of delivering a single workshop in EBM literature searching skills to medical students entering their first clinical years of study.*

Methods: *A randomized controlled trial was conducted with third-year undergraduate medical students. Participants were randomized to participate in a formal workshop in EBM literature searching skills, with EBM literature searching skills and perceived competency in EBM measured at one-week post-intervention via the Fresno tool and Clinical Effectiveness and Evidence-Based Practice Questionnaire.*

Results: *A total of 121 participants were enrolled in the study, with 97 followed-up post-intervention. There was no statistical mean difference in EBM literature searching skills between the 2 groups (mean difference=0.007 (P=0.99)). Students attending the EBM workshop were significantly more confident in their ability to construct clinical questions and had greater perceived awareness of information resources.*

Conclusions: *A single EBM workshop did not result in statistically significant changes in literature searching skills. Teaching and reinforcing EBM literature searching skills during both preclinical and clinical years may result in increased student confidence, which may facilitate student use of EBM skills as future clinicians.*

Introduction. Competency in evidence-based medicine (EBM) provides clinicians with the ability to identify, evaluate, and integrate evidence into clinical decision making. Two of the five critical steps in achieving competency in EBM are to (1) construct an answerable question from the clinical environment and (2) effectively and efficiently search the medical literature to identify the best available evidence to answer the question [1]. EBM users must be proficient in these skills before evidence can be appraised (step 3), integrated into clinical practice (step 4), and evaluated (step 5).

Various training modules and courses in EBM are now commonly implemented in medical schools worldwide [2]. The aim of such EBM programs is to provide an integration of knowledge, cognitive skills, and behaviour that promotes lifelong learning for future medical graduates [3]. There is a small, but growing evidence base evaluating how to best educate medical students and clinicians in the principles of EBM [3, 4]. The limitation of the current evidence base is that majority of these studies have focused on evaluating critical appraisal skills, with few focused on training medical undergraduates in the critical steps of constructing an answerable question and effectively searching the literature. Those studies that have been published report an improvement in the EBM skills of undergraduate medical students using a variety of interventions [5–7].

A before and after study of sixty third-year medical students in 2000 reported improvement in EBM skills following a mini-course in EBM, consisting of four sessions about writing clinical questions, searching MEDLINE, appraising articles critically, and applying evidence [5]. A 2005 non-randomized controlled trial reported the positive impact of a single MEDLINE workshop delivered to fourth-year medical students [6]. Students were provided with a clinical scenario and asked to develop a search strategy, which was assessed by a librarian using a search strategy analysis instrument. Students who attended the workshop produced higher quality search strategies, compared to those who did not attend the workshop. Similarly, a 1998 randomized controlled trial (RCT) allocating first-year medical students to a single training session on formulating questions and searching also identified improvement in question design and search skills for students receiving the intervention [7].

Highlights

- A single workshop did not improve the medical literature searching skills of third-year medical undergraduate students.
- Students taking a workshop were more confident in constructing answerable clinical questions and identifying information gaps.
- Student confidence in writing a clinical question, identifying information sources, and performing a literature search was high six-months post-workshop.

Implications

- Students' perceptions of competency may not be accurate reflections of their skills.
- Workshops may be valuable for the increase in confidence they provide.

Although these various studies have identified the positive impact of EBM workshops on students, none have identified when specific EBM skills, such as effectively searching the medical literature, should be taught—be it during a medical student's preclinical or clinical years of study. The level of "clinical maturity" of students can affect their perception of the importance and uptake of EBM principles in practice. A study of junior doctors' (postgraduate trainees in obstetrics and gynaecology) knowledge of and beliefs in EBM identified a belief that EBM was an essential skill relevant to their clinical practice, despite few having partaken in formal training in the principles of EBM [8]. Conversely, first-year medical students who have not been exposed to the clinical environment have been reported to perceive EBM as a static discipline, not relevant to clinical medicine [9].

Many medical courses have adopted the spiral curriculum, in which specific topics, skills, themes, or concepts are continuously revisited throughout the curriculum [10]. This spiral approach to learning aims to revisit past experience and promote deeper learning by building on existing knowledge. Obtaining a high level of knowledge and mastery of EBM skills requires a combination of formal education and application of these principles in a clinical context.

This RCT aimed to determine the effectiveness of delivering a single formal workshop in EBM literature searching skills to undergraduate medical students who had received prior training in EBM. The specific objectives of the study were to:

1. compare the EBM literature searching skills of medical students who participate in a single formal workshop during their first clinical year of studies, compared to medical students who have only received informal EBM training during their preclinical years of study; and

2. determine medical students' self-perceived competency in EBM literature searching skills.

Methods

Study design and setting. A single-centre, single-blinded RCT with intention-to-treat analysis was performed with third-year medical students undertaking the undergraduate bachelor of medicine/bachelor of surgery (MBBS) degree at Monash University, a five-year undergraduate course. Students spend the first two years based at the university, outside of the clinical environment. In these first two preclinical years, students undertake core subjects in anatomy, physiology, and pharmacology. During the preclinical years of the Monash MBBS degree, all students also participate in several sessions about medical information sources, using the population, intervention, comparison, outcomes (PICO) framework to write answerable clinical questions and searching the medical literature. During years three to five of the course, students are placed in a clinical learning environment. Students spend their entire third year of the degree at one clinical site but rotate between sites for the remainder of their clinical years. The Monash MBBS undergraduate degree, and by extension the students, are comparable to similar MBBS degrees in Australia and internationally that train undergraduate students in the principles of EBM across preclinical and clinical years of the degree [11].

Recruitment. Third-year medical students were recruited from three teaching hospitals associated with the course (Monash Medical Centre, Dandenong, and Casey) from the Southern Health network of hospitals. To meet eligibility, participants were required to be a third-year Monash MBBS student at the time of the study. Students who were unwilling to participate in the study or did not wish to provide consent were excluded from the study.

Randomization. Participants were randomly assigned independently by the Southern Health clinical site administrator by block randomization to either the intervention or control groups (Figure A4.1). A computer random number generator was used to generate a randomization list in blocks of four.

Intervention. Students randomized to the intervention participated in an EBM literature searching skills (EBM-LSS) workshop. The EBM-LSS workshop was two hours in duration and was delivered in the training room of the Hargrave-Andrew Library at the Clayton campus of Monash University. The EBM-LSS workshop began with a formal presentation by the subject librarian, which covered (i) how to construct an answerable question from the clinical environment, (ii) major sources of medical information, and (iii) how to effectively and efficiently search the medical literature to identify the best available evidence to answer the question.

The studies, syntheses, synopses, summaries, and systems (5S) model was used to compare and contrast the content and structure of the medical information sources and to highlight approaches to searching them effectively [12]. Students then completed an interactive, computer-based searching session and concluded the workshop by completing self-directed learning tasks (with the subject librarian providing support when requested).

Control. Students allocated to the control group did not attend the EBM-LSS workshop during the study period. These students had the opportunity to attend the EBM-LSS workshop once the study had concluded (i.e., once competency in EBM literature searching skills and self-perceived competency in EBM had been assessed).

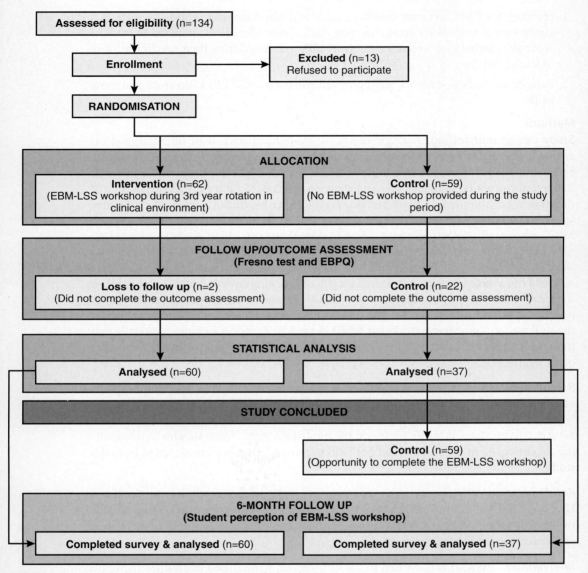

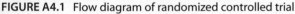

FIGURE A4.1   Flow diagram of randomized controlled trial

Outcome measures. The primary outcome to be measured in this study was competency in EBM literature searching skills, which was measured by using the previously validated Fresno tool [13]. The Fresno tool provides users with a clinical scenario and a series of open-ended questions relating to the five EBM steps. The Fresno tool evaluates skills in question formulation, knowledge of information sources, choice of study design, search strategy development, and relevance of selected evidence. Rather than using the clinical scenario in the Fresno tool, students were presented with the following scenario to avoid recall bias from previous exposure to the Fresno tool:

> Your patient is a 50 year old man with a family history of colorectal cancer. The patient recently received a pamphlet in the post advertising the National Bowel Cancer Screening program. You explain to your patient that the Screening program uses the Faecal Occult Blood Test (FOBT). Whilst understanding that no test is 100% accurate, the patient wants to know whether it would be useful for him to undertake the FOBT—will it save his life?

Based on this scenario, students were assessed for their ability to construct a clinical question (step 1 of the EBM process) and effectively search the medical literature to identify the best evidence to answer the clinical question (step 2 of the EBM process). The maximum score attainable for the Fresno tool was adjusted to reflect that only the first 2 steps of the EBM process were being evaluated in this study. Therefore, the maximum overall score possible was 29, with the maximum subcomponent scores of writing a clinical question, identifying information sources, identifying appropriate study types, and performing an effective literature search being 3, 6, 12, and 8 points, respectively.

Student self-perceived competency in EBM literature searching skills was assessed using the previously validated Clinical Effectiveness and Evidence-Based Practice Questionnaire (EBPQ) [14]. The EBPQ is a self-reported measure of implementation of EBM in the clinical environment. It can be used to evaluate educational programs as questions relate to the measurement of the practice, attitudes, and knowledge/skills associated with EBM. Only the knowledge/skills domain of the EBPQ was utilized in this study, as measuring students' practice of and attitudes toward EBM would be unnecessary since they do not practice medicine in a clinical setting.

These outcomes were measured across both intervention and control groups at 1 week post-implementation of the intervention. Control students were given the opportunity to attend the EBM-LSS workshop at the conclusion of the initial study period (study phase 1) to ensure equivalence among the student cohort. All students who attended the EBM-LSS workshop completed a questionnaire, six months after attending the workshop (study phase 2) that evaluated their confidence in (i) writing a clinical question, (ii) identifying information sources, (iii) identifying appropriate study designs to answer a clinical question, and (iv) performing a literature search efficiently. Students were asked to evaluate their confidence on a 5-point Likert scale (1=poor, 5=excellent). Students were also asked to reflect whether the EBM-LSS workshop improved their EBM competency on a 5-point Likert scale (1=strongly disagree, 5=strongly agree).

Blinding. Blinding of investigators and participants was not possible as the subject librarian and students were aware of their allocation. The outcome assessor and data analyst were blinded to the allocation.

Analyses

Sample size calculation. A previous study, which implemented the Fresno test to assess searching skills, was referred to when estimating the sample size for this trial [15]. This previous study identified a mean difference of 13 points on the Fresno test to be statistically significant in identifying competency between groups in effective EBM literature searching. A mean difference of 13 points, with a standard deviation of 10, is meaningful to discriminate between "novice" and "expert" users of EBM principles [13]. It was determined that with a power of 90%, alpha of 0.05, the required sample size per group was 21, for a total sample size of 42 participants.

Analyses. Data were analyzed using the principle of intention-to-treat. Mean difference in EBM literature searching skills competency between the intervention and control groups, as determined by the Fresno tool, were explored using a Student's *t*-test. Descriptive statistics were used to characterize participants' self-perceived competency in EBM literature searching skills at one week and six months post-intervention.

Ethical approval for this study was granted by the Monash University Human Research Ethics Committee.

Results. A total of 121 of 134 eligible students were enrolled in the study, with 62 participants (51.2%) allocated to the intervention and 59 participants (48.8%) allocated to the control group (study phase 1). There was no statistical mean difference in EBM literature searching skills between the participants who attended the formal workshop and

TABLE A4.1	Student Competency Scores Across Evidence-Based Medicine (EBM) Literature Searching Skills as Identified by the Fresno Tool					
	MEAN (SD) SCORE					
	Intervention		Control		Mean	P
Component	(n=60)		(n=37)		Difference	Value
Overall EBM literature searching skills	10.51	(5.10)	10.50	(4.53)	0.007	0.99
Subcomponents						
Writing a focused clinical question	1.73	(0.66)	1.76	(0.76)	−0.029	0.82
Identifying information sources	2.31	(1.84)	2.78	(1.77)	−0.478	0.15
Identifying an appropriate study type	4.33	(2.85)	3.80	(2.77)	0.535	0.30
Performing a literature search	2.12	(2.39)	2.14	(2.51)	−0.019	0.96

participants who did not (mean difference=0.007 (P=0.99). There was no statistically significant difference between the 2 groups with respect to writing a focused clinical question (step 1 of the EBM process), identifying information sources, or performing a structured literature search (step 2 of the EBM process) (Table A4.1). Students who received the EBM-LSS workshop were more likely to choose a systematic review (as it is perceived to offer the best level of evidence) to answer the question in the clinical scenario; however, this was not a significantly statistical difference between groups (RR=1.26, 95% CI 0.91, 1.74).

Participants in the EBM-LSS workshop were significantly more confident in completing step 1 of the EBM process (converting a clinical scenario into a question) and had a greater perceived awareness of information resources (step 2 of the EBM process) (Table A4.2). Students in the EBM-LSS workshop also had a greater confidence in identifying gaps in their professional practice.

A total of 97 (80.2%) participants were followed-up post-intervention (60 in the intervention group and 37 in the control group) (study phase 2). Twenty-four participants

TABLE A4.2	Student Self-Perceived Competency Across EBM Literature Searching Skills as Identified by the Clinical Effectiveness and Evidence-Based Practice Questionnaire					
	MEAN (SD) SCORE				Mean	
Component	Intervention (n=60)		Control (n=37)		Difference	P Value
Research skills	4.72	(0.94)	4.45	(1.14)	0.269	0.21
Information technology skills	5.08	(1.10)	4.83	(1.34)	0.245	0.33
Monitoring and reviewing of practice skills	4.53	(1.01)	4.33	(1.17)	0.201	0.38
Conversion of your information needs into a research question	5.15	(1.02)	4.56	(1.32)	0.582	0.01
Awareness of major information types and sources	5.20	(0.90)	4.73	(1.42)	0.473	0.04
Ability to identify gaps in your professional practice	5.10	(0.98)	4.63	(1.12)	0.461	0.03
Knowledge of how to retrieve evidence	5.10	(1.03)	4.86	(1.15)	0.235	0.30
Ability to critically analyze evidence against set standards	4.67	(1.14)	4.72	(1.16)	−0.055	0.81
Ability to determine how valid (close to the truth) the material is	4.68	(1.18)	4.61	(1.27)	0.072	0.77
Ability to determine how useful (clinically applicable) the material is	4.88	(1.09)	4.91	(1.22)	−0.033	0.89
Ability to apply information to individual cases	5.08	(1.02)	4.75	(1.05)	0.334	0.12
Sharing of ideas and information with colleagues	5.45	(1.01)	5.38	(1.12)	0.061	0.78
Dissemination of new ideas about care to colleagues	5.16	(1.10)	5.02	(1.20)	0.138	0.57
Ability to review your own practice	5.05	(1.09)	4.71	(1.17)	0.336	0.16

TABLE A4.3	Student Confidence in EBM Literature Searching at 6 Month After the EBM Literature Searching Skills (EBM-LSS) Workshop Attendance (n=97)									

	CONFIDENCE IN EBM LITERATURE SEARCHING SKILLS									
	Poor	Below Average		Average		Very Good		Excellent	
	n	n	(%)	n	(%)	n	(%)	n	(%)
Writing a focused clinical question	0	1	(1.0%)	9	(9.3%)	43	(44.3%)	44	(45.4%)
Identifying information sources	0	2	(2.1%)	14	(14.4%)	51	(52.6%)	30	(30.9%)
Identifying an appropriate study type	0	2	(2.1%)	19	(19.6%)	53	(54.6%)	23	(23.7%)
Performing a literature search	0	3	(3.1%)	19	(19.6%)	50	(51.5%)	25	(25.8%)

(2 intervention and 22 control group) declined to complete the follow-up survey. The remaining students completed a 6-month post-workshop follow-up survey, which assessed their confidence in EBM skills such as preparing an answerable clinical question and literature searching skills. More than 75% of respondents believed that their EBM literature searching skills were very good or excellent across the 4 measured competencies (Table A4.3). This contrasts with the scores obtained from the Fresno tool 6 months earlier, which indicated that students in both groups exhibited "novice" rather than "intermediate" or "expert" skill in EBM literature searching. Despite the absence of any measureable improvement after the EBM-LSS workshop, more than 70% of participants (both intervention and control groups) agreed that the EBM-LSS workshop was effective in improving their EBM literature searching skills (Table A4.4).

Discussion. This study indicated that the delivery of a single EBM-LSS workshop to third-year undergraduate medical students did not significantly improve student ability to perform the first two steps of the EBM process. Students who had been randomized to an EBM-LSS workshop had greater confidence in their ability to write answerable clinical questions and in their awareness of relevant information sources, compared to students who did not receive the EBM-LSS workshop. Although no data were collected before the implementation of the EBM-LSS workshop, student confidence in performing critical EBM literature searching was significantly higher immediately after the intervention group took the workshop in the intervention group than in the controls. However, this self-perceived increase in confidence should be viewed with caution, since it does not necessarily correlate with a higher competency in practicing EBM [16].

A recently published study documented the effectiveness of combining an online educational intervention with clinical rotations in a cohort of third-year undergraduate medical students [17] and involved extended, faculty mentored instruction throughout the year. The authors concluded that there was a significant improvement in EBM skills after the educational intervention (as measured by the Fresno tool). The results of our study might differ from this and previously published studies for a variety of reasons. Our study evaluated the impact of a single workshop, while other studies evaluated the impact of a series of workshops [5, 17]. Delivering a series of workshops, rather than a single workshop, would promote reinforcement and development of student skills over a period of time and, therefore, be more likely to result in significant improvements.

TABLE A4.4	Student Perceived Worth of the EBM-LSS Workshop at 6 Month Post-EBM-LSS Workshop Attendance (n=97)								

	STRONGLY DISAGREE	DISAGREE		NEITHER AGREE OR DISAGREE		AGREE		STRONGLY AGREE	
	n	n	(%)	n	(%)	n	(%)	n	(%)
EBM-LSS workshop improved EBM competency	0	8	(8.2%)	20	(20.6%)	34	(35.1%)	35	(36.1%)

The EBM-LSS workshop in our study did not focus solely on MEDLINE, as a number of other studies reported [5, 6], but highlighted a range of different information sources. Focusing on more than one source limits the time available to explore specific sources in depth, which may also have limited the potential for significant improvements in student literature searching skills. However, this approach was used to highlight to students that it is not always necessary to start their search with MEDLINE, as they may be able to locate reliable evidence using another source, such as the Cochrane Library. The different approaches to practicing EBM—the "doing," "using," and "replicating" modes [18]—were also highlighted as this may influence which source they choose to search first.

Previous research has indicated that clinical maturity, perceived relevance of EBM in the clinical environment, and continued practice of evidence-based skills in this context may influence a medical student's competence in EBM skills [8, 9, 19, 20]. Whilst there is no significant difference in EBM skills between the intervention and control groups in this study, the results indicate that students who are taught these skills during the clinical years of their study demonstrate greater self-confidence in adopting the first two EBM steps. This increased confidence may be attributed to observing how practicing clinicians use these skills in the clinical environment and positively influence the manner in which these students implement EBM skills during their clinical years of study and beyond [21].

Integrating a formal workshop during the clinical years of study provides students with opportunities to practice searching for and identifying evidence that can be directly related to the clinical context. It is important that students are aware that they can adjust their approach to suit the clinical environment and do not always have to carry out all five steps of EBM, the "doing" mode [18]. They may also incorporate evidence in a "using" or "replicating" mode, in which one or more of the five steps are not carried out by them directly [18].

Limitations. There was no assessment of EBM literature searching skills before and after the intervention. This is important to note as the authors were not able to measure the impact of previous training programs implemented during the preclinical years of student training and the potential confounding effect on this trial. Given that it was not possible to blind the students in this study, it is possible that contamination between the two arms of the study (with students sharing knowledge about the EBM-LSS workshop intentionally or indirectly) might have been a confounding factor in this study. Whilst it did not affect the power of the study, it must also be noted that twenty-two students from the control arm did not complete the outcome assessment.

The Fresno tool evaluates skills in question formulation, knowledge of information sources, choice of study design, search strategy development, and relevance of selected evidence. Students were not directed to use MEDLINE but were given the choice to select a relevant source. The Fresno tool assigns an "excellent" score if three PICO elements are used in the search strategy. However, for the scenario that the students completed in the intervention, a relevant Cochrane systematic review was able to be located in the Cochrane Library with a basic search using only one PICO element. This may have resulted in students obtaining low scores in the "performing a literature search" component of the Fresno tool, even though they might have located a Cochrane systematic review.

It can be argued that the most important outcome is to ensure that students can locate and identify the best evidence; how many PICO elements they include or where they look may be secondary to this. A clinical scenario in which there was limited evidence (i.e., no Cochrane systematic review) might have been better at discriminating skill levels between the students. It should also be noted that the authors used adapted versions of the Fresno and EBPQ tools, both of which have been validated on practicing health professionals, rather than undergraduate medical students.

Conclusions. Medical students may develop effective, if not efficient, skills in searching the medical literature and finding evidence during the preclinical years. However, as students transfer into the clinical years of their medical education, it is valuable to reinforce and develop these skills further in the clinical environment. Increased confidence may be an important factor in students continuing to search for and use evidence effectively and efficiently in their practice in the future.

Acknowledgments. The authors thank the involvement of the third-year Monash University MBBS students for their participation in this study. The authors also thank Dominic Upton and Penelope Upton for the use of the EBPQ.

References

1. Straus S, Glasziou P, Richardson W, Haynes B. *Evidence-based medicine: how to practice and teach it.* Edinburgh, UK: Churchill Livingstone, Elsevier; 2011.
2. Dinkevich E, Marksinson A, Ahsan S, Lawrence B. Effect of a brief intervention on evidence-based medicine skills of pediatric residents. *BMC Med Educ.* 2006;6:1.
3. Ilic D. Teaching evidence based practice: perspectives from the undergraduate and post-graduate viewpoint. *Ann Acad Med Singapore.* 2009;38(6):559–63.
4. Coomarasamy A, Khan K. What is the evidence that postgraduate teaching in evidence based medicine changes anything? a systematic review. *BMJ.* 2004 Oct 30;329(7473): 1017.
5. Ghali W, Saitz R, Eskew A, Gupta M, Quan H, Hershman W. Successful teaching in evidence-based medicine. *Med Educ.* 2000 Jan;34(1):18–22.
6. Gruppen L, Rana G, Arndt T. A controlled comparison study of the efficacy of training medical students in evidence-based medicine literature searching skills. *Acad Med.* 2005 Oct;80(10):940–4.
7. Rosenberg W, Deeks J, Lusher A, Snowball R, Dooley G, Sackett D. Improving searching skills and evidence retrieval. *J R Coll Physicians Lond.* 1998 Nov–Dec;32(6):557–63.
8. Hadley J, Wall D, Khan K. Learning needs analysis to guide teaching evidence-based medicine: knowledge and beliefs amongst trainees from various specialities. *BMC Med Educ.* 2007;7:11.
9. Astin J, Jenkins T, Moore L. Medical students' perspective on the teaching of medical statistics in the undergraduate medical curriculum. *Stat Med.* 2002 Apr 15;21(7): 1003–6.
10. Bruner J. *The process of education.* Cambridge, MA: Harvard University Press; 1960.
11. Finkel M, Brown H, Gerber L, Supino P. Teaching evidence-based medicine to medical students. *Med Teach.* 2003 Mar;25(2):202–9.
12. Haynes RB. Of studies, syntheses, synopses, summaries, and systems: the "5S" evolution of information services for evidence-based health care decisions. *ACP J Club.* 2006 Nov–Dec;145:A8.
13. Ramos K, Schafer S, Tracz S. Validation of the Fresno test of competence in evidence based medicine. *BMJ.* 2003 Feb 8;326(7384):319.
14. Upton D, Upton P. Development of an evidence-based practice questionnaire for nurses. *J Adv Nurs.* 2006 Feb; 53(4):454–8.
15. Kim S, Willett L, Murphy D, O'Rourke K, Sharma R, Shea J. Impact of an evidence-based medicine curriculum on resident use of electronic resources: a randomized controlled study. *J Gen Intern Med.* 2008 Nov;23(11):1804–8.
16. Lai N, Teng C. Self-perceived competence correlates poorly with objectively measured competence in evidence based medicine among medical students. *BMC Med Educ.* 2011;11:25.
17. Aronoff SC, Evans B, Fleece D, Lyons P, Kaplan L, Rojos R. Integrating evidence based medicine into undergraduate medical education: combining online instruction with clinical clerkships. *Teach Learn Med.* 2010 Jul;22(3): 219–23.
18. Straus SE, Green ML, Bell DS, Badgett R, Davis D, Gerrity M, Ortiz E, Shaneyfelt TM, Whelan C, Mangrulkar R. Evaluating the teaching of evidence based medicine: conceptual framework. *BMJ.* 2004 Oct 30;329(7473):1029–32.
19. Bradley P, Oterholt C, Nordheim L, Bjorndal A. Medical students' and tutors' experiences of directed and self-directed learning programs in evidence-based medicine: a qualitative evaluation accompanying a randomized controlled trial. *Eval Rev.* 2005 Apr;29(2):149–77.
20. Dorsch JL, Aiyer MK, Meyer LE. Impact of an evidence-based medicine curriculum on medical students' attitudes and skills. *J Med Lib Assoc.* 2004 Oct;92(4):397–406.
21. Ilic D, Forbes K. Undergraduate medical student perceptions and use of evidence based medicine: a qualitative study. *BMC Med Educ.* 2010;10:58.

Authors' Affiliations

Dragan Ilic, PhD (corresponding author), Senior Lecturer, Level 6, Department of Epidemiology and Preventive Medicine, School of Public Health and Preventive Medicine, The Alfred Centre, Monash University, 99 Commercial Road, Melbourne VIC3004, Australia; **Katrina Tepper, BSc (Hons),** Research and Learning Coordinator, Hargrave-Andrew Library (Building 30), Monash University, Clayton, VIC 3800, Australia; **Marie Misso, PhD,** Senior Evidence Officer, Jean Hailes for Women's Health, School of Public Health and Preventive Medicine, Monash Site, 43-51 Kanooka Grove, Clayton VIC 3168, Australia

Received September 2011; accepted December 2011

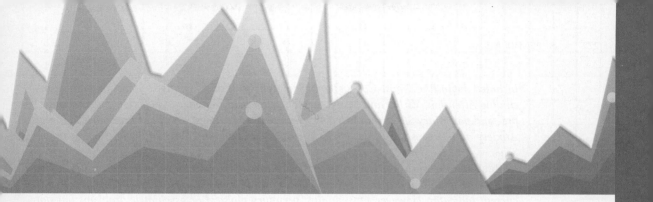

Appendix A-5

Predictors of Postconcussive Symptoms
3 Months After Mild Traumatic Brain Injury

Jennie Ponsford
Monash University; Monash-Epworth Rehabilitation Research Centre, Epworth Hospital; and National Trauma Research Institute, Melbourne, Australia

Peter Cameron and Mark Fitzgerald
Monash University; Alfred Hospital; and National Trauma Research Institute, Melbourne, Australia

Michele Grant
Monash University; Monash-Epworth Rehabilitation Research Centre, Epworth Hospital; and National Trauma Research Institute, Melbourne, Australia

Antonina Mikocka-Walus
Monash University, National Trauma Research Institute and University of South Australia

Michael Schönberger
Monash University; Monash-Epworth Rehabilitation Research Centre, Epworth Hospital; and University of Freiburg

Objective: *There is continuing controversy regarding predictors of poor outcome following mild traumatic brain injury (mTBI). This study aimed to prospectively examine the influence of preinjury factors, injury-related factors, and postinjury factors on outcome following mTBI.*

Method: *Participants were 123 patients with mTBI and 100 trauma patient controls recruited and assessed in the emergency department and followed up 1 week and 3 months postinjury. Outcome was measured in terms of reported postconcussional symptoms. Measures*

This article was published Online First April 2, 2012.
Jennie Ponsford and Michele Grant, Monash University, Monash-Epworth Rehabilitation Research Centre, Epworth Hospital, and National Trauma Research Institute, Melbourne, Australia; Peter Cameron, Monash University, Alfred Hospital, and National Trauma Research Institute, Melbourne, Australia; Mark Fitzgerald, Monash University, Alfred Hospital, and National Trauma Research Institute, Melbourne, Australia; Antonina Mikocka-Walus, Monash University, School of Nursing and Midwifery, University of South Australia, National Trauma Research Institute, Melbourne, Australia; and Michael Schönberger, Monash University, Monash-Epworth Rehabilitation Research Centre, Epworth Hospital, and Department of Rehabilitation Psychology, Institute of Psychology, University of Freiburg, Germany.
This research was funded by a grant from the Victorian Neurotrauma Initiative. The authors also gratefully acknowledge the assistance of staff in the Alfred Hospital Emergency and Trauma Care Department.
© 2012 American Psychological Association 0894-4105/12 DOI: 10.1037/a0027888

included the ImPACT Post-Concussional Symptom Scale and cognitive concussion battery, including Attention, Verbal and Visual memory, Processing Speed and Reaction Time modules, pre- and postinjury SF-36 and MINI Psychiatric status ratings, VAS Pain Inventory, Hospital Anxiety and Depression Scale, PTSD Checklist–Specific, and Revised Social Readjustment Scale.

Results: *Presence of mTBI predicted postconcussional symptoms 1 week postinjury, along with being female and premorbid psychiatric history, with elevated HADS anxiety a concurrent indicator. However, at 3 months, preinjury physical or psychiatric problems but not mTBI most strongly predicted continuing symptoms, with concurrent indicators including HADS anxiety, PTSD symptoms, other life stressors and pain. HADS anxiety and age predicted 3-month PCS in the mTBI group, whereas PTSD symptoms and other life stressors were most significant for the controls. Cognitive measures were not predictive of PCS at 1 week or 3 months.*

Conclusions: *Given the evident influence of both premorbid and concurrent psychiatric problems, especially anxiety, on postinjury symptoms, managing the anxiety response in vulnerable individuals with mTBI may be important to minimize ongoing sequelae.*

Keywords: *traumatic brain injury, concussion, outcome assessment*

Mild traumatic brain injury (mTBI) is a prevalent neurological condition, affecting 100–300 out of 100,000 annually (Cassidy et al., 2004; Hirtz et al., 2007). Although studies have shown that most cases make a full recovery within 3 months of injury, approximately 15%–25% of cases experience ongoing symptoms, which may cause significant disability (Carroll et al., 2004; Ponsford et al., 2000), with frequencies varying according to population studied, setting, and timing of recruitment (Belanger, Curtiss, Demery, Lebowitz, & Vanderploeg, 2005). The term *postconcus-sion syndrome* (PCS) refers to the somatic, cognitive, emotional, motor, or sensory symptoms ascribed to a concussion or head injury (Benton, 1989). These symptoms commonly include headaches, dizziness, visual disturbance, memory difficulties, poor concentration, mental slowness, difficulty dividing attention, alcohol intolerance, fatigue, irritability, depression, and anxiety (Carroll et al., 2004; Kraus et al., 2005; Lundin, de Boussard, Edman, & Borg, 2006; Ponsford et al., 2000; Yang, Tu, Hua, & Huang, 2007). Given the high frequency of mTBI, it is neither realistic nor necessary to provide comprehensive treatment to all people with these injuries. However, single-session therapies applied to at-risk individuals with mTBI may be efficacious (Mittenberg, Canyock, Condit, & Patton, 2001). Currently, clinicians assessing these patients do not have clear guidelines as to how to predict who is likely to experience ongoing symptoms. The early identification of such cases might allow for the early provision of management strategies to circumvent ongoing problems. Understanding the causes of ongoing PCS may also guide treatment.

Although numerous injury-related factors have been associated with continuing symptoms following mTBI, findings have been inconsistent (Carroll et al., 2004). The strongest predictors of outcome in moderate to severe TBI—namely, duration of loss of consciousness, initial Glasgow Coma Scores (GCS), and duration of posttraumatic amnesia (PTA), which are measures of injury severity— have not been shown to be significant predictors of ongoing sequelae following mTBI (Carroll et al., 2004; Ponsford et al., 2000). The reasons for this are unclear, but measurement issues may contribute to this (Ponsford et al., 2004). Although presence of intracranial abnormalities has been associated with poorer cognitive performance or persistent PCS in some studies (Lange, Iverson, & Franzen, 2009; Lewine et al., 2007; Lo, Shifteh, Gold, Bello, & Lipton, 2009; Sadowski-Cron et al., 2006; Williams, Levin, & Eisenberg, 1990), patients with uncomplicated mTBI do not show intracranial abnormalities. Poorer performances on cognitive tests of reaction time (RT), processing speed, immediate memory, verbal memory, and visual memory have also been documented in mTBI patients in relation to trauma controls early after injury (Landre, Poppe, Davis, Schmaus, & Hobbs, 2006; Peterson, Stull, Collins, & Wang, 2009; Ponsford et al., 2000;

Sheedy, Geffen, Donnelly, & Faux, 2006; Shores et al., 2008), although there have been mixed findings regarding the relationship of cognitive impairments with PCS (Landre et al., 2006; Meares et al., 2008; Ponsford et al., 2000).

Of possible demographic predictors, female gender has been associated with greater reporting of PCS (Dischinger, Ryb, Kufera, & Auman, 2009; Meares et al., 2008; Ponsford et al., 2000). Age over 40 years was a negative prognostic factor in one study (Thornhill et al., 2000), but not other studies of mTBI, despite being a strong predictor of poorer outcome following moderate to severe TBI (Hukkelhoven et al., 2003). One study (Stulemeijer, Vos, Bleijenberg, & van der Werf, 2007) found that lower education predicted cognitive complaints 6 months postinjury. Findings regarding the effects of multiple concussive head injuries have been mixed. Results of a recent meta-analysis suggested that multiple self-reported concussions were associated with poorer performances on tests of delayed memory and executive function (Belanger, Spiegel, & Vanderploeg, 2010). However, the clinical significance of these differences was unclear.

The presence of preinjury psychiatric or other health problems and other life stressors have emerged as significant predictors of poorer mTBI outcomes in several studies (Carroll et al., 2004; Kashluba, Paniak, & Casey, 2008; McLean et al., 2009; Meares et al., 2008; Ruff, 2005; Wood, 2004). Concurrent anxiety, depression, and posttraumatic stress may contribute to symptoms (Bryant, 2008; Hoge et al., 2008; Stulemeijer et al., 2007), as may other injuries, pain, and medications (Carroll et al., 2004; Meares et al., 2006, 2008; Ponsford, 2005). Meares et al. (2006, 2008) found that a diagnosis of PCS an average of 4.9 days postinjury was just as likely in trauma controls as it was in patients with mTBI, in patients admitted to hospital with major trauma, with PCS predicted by previous affective or anxiety disorder, female gender, IQ, processing speed, and acute posttraumatic stress symptoms, but not presence of mTBI. Meares and colleagues (2008) raised doubts as to whether mild TBI contributes anything to symptoms over and above these factors. However, it is possible that the effects of anesthesia and analgesia impacted on findings in this group.

Increased reporting of symptoms may be associated with litigation or compensation-seeking (Binder & Rohling, 1996; Kashluba et al., 2008; Paniak et al., 2002). This will in turn depend upon the cause of injury and context of assessment. In a study focusing on mTBI cases with disappointing recoveries mostly in a litigation or compensation context, the variables most strongly related to outcome were depression, pain, and symptom invalidity on measures of response bias (Mooney, Speed, & Sheppard, 2005).

Thus it appears that mTBI is a complex condition. Potential contributing factors relate to preinjury factors (demographic variables including gender, age, and education; preinjury physical and psychiatric status; and history of previous head injury), injury-related factors (presence and severity of mTBI in terms of PTA duration and GCS, associated cognitive impairments), and the postinjury coexistence of pain, posttraumatic stress disorder (PTSD), other forms of anxiety, depression, other life stressors, and litigation. However, no study has prospectively examined the relative influence of all these factors in patients with uncomplicated mTBI and a general trauma sample recruited in the emergency department (ED) soon after injury not requiring general anesthesia. Therefore, the aim of this study was to prospectively examine the influence of the above-mentioned factors on outcome measured in terms of PCS 1 week and 3 months postinjury. It was hypothesized, on the basis of previous studies, that injury-related factors, including presence and severity of a mTBI, would have the strongest influence on outcome measured in terms of postconcus-sive symptoms at 1 week postinjury and that ongoing problems at 3 months postinjury would be predicted by a combination of mTBI presence and severity; psychological factors including anxiety, depression, pain, and PTSD; and other life stressors. It was considered important for clinicians to be able to predict, on the basis of factors known in the ED (i.e., preinjury and injury-related factors), what the outcome would be at both 1 week and 3 months postinjury. It was also considered important to be able to identify, on the basis of status at 1 week postinjury, when patients may be reviewed clinically, what factors predicted ongoing PCS at 3 months postinjury. Concurrent predictors were examined at each time point to identify causative factors relating to PCS at each time point.

Method. The study was conducted as part of a study examining outcome and the use of a revised version of the Westmead PTA Scale as a screening tool in patients with mTBI. It was approved by the Alfred Hospital and Monash University Research Ethics Committees.

Participants. Participants were recruited consecutively from the Alfred Emergency & Trauma Centre (E&TC) in Melbourne, Australia. Inclusion criteria for the mTBI group included (1) recent (<24 hr) history of trauma to the head, resulting in loss of consciousness (LOC) <30 minutes, PTA <24 hours, and a GCS score of 13–15 on presentation to the ED; (2) age 18 years or over; and (3) English speaking. Participants were excluded if they (1) were intubated or required general anesthesia following injury; (2) had a breath alcohol reading >.05 at time of recruitment; (3) were under the influence of illicit substances at the time of injury; (4) had focal neurological signs, seizures, or intracerebral abnormality on computed tomography (CT); (5) had a dominant upper-limb injury that precluded use of a computer mouse; (6) were under spinal precautions and not able to sit upright; (7) had a history of previous cognitive impairment, neurological illness, significant alcohol or drug abuse or other psychiatric impairment currently affecting daily functioning; or (8) were unavailable for follow-up. The trauma control (TC) group comprised patients presenting with minor injuries not involving the head and no LOC or PTA following their injury. Other inclusion and exclusion criteria were the same as for the mTBI group. Individuals with a medical history of nonneurological illness (e.g., cardiac disease, hypertension, cancer, diabetes), psychiatric history (excluding psychosis), prior mTBI, and reported alcohol or cannabis use were included in the study if they did not report any significant preinjury cognitive difficulties.

Measures. The dependent variable, PCS, was measured using the ImPACT Post-Concussion Symptom Inventory (Lovell & Collins, 1998) comprising 22 common concussion symptoms (e.g., headache, dizziness) with the severity ranging from 0 = *none* to 6 = *severe*. The list is more expansive than the criteria included in ICD-10. The symptoms were added into a total Post-Concussive Symptoms summary score, reflecting the number and severity of symptoms.

The following measures were examined as potential predictors of PCS:

Preinjury Factors. Preinjury factors included age in years, gender, education in years, and previous head injury (yes/no; number of previous head injuries). Preinjury physical and mental health was assessed with the SF-36 Health Survey (SF-36; Jen-kinson, Coulter, & Wright, 1993; Ware & Sherbourne, 1992), comprising a 36-item questionnaire, yielding an 8-scale health profile and two summary measures—a Physical Component Score and a Mental Component Score. Preinjury psychiatric history was assessed with the Mini-International Neuropsychiatric Interview (MINI; Sheehan et al., 1998), a brief, reliable and valid structured diagnostic interview comprising 130 questions, screening for 16 Axis I *Diagnostic and Statistical Manual of Mental Disorders* (4th ed.; *DSM-IV*) disorders and 1 personality disorder. Presence or absence of a diagnosis in each category was documented.

Injury-Related Factors. The Glasgow Coma Scale score (Te-asdale & Jennett, 1976) utilizes the injured person's best eye-opening, verbal, and motor responses to assess the conscious state, with a total score between 3 (showing no response) and 15 (alert and well oriented).

The PTA duration in days was determined by asking the patient what his or her first memory was after the injury and what had happened after that, until the patient could provide detailed and continuous recall of events after the injury. This was verified by examination of ambulance and hospital admission notes and discussion with accompanying persons. Patients were also screened using the revised Westmead PTA Scale (Ponsford et al.,

2000), and if still in PTA on admission to the ED also had their orientation and ability to lay down new memories assessed prospectively at hourly intervals using this measure.

Cognitive performance was determined with the ImPACT concussion battery (Iverson, Lovell, & Collins, 2005), a computer-administered neuropsychological test battery consisting of five test modules, testing attention, verbal and visual memory, processing speed, and RT. Summary scores for each module were used in analyses.

Postinjury Factors

Pain. The Visual Analogue Scale (VAS) is a brief scale ranging from 0 (*no pain*) to 10 (*extreme pain*) used to measure pain. The VAS has been commonly used as a brief and convenient measure of pain for more than 30 years (Huskisson, 1974).

Use of narcotic analgesia.   Yes/No

Posttraumatic Stress Symptoms. The PTSD Checklist— Specific (PCLS) is a self-report rating scale for assessing the 17 *DSM-IV* symptoms of PTSD on a 5-point scale from *not at all* to *extremely*. A total symptom severity score (range 17–85) is obtained by summing scores from the 17 items. The scale has been comprehensively validated (Blanchard, Jones-Alexander, Buckley, & Forneris, 1996; Forbes, Creamer, & Biddle, 2001).

Anxiety and Depression. The Hospital Anxiety and Depression Scale (HADS) is a validated self-assessment scale of current anxiety and depression symptoms, with 14 questions graded on a 4-point Likert scale (0–3), yielding separate anxiety and depression subscale scores of 0–21. The scale minimizes use of physical symptoms of mood disorders, which may be present in the medically ill (Snaith & Zigmond, 1986). The validity and reliability of the HADS has been established in patients with TBI (Schönberger & Ponsford, 2010; Whelan-Goodinson, Ponsford, & Schönberger, 2009).

Other Life Stressors. The Revised Social Readjustment Rating Scale (RSRRS) measures 43 stressful events that happened in the last 12 months (Holmes & Rahe, 1967; Horowitz, Schaefer, Hi-roto, Wilner, & Levin, 1977). The total score was recorded. These scores are interpreted as follows: low stress <149; mild stress = 150–200; moderate stress = 200–299; major stress >300.

Litigation (yes/no). Participants were asked to indicate whether (1) they were seeking compensation, (2) claims or charges had been made against them, and (3) any litigation had been resolved.

Procedure. Potential mTBI and TC participants were identified on the computerized E&TC patient list. Patients with mTBI were recruited after they had emerged from PTA, as assessed using the revised Westmead PTA Scale. After providing informed consent and demographic information, participants completed the acute assessment at the hospital prior to discharge or, in a few cases, at home, but within 48 hours of injury. The acute assessment comprised a computerized concussion assessment battery (ImPACT) that also included the PCS to document current symptoms. The SF-36 was completed because it pertained to their general health and wellbeing prior to injury. This assessment took 45 min.

At 1 week follow-up, participants in both mTBI and TC groups completed the ImPACT cognitive battery, PCS measure, SF-36, HADS, and VAS as they pertained to current functioning. Information regarding current capacity for work, study, and functional activities was also collected. The MINI diagnostic interview was completed with respect to prevalence of lifetime preinjury psychiatric disorders. At the 3-month follow-up, participants repeated the same assessments. However, the SF-36 examined the participants' general health over the preceding 4-week period, and the MINI examined psychiatric status within the 3 months since injury. Participants also completed the PCL-S to assess postinjury PTSD symptoms and the RSRRS to measure concurrent life stressors and reported on current employment status. These assessments took 1 hr.

Analysis. Data analysis was undertaken with SPSS17 (SPSS, Inc., Chicago, IL), and statistical significance was reported at the 0.05 level. Missing values, of which there were very few, were excluded from descriptive statistics. Categorical variables were presented as percentages and continuous variables as medians and ranges. The main outcome was PCS. Preliminary correlational analyses were conducted using Spearman's rho to examine both the correlations between the variables and PCS and the intercor-relations of the variables, because only a limited number of variables could be included in each model, and there was a need to avoid multicollinearity. Following these analyses, a series of generalized linear models (GLM) were computed to identify predictors of postconcussive symptoms at 1 week and 3 months postinjury. Because GLMs do not exclude cases with missing values, the only variables excluded were those that contributed to multicollinearity. Because the PCS scores were skewed, for use in regression analysis, PCS scores were grouped into three categories with equal frequencies. Because the PCS scores declined over time, the grouping was done separately for PCS scores at 1 week and 3 months as follows: The baseline PCS scores were divided into ≤16, 17–35, and ≥36. The PCS scores at 1 week were split into ≤5, 6–23, and ≥24. The PCS scores at 3 months were divided into 0, 1–8, and >09. GLM is a flexible approach to multiple regression that allows it to predict ordinal dependent variables. In order to do so, ordinal logistic regression was chosen as the link function in the GLMs.

The GLMs were conducted in three models. Table A5.1 shows the predictors that were used in each model. The first model used information from time of injury to predict outcome, first at 1 week postinjury and separately at 3 months postinjury. The SF-36 Mental Health scale was removed to avoid collinearity with preinjury psychiatric status. The second model examined prediction of PCS, first at 1 week and second at 3 months postinjury on the basis of information known at 1 week postinjury. SF-36 Mental quality of life and HADS depression were removed from the model to avoid collinearity with other variables.

TABLE A5.1	Predictor Variables for GLM Models			
DATA PHASE	**VARIABLE**	**MODEL 1**[a]	**MODEL 2**[a]	**MODEL 3**[b]
Preinjury	Gender	✓	✓	✓
	Age	✓	✓	✓
	Psychiatric history (MINI)	✓		
	Physical health (SF-36)	✓		✓
Acute	PTA duration	✓	✓	✓
	Verbal memory (ImPACT)	✓		
	Visual memory (ImPACT)	✓		
	Group (mTBI/control)	✓	✓	✓
1 week	Verbal memory (ImPACT)		✓	
	Visual memory (ImPACT)		✓	
	Pain (VAS)		✓	
	Physical health (SF-36)		✓	
	Anxiety (HADS)		✓	
	Narcotic/analgesics		✓[c]	
3 months	Verbal memory (ImPACT)			✓
	Visual memory (ImPACT)			✓
	Pain (VAS)			✓
	PTSD symptoms (PCLS)			✓
	Stressful life events (RSRRS)			✓
	Anxiety (HADS)			✓

Note: GLM = generalized linear models; MINI = Mini-International Neuropsychiatric Interview; SF-36 = Short-Form 36; PTA = posttraumatic amnesia; mTBI = mild traumatic brain injury; VAS = Visual Analogue Scale; HADS = Hospital Anxiety and Depression Scale; PTSD = posttraumatic stress disorder; PCLS = PTSD Checklist—Specific; RSRRS = Revised Social Readjustment Rating Scale.
[a] Developed to predict PCS at 1 week and 3 months. [b] Developed to predict PCS at 3 months. [c] Adjusted for only in the PCS at 1-week model.

Narcotics/analgesics were adjusted for only in the PCS 1-week model, because a significant number of participants were still using these. The third model examined the influence of both preinjury demographic and health factors and concurrent factors relating to cognitive function, pain, PTSD symptoms, general anxiety symptoms, and other life stres-sors on reported PCS at 3 months postinjury. The model was conducted to predict PCS at 3 months only. In order to examine whether the variables predicting outcome differed between mTBI and TC groups, models predicting 3-month PCS were conducted for mTBI and TC groups separately, using the same variables as in the previous models. The relationship between the presence of preinjury psychiatric disorders and HADS scores 1 week and 3 months postinjury was examined with Student t test. Group differences and changes over time in PCS and HADS were calculated with Mann–Whitney test, Wilcoxon signed-ranks test, and Friedman test because the variables were not normally distributed.

Results. Participants were recruited between January 2007 and January 2009. During this period, 882 potential mTBI participants were admitted to the E&TC while it was staffed by a mTBI researcher, including evenings and weekends. Of these, 196 were eligible, and 123 were recruited into the study. Of 1404 potential TC participants, 338 were eligible and 100 were recruited and completed the acute assessment. The participant profiles are described in Table A5.2. Patients were predominantly young single men injured in motor vehicle collisions. There were no significant group differences in terms of gender, age, education, marital status, or employment status, or in history of previous mTBI. The mTBI group more commonly sustained assault-related injuries than did controls. More mTBI participants than controls had soft tissue injuries/ lacerations.

TABLE A5.2   Profile of Patients by Group

DEMOGRAPHICS	MTBI (N = 123)	TC (N = 100)
Age (years)[a]	31 (18–72)	32 (19–66)
Education (years)[a]	13 (14–22)	14 (9–20)
Gender (male)[b]	91 (74)	64 (64)
Married/de facto[b]	47 (38.2)	41 (40)
Employment status[b]		
Full time	96 (78)	84 (84)
Part time	9 (7.3)	2 (2)
Casual	4 (3.3)	9 (9)
Student	3 (2.4)	2 (2)
Not working	11 (8.9)	3 (3)
Cause of injury[b]		
Assault	16 (13.3)*	2 (2)
Motor vehicle collision[c]	49 (40.9)	28 (28)
Bicycle collision	24 (20)	18 (18)
Fall	15 (12.5)	23 (23)
Sport injury	10 (8.3)	11 (11)
Other	9 (7.3)	18 (18)
Type of injury[b]		
Soft tissue/laceration	97 (78.9)**	59 (59)
Fracture	21 (17.1)	21 (21)
Ligamentous	5 (4.1)	19 (19)
Dislocation	0 (0)	1 (1)
Involved in litigation[b]	15 (17.2)	7 (8.9)
History of head injury[b]	51 (41.5)	28 (28)

Note: Chi-square tests. TC = trauma control; mTBI = mild traumatic brain injury.
[a] Values are given as median (range). [b] Values are given as N (percentage). [c] This category includes motor vehicle, motorcycle, and pedestrian hit by vehicle collisions.
*p = .001.
**p < .001.

At acute ED assessment, 77 (62.6%) TBI and 44 (44%) controls reported taking narcotic analgesics ($p = .006$). At 1 week, these numbers dropped to 20 (18.2%) in the TBI group and 19 (21.1%) in controls without any statistical group difference ($p = .603$). At 3 months the use of narcotic analgesics dropped to 2 patients in each group ($p = .905$).

Of the 120 mTBI participants with a known LOC status, 111 (92.5%) had a loss of consciousness (LOC) with the median LOC being 7 s, a mean of 61.44 ($SD = 110$) s, and a range of 0–10 min. Overall, 118 (96.7%) TBI participants had a reported period of PTA, with the median PTA being 15 min, a mean of 103 ($SD = 191$) min, and the range being 0–24 hr.

Of the 123 mTBI participants, 111 (90.24%) completed the 1-week assessment, and 90 (73.17%) completed the 3-month follow-up. Of the 100 TCs, 90 (90%) completed the 1-week follow-up and 80 (80%) the 3-month follow-up. There was no significant difference in gender between participants who consented to participate in the study and those who declined ($p = .369$). However, those who consented to participate were significantly older, with a median age of 32 years in comparison with 29 years for decliners ($p = .008$). The subsequent results are presented for those participants completing the 3-month follow-up only. The scores for PCS and HADS at each time point at which they were assessed are set out in Table A5.3. The groups differed significantly in terms of reported PCS, both on acute assessment in the ED and 1-week postinjury, with the mTBI group having more than double the Post-Concussive Symptom Inventory score of the control group at both time points. There was a significant decline in PCS over time. There were no significant differences in overall reporting of PCS at 3 months postinjury, nor did any particular symptom differentiate the groups. Applying the ICD-10 criteria used by Meares et al. (2008), 45.5% of mTBI participants and 14.0% of TCs reported a score of 4 or more on three or more of the ICD-10 symptoms at acute assessment in the ED ($p < .001$). However, neither these criteria nor any other cut-off score for PCS significantly differentiated the mTBI and TC groups at 1 week or 3 months postinjury. Groups did not differ on the HADS at acute assessment, 1 week, or 3 months postinjury. There was a significant reduction in anxiety and depression symptoms in both groups over time. More detailed results obtained by the mTBI and TC participants on each of the variables are detailed in another article (Ponsford, Cameron, Fitzgerald, Grant, & Mikocka-Walus, 2011).

Predictors of Postconcussive Symptoms. Preliminary correlational analyses revealed no significant association between education and PCS at 1 week ($r = -.036$, $p = .618$) or 3 months postinjury ($r = -.074$, $p = .345$). History of previous head injury was not significantly associated with PCS at 1 week ($r = .052$, $p = .469$) or 3 months postinjury ($r = -.048$,

TABLE A5.3	Postconcussive Symptom (PCS) Scores and HADS Scores by Group at Each Time Point					
		MTBI ($N = 90$)		TC ($N = 80$)		
Measure	Time point	Median[a] (min-max)	Mean	Median[a] (min-max)	Mean	P
PCS total	Acute	32.5 (0–86)	37.88	13.5 (0–97)	19.1	<.001
	1 week	16 (0–97)	22.13	7.5 (0–78)	15.85	.019
	3 months	4 (0–81)[b]	10.36	4 (0–81)[c]	9.57	.424
HADS Anxiety	1 week	5 (0–17)	5.28	4 (0–16)	5.04	.527
	3 months	3 (0–16)[d]	4.02	2 (0–16)[e]	3.38	.407
HADS Depression	1 week	3 (0–18)	4.35	3 (0–14)	3.75	.267
	3 months	1 (0–16)[f]	2.4	1 (0–11)[g]	1.59	.058

Note: Probability values for the group comparisons are presented in the last column, and within-subject comparison results are provided in superscript below the tables. HADS = Hospital Anxiety and Depression Scale; TC = trauma control; mTBI = mild traumatic brain injury.
[a] Median is given as minimum-maximum. [b] $p < .001$ Friedman test showing decline in PCS over time in mTBI patients. [c] $p < .001$ Friedman test showing decline in PCS overtime in controls. [d] $p = .002$ Wilcoxon signed-rank test showing a drop in HADS Anxiety over time in mTBI patients. [e] $p < .001$ Wilcoxon signed-rank test showing a drop in HADS Anxiety over time in controls. [f] $p < .001$ Wilcoxon signed-rank test showing decline in HADS Depression over time in mTBI patients. [g] $p < .001$ Wilcoxon signed-rank test showing decline in HADS Depression over time in mTBI patients.

$p = .540$). Nor was there a significant association between seeking compensation/ litigation and reported PCS at 3 months postinjury ($r = .081, p = .298$), with few participants seeking compensation. These variables were therefore not included in the predictive models.

Regarding the cognitive variables, as described by Ponsford et al. (2011), the mTBI participants differed significantly from TCs in performance on the ImPACT Visual Memory index only, whereas the group difference on Verbal Memory approached significance. There were no group differences apparent on the other scales. Moreover, these two variables showed the strongest correlations with PCS of each of the ImPACT summary scores (1-week Verbal Memory composite with 3-month total PCS: $r = -.206, p = .007$; 1-week Visual Memory composite with 3-month total PCS: $r = -.129, p = .097$). Therefore, giving consideration to the potential for multicollinearity and the limitations on the number of variables that could be included in the regression analyses, these were the two cognitive measures from ImPACT selected for use in the regressions.

Examination of the intercorrelations of predictor variables revealed that initial GCS was significantly associated with PTA duration ($r = .572, p < .001$). To avoid multicollinearity, we did not include GCS in the analyses, because PTA showed a stronger association with PCS. The preinjury SF-36 Mental Component score was significantly correlated with the SF-36 Physical Component score ($-.328, p < .001$) and with preinjury MINI neuro-psychiatric status ($-.377, p < .001$). Because the latter showed a stronger correlation with PCS, the SF-36 Mental Component score was excluded from the regressions. Additionally, there were significant correlations between the HADS anxiety and depression scores ($r = .670, p < .001$). Because HADS anxiety was more strongly associated with PCS, to avoid multicollinearity, we included only the HADS anxiety score as a predictor.

Prediction of 1-Week PCS From Preinjury and Acute Injury Predictors. For Model 1a (ED/ acute predictors), the significant predictors of a higher PCS score at 1-week postinjury were having had a mTBI, gender and preinjury psychiatric history, with participants with mTBI (odds ratio [OR] = 3.25, $p = .001$), women (OR = 2.56, $p = .004$), and those with psychiatric history (OR = 3.7, $p < .001$) at a higher risk of PCS at 1 week. Other variables used in the model that were not significantly predictive were acute cognitive memory measures (ImPACT Verbal Memory score, acute ImPACT Visual Memory score), as well as PTA duration, age, and preinjury SF-36 Physical Health.

Prediction of 3-Month PCS From Preinjury and Acute Injury Predictors. For Model 1b (ED/acute predictors), the significant predictors of higher PCS score at 3 months postinjury were presence of preinjury psychiatric history (OR = 2.56, $p = .006$) and lower preinjury Physical Health on the SF-36 (OR = 1.09, $p = .004$), with mTBI no longer a significant predictor. Again, acute cognitive measures of memory as well as Group (mTBI vs. TC), gender, age, and PTA duration were not associated with PCS at 3 months.

Prediction of PCS at 1 Week From Injury-Related and Concurrent Measures at 1 Week. For Model 2a (1-week variables), the significant predictor of a higher PCS score at 1 week were having had a mTBI (OR = 3.30, $p < .001$), more anxiety symptoms on the HADS (OR = 1.32, $p < .001$), and greater pain severity on the VAS (OR = 1.03, $p < .001$). Again, 1-week ImPACT Verbal Memory and Visual Memory scores—as well as gender, age, preinjury SF-36 Physical Health, PTA duration, and 1-week narcotic analgesia—were not significantly predictive.

Prediction of PCS at 3 Months From Injury-Related and 1-Week Variables. For Model 2b (1-week variables predicting outcome at 3 months), having a mTBI was no longer a significant predictor of higher PCS score at 3 months postinjury. However, presence of more anxiety symptoms on the HADS at 1 week remained a highly significant predictor of 3-month PCS (OR = 1.18, $p < .001$). One-week assessments on ImPACT Verbal and Visual Memory measures as well as gender, age, preinjury SF-36 Physical Health, PTA duration, and VAS pain at 1 week were not significant predictors of 3-month PCS.

Prediction of PCS at 3 Months From Injury-Related and Concurrent 3-Month Variables. For Model 3 (3-month variables), again having a mTBI was no longer a significant predictor of 3-month PCS, nor were 3-month ImPACT Verbal and Visual Memory scores, gender, age, preinjury SF36 Physical Health, or PTA duration. The significant concurrent predictors or indicators were a higher anxiety symptom score on the HADS (OR = 1.31, p = .002), greater VAS pain severity (OR = 1.04, p = .04), presence of more PTSD symptoms on the PCLS (OR = 1.09, p = .03), and other stressful life events on the RSRRS (OR = 1.001, p = .02).

Prediction of PCS at 3 Months for mTBI and Trauma Control Groups Separately. The final models examined predictors of PCS at 3 months postinjury for each group separately. In the model including only mTBI participants, the significant predictors were HADS anxiety symptoms (OR = 1.42, p = .01) and higher age (OR = 1.07, p = .04). In the model including only TC participants, the significant predictors were presence of PTSD symptoms on PCLS (OR = 1.23, p = .04) and other life stressors on the RSRRS (OR = 1.001, p = .02). Three-month ImPACT Verbal and Visual Memory scores, along with gender, preinjury SF-36 Physical health, PTA duration, and 3-month VAS pain, were not significant predictors of 3-month PCS in either group.

An analysis of the bivariate relationship between the presence of preinjury psychiatric disorders and HADS scores 1 week and 3 months postinjury revealed that HADS anxiety scores at 1 week were associated with greater likelihood of a preinjury psychiatric disorder, $t(1, 75) = -2.500, p = .013$, whereas HADS Depression scores did not show such an association. HADS anxiety and depression scores at 3 months postinjury were not significantly associated with preinjury psychiatric disturbances.

Discussion. This study of predictors of outcome in individuals with uncomplicated mTBI and general trauma not requiring surgery found that mTBI predicted PCS during the acute phase after injury, but not at 3 months postinjury. It also found that premorbid psychiatric factors and postinjury anxiety were the strongest predictors of persistent symptoms at 3 months postinjury.

Three factors contributed uniquely to reporting of PCS at 1 week after injury—namely, having experienced a mTBI, presence of a preinjury psychiatric disorder, and being female. The finding is in some respects consistent with the findings of Meares and colleagues (2008) in identifying the association between preinjury psychiatric disturbance, female gender, and reported PCS soon after injury. However, the present study, by focusing on trauma groups who were well-matched but had less-complex injuries and had had no surgery since injury, has identified that the experience of a mTBI also renders the person more than three times as likely to experience PCS in the first week postinjury than a general trauma patient without mTBI. Therefore it would seem erroneous to conclude that mTBI does not cause PCS in the early days after injury. As has been found in some previous studies, one of the traditional markers of injury severity, namely, duration of PTA, was not associated with reported PCS either at 1 week or 3 months after injury. Moreover, performance on the ImPACT cognitive concussion battery, specifically the Verbal and Visual memory modules, also failed to predict PCS both at 1 week and 3 months postinjury (Carroll et al., 2004; Meares et al., 2006, 2008; Ponsford et al., 2000; Stulemeijer, van der Werf, Borm, & Vos, 2008), despite the fact that mTBI participants did perform more poorly on the ImPACT Visual Memory index at both of these time points. Some previous studies have found other neuropsychological tests to be sensitive to effects of mTBI in the early stages after injury, including tests of visual RT, Digit Symbol Coding, the Speed of Comprehension Task, and Paced Auditory Serial Addition Task when administered in the early days after injury, with some studies also showing impairment on tests of visual or verbal memory (Carroll et al., 2004; Kwok, Lee, Leung, & Poon, 2008; Malojcic, Mubrin, Coric, Susnic & Spilich, 2008; Peterson et al., 2009; Ponsford et al., 2000; Vanderploeg, Curtiss, & Belanger, 2005). However, there is limited evidence that administration of these tests is predictive of PCS in either the short or the long term. The administration of computerized neuropsychological tests in the acute setting does not appear to be helpful in the management of patients with uncomplicated mTBI.

Neither education nor history of previous head injury was associated with PCS at 1 week or 3 months postinjury. Older age emerged as a predictor in the mTBI group only at 3 months postinjury. It was also clear that litigation was not a factor that contributed to reporting of PCS. This possibly reflects the low proportion of participants engaged in litigation. The influence of litigation may only appear when recruitment occurs in that context, as was the case in the study by Mooney and colleagues (2005).

PCS reporting was more strongly associated with the injured person's anxiety levels at 1 week postinjury, which was in turn associated with preinjury psychiatric history. It is possible that the experience of PCS resulted in heightened anxiety in individuals with a psychiatric history, who may have greater anxiety sensitivity and less adaptive coping mechanisms or stress tolerance. The symptoms experienced then caused anxiety, which might have further exacerbated symptoms. In support of this contention is the finding that reporting more anxiety symptoms on the HADS at 1 week postinjury was associated with greater likelihood of persisting PCS 3 months postinjury.

This finding supports that of previous studies by Dischinger et al. (2009) in which early symptoms of anxiety, noise sensitivity, and trouble thinking predicted long-term PCS 3 months postinjury, with women who reported anxiety early after injury being most likely to develop ongoing PCS. Stulemeijer and colleagues (2008) also found that emotional distress was significantly associated with continuing cognitive complaints 6 months postinjury, along with lower education, personality, and poor physical functioning, especially fatigue. This suggests that individuals showing high levels of anxiety symptoms early after injury may be targeted for preventative intervention. As suggested by Mttenberg, Tremont, Zielin-ski, Fichera, and Rayles (1996), the injured person's appraisal or attribution of symptoms may play a role in perpetuating them. Mittenberg and colleagues (1996) and Cicerone (2002) have advocated for the use of cognitive behavior therapy (CBT) to encourage patients to change their inner dialogue to develop a sense of mastery over symptoms and take control of their lifestyle, by using thought stopping, replacing negatively biased thoughts, and encouraging return to rewarding activities. Hodgson and colleagues (Hodgson, McDonald, Tate, & Gertler, 2005) showed that CBT may reduce social anxiety following mTBI. While Ghaffar, McCullagh, Ouchterlony, and Feinstein (2006) found no significant overall advantage in the provision of routine multidisciplinary treatment and follow-up to all individuals with mTBI, individuals with preexisting psychiatric problems did benefit from the intervention. We would therefore propose that individuals with a history of psychiatric disorder and those showing high levels of anxiety at 1 week after mTBI may be targeted for cognitive-behavioral interventions. There is a need for further evaluation of such intervention models, however.

By 3 months postinjury the experience of a mTBI did not contribute uniquely to reported PCS, which was most strongly associated with the experience of PTSD symptoms and other stressors, anxiety, and pain. However, it should be noted that the frequency of a score indicative of a formal diagnosis of PTSD was not high in either group ($n = 7$ in mTBI and 3 in TC group). Moreover, the fact that the predictors of PCS differed between the mTBI and TC groups at 3 months postinjury suggests that there may have been differing sources of anxiety, with PTSD symptoms and other life stressors most significant for the TCs, but older age and the presence of anxiety on the HADS showing a stronger association for mTBI participants. The higher HADS anxiety scores may have been a response to the experience of injury-related symptoms. This is also supported by the finding of greater self-reported concentration and memory difficulties affecting daily activities in the mTBI group in relation to TCs, as reported by Ponsford and colleagues (2011). However, one cannot be sure of the direction of this association, and further investigation of this is warranted.

This study focused on individuals with mTBI with no focal neurological signs, nor evidence of injury on CT scan and who were not under the influence of illicit substances or requiring general anesthesia. We did this to exclude extraneous causes of cognitive impairment. This sample represents the very mildest end of the mTBI spectrum and cannot be said to represent individuals with complicated mTBI for whom predictors of outcome may differ. The sample who participated was also slightly older than the group that did not agree to participate, and one cannot rule out the possibility that this in some way influenced the findings, given that age proved to be a significant predictor in the model predicting 3-month outcome in the TBI group. Moreover, given the number of statistical comparisons, we cannot rule out the possibility of Type I error.

Taking into account these factors, we believe that this study has demonstrated that the presence of a mTBI does contribute significantly to PCS within the acute stages after injury in patients with uncomplicated trauma, but not to longer-term PCS, which were more strongly predicted by premorbid psychiatric factors and postinjury anxiety. Individuals with a preinjury psychiatric history appear to respond to the experience of mTBI and PCS with greater anxiety, which may, in turn, exacerbate their PCS. The effects of mTBI are thus complex and multifactorial. If we are to improve management of this condition, we need to acknowledge this complexity, and equip individuals with information and coping strategies to minimize the development of anxiety.

References

Belanger, H. G., Curtiss, G., Demery, J. A., Lebowitz, B. K., & Vander-ploeg, R. D. (2005). Factors moderating neuropsychological outcomes following mild traumatic brain injury: A meta-analysis. *Journal of the International Neuropsychological Society*, 11, 215–227. doi:10.1017/ S1355617705050277

Belanger, H. G., Spiegel, E., & Vanderploeg, R. D. (2010). Neuropsycho-logical performance following a history of multiple self-reported concussions. *Journal of the International Neuropsychological Society*, 16, 262–267. doi:10.1017/S1355617709991287

Benton, A. L. (1989). Historical notes on the postconcussion syndrome. In H. S. Levin, H. Eisenberg, & A. L. Benton (Eds.), *Mild head injury* (pp. 3–7). New York, NY: Oxford University Press.

Binder, L. M., & Rohling, M. L. (1996). Money matters: A meta-analytic review of the effects of financial incentives on recovery after closed-head injury. *American Journal of Psychiatry*, 153, 7–10.

Blanchard, E. B., Jones-Alexander, J., Buckley, T. C., & Forneris, C. A. (1996). Psychometric properties of the PTSD Checklist (PCL). *Behaviour Research and Therapy*, 34, 669–673. doi:0005-7967(96)00033-2

Bryant, R. A. (2008). Disentangling mild traumatic brain injury and stress reactions. *New England Journal of Medicine*, 358, 525–527. doi: 10.1056/NEJMe078235

Carroll, L. J., Cassidy, J. D., Peloso, P. M., Borg, J., von Holst, H., Holm, L., ... W.H.O. Collaborating Centre Task Force on Mild Traumatic Brain Injury. (2004). Prognosis for mild traumatic brain injury: Results of the WHO Collaborating Centre Task Force on Mild Traumatic Brain Injury. *Journal of Rehabilitation Medicine*, 43(Suppl), 84–105. doi: 10.1080/16501960410023859

Cassidy, J. D., Carroll, L. J., Peloso, P. M., Borg, J., Holst, H. v., Holm, L., ... Coronado, V. (2004). Incidence, risk factors and prevention of mild traumatic brain injury: Results of the WHO Collaborative Centre Task Force on Mild Traumatic Brain Injury. *Journal of Rehabilitation Medicine, 36*(Suppl), 28–60. doi:10.1080/16501960410023732

Cicerone, K. D. (2002). Remediation of 'working attention' in mild traumatic brain injury. *Brain Injury*, 16, 185–195. doi:10.1080/ 02699050110103959

Dischinger, P. C., Ryb, G. E., Kufera, J. A., & Auman, K. M. (2009). Early predictors of postconcussive syndrome in a population of trauma patients with mild traumatic brain injury. *Journal of Trauma-Injury Infection & Critical Care*, 66, 289–296.

Forbes, D., Creamer, M., & Biddle, D. (2001). The validity of the PTSD checklist as a measure of symptomatic change in combat-related PTSD. *Behaviour Research and Therapy*, 39, 977–986. doi:10.1016/S0005-7967(00)00084-X

Ghaffar, O., McCullagh, S., Ouchterlony, D., & Feinstein, A. (2006). Randomized treatment trial in mild traumatic brain injury. *Journal of Psychosomatic Research, 61*, 153–160. doi:10.1016/j.jpsychores .2005.07.018

Hirtz, D., Thurman, D. J., Gwinn-Hardy, K., Mohamed, M., Chaudhuri, A. R., & Zalutsky, R. (2007). How common are the "common" neurologic disorders? *Neurology, 68*, 326–337. doi:10.1212/ 01.wnl.0000252807.38124.a3

Hodgson, J., McDonald, S., Tate, R., & Gertler, P. (2005). A randomised controlled trial of a cognitive behavioural therapy program for managing social anxiety after acquired brain injury. *Brain Impairment, 6*, 169– 180. doi:10.1375/brim.2005.6.3.169

Hoge, C. W., McGurk, D., Thomas, J. L., Cox, A. L., Engel, C. C., & Castro, C. A. (2008). Mild traumatic brain injury in U.S. soldiers returning from Iraq. *New England Journal of Medicine, 358*, 453–463. doi:10.1056/NEJMoa072972

Holmes, T. H., & Rahe, R. H. (1967). The Social Readjustment Rating Scale. *Journal of Psychosomatic Research, 11*, 213–218. doi:10.1016/ 0022-3999(67)90010-4

Horowitz, M., Schaefer, C., Hiroto, D., Wilner, N., & Levin, B. (1977). Life event questionnaires for measuring presumptive stress. *Psychosomatic Medicine, 39*, 413–431.

Hukkelhoven, C. W., Steyerberg, E. W., Rampen, A. J., Farace, E., Habbema, J. D., Marshall, L. F., … Maas, A. I. R. (2003). Patient age and outcome following severe traumatic brain injury: An analysis of 5600 patients. *Journal of Neurosurgery, 99*, 666–673. doi:10.3171/ jns.2003.99.4.0666

Huskisson, E. C. (1974). Measurement of pain. *Lancet, 304*, 1127–1131. doi:10.1016/ S0140-6736(74)90884-8

Iverson, G. L., Lovell, M. R., & Collins, M. W. (2005). Validity of ImPACT for measuring processing speed following sports-related concussion. *Journal of Clinical and Experimental Neuropsychology, 27*, 683–689. doi:10.1081/13803390490918435

Jenkinson, C., Coulter, A., & Wright, L. (1993). Short form 36 (SF36) health survey questionnaire: Normative data for adults of working age. *British Medical Journal, 306*, 1437–1440. doi:10.1136/ bmj.306.6890.1437

Kashluba, S., Paniak, C., & Casey, J. E. (2008). Persistent symptoms associated with factors identified by the WHO Task Force on mild traumatic brain injury. *Clinical Neuropsychologist, 22*, 195–208. doi: 10.1080/13854040701263655

Kraus, J., Schaffer, K., Ayers, K., Stenehjem, J., Shen, H., & Afifi, A. (2005). Physical complaints, medical service use, and social and employment changes following mild traumatic brain injury: A 6-month longitudinal study. *Journal of Head Trauma Rehabilitation, 20*, 239– 256. doi:10.1097/00001199-200505000-00007

Kwok, F. Y., Lee, T. M., Leung, C. H., & Poon, W. S. (2008). Changes of cognitive functioning following mild traumatic brain injury over a 3-month period. *Brain Injury, 22*, 740 –751. doi:org/10.1080/ 02699050802336989

Landre, N., Poppe, C. J., Davis, N., Schmaus, B., & Hobbs, S. E. (2006). Cognitive functioning and postconcussive symptoms in trauma patients with and without mild TBI. *Archives of Clinical Neuropsychology, 21*, 255–273. doi:10.1016/j.acn.2005.12.007

Lange, R. T., Iverson, G. L., & Franzen, M. D. (2009). Neuropsychological functioning following complicated vs. uncomplicated mild traumatic brain injury. *Brain Injury, 23*, 83–91. doi:10.1080/02699050802635281

Lewine, J. D., Davis, J. T., Bigler, E. D., Thoma, R., Hill, D., Funke, M., … Orrison, W. (2007). Objective documentation of traumatic brain injury subsequent to mild head trauma: Multimodal brain imaging with MEG, SPECT, and MRI. *Journal of Head Trauma Rehabilitation, 22*, 141–155. doi:10.1097/01.HTR.0000271115.29954.27

Lo, C., Shifteh, K., Gold, T., Bello, J. A., & Lipton, M. L. (2009). Diffusion tensor imaging abnormalities in patients with mild traumatic brain injury and neurocognitive impairment. *Journal of Computer Assisted Tomography, 33*, 293–297. doi:10.1097/RCT.0b013e31817579d1

Lovell, M. R., & Collins, M. W. (1998). Neuropsychological assessment of the college football player. *Journal of Head Trauma Rehabilitation, 13*, 9–26. doi:10.1097/00001199-199804000-00004

Lundin, A., de Boussard, C., Edman, G., & Borg, J. (2006). Symptoms and disability until 3 months after mild TBI. *Brain Injury, 20*, 799–806. doi:10.1080/02699050600744327

Malojcic, B., Mubrin, Z., Coric, B., Susnic, M., & Spilich, G. J. (2008). Consequences of mild traumatic brain injury on information processing assessed with attention and short-term memory tasks. *Journal of Neu-rotrauma, 25*, 30–37. doi:org/10.1089/neu.2007.0384

McLean, S. A., Kirsch, N. L., Tabn-Schriner, C. U., Sen, A., Frederiksen, S., Harris, R. E., … Maio, R. F. (2009). Health status not head injury predicts concussion symptoms after minor injury. *American Journal of Emergency Medicine, 27,* 182–190. doi:10.1016/j.ajem.2008.01.054

Meares, S., Shores, E., Batchelor, J., Baguley, I. J., Chapman, J., Gurka, J., & Marosszeky, J. E. (2006). The relationship of psychological and cognitive factors and opioids in the development of the postconcussion syndrome in general trauma patients with mild traumatic brain injury. *Journal of the International Neuropsychological Society, 12,* 792–801. doi:10.1017/S1355617706060978

Meares, S., Shores, E., Taylor, A., Batchelor, J., Bryant, R., Baguley, I., … Marosszeky, J. (2008). Mild traumatic brain injury does not predict acute postconcussion syndrome. *Journal of Neurology, Neurosurgery & Psychiatry, 79,* 300–306. doi:10.1136/jnnp.2007.126565

Mittenberg, W., Canyock, E. M., Condit, D., & Patton, C. (2001). Treatment of post-concussion syndrome following mild head injury. *Journal of Clinical and Experimental Neuropsychology, 23,* 829–836. doi:10.1076/ jcen.23.6.829.1022

Mittenberg, W., Tremont, G., Zielinski, R. E., Fichera, S., & Rayles, K. R. (1996). Cognitive–behavioural prevention of postconcussion syndrome. *Archives of Clinical Neuropsychology, 11,* 139–145.

Mooney, G., Speed, J., & Sheppard, S. (2005). Factors related to recovery after mild traumatic brain injury. *Brain Injury, 19,* 975–987. doi: 10.1080/02699050500110264

Paniak, C., Reynolds, S., Toller-Lobe, G., Melnyk, A., Nagy, J., & Schmidt, D. (2002). A longitudinal study of the relationship between financial compensation and symptoms after treated mild traumatic brain injury. *Journal of Clinical and Experimental Neuropsychology, 24,* 187–193. doi:10.1076/ jcen.24.2.187.999

Peterson, S., Stull, M. J., Collins, M. W., & Wang, H. E. (2009). Neuro-cognitive function of emergency department patients with mild traumatic brain injury. *Annals of Emergency Medicine, 53,* 796–803.

Ponsford, J. (2005). Rehabilitation interventions after mild head injury. *Current Opinion in Neurology, 18,* 692–697. doi:10.1097/ 01.wco.0000186840.61431.44

Ponsford, J., Cameron, P., Fitzgerald, M., Grant, M., & Mikocka-Walus, A. (2011). Long term outcomes after uncomplicated mild traumatic brain injury: A comparison with trauma controls. *Journal of Neurotrauma, 28,* 937–948.

Ponsford, J., Cameron, P., Willmott, C., Rothwell, A., Kelly, A.-M., Nelms, R., & Ng, K. (2004). Use of the Westmead PTA Scale to monitor recovery of memory after mild head injury. *Brain Injury, 18,* 603–614. doi:10.1080/02699050310001646152

Ponsford, J., Willmott, C., Rothwell, A., Cameron, P., Kelly, A. M., Nelms, R., … Ng, K. (2000). Factors influencing outcome following mild traumatic brain injury in adults. *Journal of the International Neuropsy-chological Society, 6,* 568–579. doi:10.1017/S1355617700655066

Ruff, R. (2005). Two decades of advances in understanding of mild traumatic brain injury. *Journal of Head Trauma Rehabilitation, 20,* 5–18. doi:10.1097/00001199-200501000-00003

Sadowski-Cron, C., Schneider, J., Senn, P., Radanov, B. P., Ballinari, P., & Zimmermann, H. (2006). Patients with mild traumatic brain injury: Immediate and long-term outcome compared to intracranial injuries on CT scan. *Brain Injury, 20,* 1131–1137. doi:10.1080/02699050600832569

Schönberger, M., & Ponsford, J. (2010). The factor structure of the Hospital Anxiety and Depression Scale in individuals with traumatic brain injury. *Psychiatry Research, 179,* 342–349.

Sheedy, J., Geffen, G., Donnelly, J., & Faux, S. (2006). Emergency department assessment of mild traumatic brain injury and prediction of post-concussion symptoms at one month post injury. *Journal of Clinical and Experimental Neuropsychology, 28,* 755–772. doi:10.1080/13803390591000864

Sheehan, D. V., Lecrubier, Y., Sheehan, K. H., Amorim, P., Janavs, J., & Weiller, E. (1998). The Mini-International Neuropsychiatric Interview (M. I. N. I.): The development and validation of a structured diagnostic psychiatric interview for *DSM–IV* and ICD-10. *Journal of Clinical Psychiatry, 59*(Suppl 20), 22–33.

Shores, E. A., Lammel, A., Hullick, C., Sheedy, J., Flynn, M., Levick, W., & Batchelor, J. (2008). The diagnostic accuracy of the Revised West-mead PTA Scale as an adjunct to the Glasgow Coma Scale in the early identification of cognitive impairment in patients with mild traumatic brain injury. *Journal of Neurology, Neurosurgery & Psychiatry, 79,* 1100–1106. doi:10.1136/jnnp.2007.132571

Snaith, R. P., & Zigmond, A. S. (1986). The hospital anxiety and depression scale. *British Medical Journal (Clinical Research Edition), 292,* 344. doi:10.1136/bmj.292.6516.344

Stulemeijer, M., van der Werf, S., Borm, G., & Vos, P. (2008). Early prediction of favourable recovery 6 months after mild traumatic brain injury. *Journal of Neurology, Neurosurgery & Psychiatry, 79*, 936–942. doi:10.1136/jnnp.2007.131250

Stulemeijer, M., Vos, P. E., Bleijenberg, G., & van der Werf, S. P. (2007). Cognitive complaints after mild traumatic brain injury: Things are not always what they seem. *Journal of Psychosomatic Research, 63*, 637– 645. doi:10.1016/j.jpsychores.2007.06.023

Teasdale, G., & Jennett, B. (1976). Assessment and prognosis of coma after head injury. *Acta Neurochirurgica, 34*, 45–55. doi:10.1007/ BF01405862

Thornhill, S., Teasdale, G. M., Murray, G. D., McEwen, J., Roy, C. W., & Penny, K. I. (2000). Disability in young people and adults one year after head injury: Prospective cohort study. *British Medical Journal, 320*, 1631–1635. doi:10.1136/bmj.320.7250.1631

Vanderploeg, R. D., Curtiss, G., & Belanger, H. G. (2005). Long-term neuropsychological outcomes following mild traumatic brain injury. *Journal of the International Neuropsychological Society, 11*, 228–236. doi:org/10.1017/S1355617705050289

Ware, J. E., & Sherbourne, C. D. (1992). The MOS 36-item short-form health survey (SF-36). I. Conceptual framework and item selection. *Medical Care, 30*, 473–483. doi:10.1097/00005650-199206000-00002

Whelan-Goodinson, R., Ponsford, J., & Schönberger, M. (2009). Validity of the Hospital Anxiety and Depression Scale to assess depression and anxiety following traumatic brain injury as compared with the Structured Clinical Interview for *DSM–IV*. *Journal of Affective Disorders, 114*, 94–102. doi:10.1016/j.jad.2008.06.007

Williams, D. H., Levin, H. S., & Eisenberg, H. M. (1990). Mild head injury classification. *Neurosurgery, 27*, 422–428. doi:10.1227/00006123-199009000-00014

Wood, R. L. (2004). Understanding the 'miserable minority': A diasthesis– stress paradigm for post-concussional syndrome. *Brain Injury, 18*, 1135– 1153. doi:10.1080/02699050410001675906

Yang, C.-C., Tu, Y.-K., Hua, M.-S., & Huang, S.-J. (2007). The association between the postconcussion symptoms and clinical outcomes for patients with mild traumatic brain injury. *Journal of Trauma: Injury, Infection, & Critical Care, 62*, 657–663. doi:10.1097/01.ta.0000203577.68764.b8

Received September 7, 2010

Revision received September 9, 2011

Accepted September 12, 2011

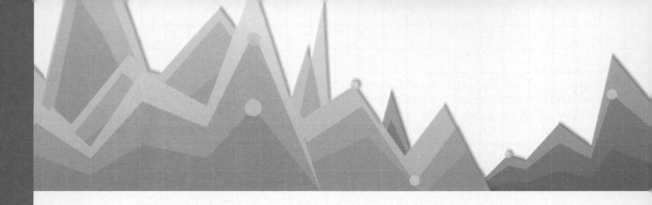

Appendix A-6

The Affects of a Single Bout of Exercise on Mood and Self-Esteem in Clinically Diagnosed Mental Health Patients

Naomi J. Ellis, Jason A. Randall*, Grant Punnett

Open Journal of Medical Psychology, 2013, 2, 81-85 http://dx.doi.org/10.4236/ojmp.2013. 23013 Published Online July 2013 (http://www.scirp.org/journal/ojmp)

Received March 15, 2013; revised April 30, 2013; accepted May 9, 2013

Abstract

Objectives: *Research has highlighted the importance of regular exercise within the general population and mental health groups in regard to mood and self-esteem, as well as single bout exercise within the general population. However, research into single bout exercise in mental health population is lacking. This study investigated the impact of a single bout of exercise, on mood and self-esteem, in patients with a wider clinical mental health diagnosis.*

Design: *A quantitative questionnaire was completed immediately pre and post a single, 45 minute bout of moderate intensity exercise, consisting of the Brunel Universal Mood States (BRUMS) questionnaire and the Rosenberg Self Esteem Scale (RSE).*

Methods: *Participants attending a mental health hospital with a clinical mental health diagnosis (N = 54) completed the questionnaire. Information regarding physical activity levels, mental health diagnosis and length of hospital stay were collated.*

Results: *A significant improvement was identified on the RSE as well as the BRUMS (depression, anger, confusion, anxious tension and vigour) over time.*

Conclusion: *The significant findings highlight the importance of exercise promotion within this population group, and the potentially beneficial role that a single bout of exercise can have on mood and self-esteem in patients experiencing mental health problems.*

Keywords: Clinical; Exercise; Health; Mental Health; Mood; Self-Esteem

*Corresponding author

1. Introduction. Mental health is currently at the forefront of government policy and is receiving ever increasing interest from researchers, the general public and policy makers [1]. The most recent figures suggest that in the UK 1 in 4 people report at least one diagnosable mental health condition during their lifetime [2,3] costing the UK an estimated £77 billion in 2002/03 [3,4].

There is a growing recognition surrounding the mental health benefits of regular physical activity in the general population [5]. Research suggests it can reduce stress, [5,6] anxiety [7] and depression [8] whilst improving mood [5,9,10]. A number of reviews have explored psychological outcomes and regular exercise within the general population [9-11]. Findings suggest that regular exercise improves various psychological characteristics (e.g., mood). Whilst regular exercise appears to be preferable, it is not always practical. Research indicates that a single bout of exercise can enhance mood and well-being in the general population [9,12-15]. This highlights potential benefits for groups where attrition is high or attendance to multiple bouts is difficult, such as some clinical mental health populations [16].

Research into regular exercise and psychological benefits within mental health populations is by no means lacking and has further strengthened our understanding of the relationship between mental health and exercise [17-19]. There are a variety of recent reviews and meta-analyses on anxiety [20,21], depression [22,20] and psychosis [23] highlighting the relationship between exercise and psychological benefits within these populations.

Research specifically investigating the effect of a single bout of exercise with individuals experiencing mental health difficulties is limited [24,25]. Significant improvements in psychological outcomes were reported in people with depressive disorders [24-26]. Similar findings were also reported by Weinstein [25], although these reductions in depressive symptoms were not maintained over time (one hour post).

Given that evidence suggests a single bout of exercise can promote a change in mood and self-esteem within the general population [14], and in individuals with depression [24], the potential of such immediate benefits in mental health population groups, in whom the need is often greatest, warrants further investigation. Therefore, the aim of this research is to examine whether a single bout of exercise has an effect on mood and self-esteem in clinically diagnosed patients experiencing a range mental health problems.

2. Method

2.1 Participants. A total of 65 participants, 45 males (69.2%) and 20 females (30.8%), engaged with the research consisting of 40 (61.5%) inpatients, 22 (35.5%) outpatients and 3 (4.6%) who did not specify. Overall 59 (90.8%) described themselves as white British, 2 (3.2%) as black British, 1 (1.5%) as "other" with 3 (4.6%) not disclosing. The mean age was 44.6 (SD = 11.7) years, minimum 19 years and maximum 70 years. Length of inpatient stay varied from 2 days to 2 years 9 months, with a mean stay of 59.22 (SD = 204.01) days. The primary diagnosis, based on staff information, was anxiety (52.3%), with additional diagnoses of depression (32.3%), schizophrenia (6.1%), bipolar (4.6%), alcoholism (3.1%) and other (1.5%). Physical activity levels were reported as being below the recommended amounts of 30 minutes at a moderate intensity on a minimum of 5 days per week. Participants reported, a mean of 2.8 days of activity (SD = 2.2) in the previous week with no difference between inpatients and outpatient responses.

2.2 Effect Size. Of the two studies undertaken within this area effect size varies. Bartholomew [24] reported a medium effect size (n = 40), while Weinstein [25] found a small effect size (n = 14). Research in the general population relating to single bout exercise and mental health has typically also found a medium effect size [14,15]. Therefore using a medium effect size of d = 0.6 and a power of 0.8 [27] 45 participants were required for this research.

2.3 Measures. Participants completed a self report questionnaire comprising of demographic information, a single item measure of physical activity, the Brunel Universal Mood States (BRUMS) questionnaire and the Rosenberg Self-esteem scale.

The physical activity single item measure has been taken from the Outdoor Health Questionnaire used in the national Walking for Health scheme. The measure has been validated [28] and the single item physical activity question has been used independently as a self-reported method of obtaining levels of physical activity [29].

The BRUMS has been regularly used to assess mood [30]. The original POMS [31] has been adapted to create a shorter 24 item version, BRUMS, that has been tested for validity and reliability [32,33]. The BRUMS has 6 mood dimensions; tension, depression, anger, vigour, fatigue and confusion. Answers are on a five point Likert scale, ranging from "not at all" to "extremely".

The Rosenberg Self Esteem scale [34] assesses global self-esteem and is one of the most widely used tests by psychologists for this purpose. The scale has ten items on a four point Likert-type scale ranging from "strongly agree" to "strongly disagree", and has been used within this population group [35].

2.4 Procedure. A questionnaire was developed in conjunction with the mental health Hospital ensuring it was appropriate for their patient group. Potential participants were initially approached by a member of staff, and the study explained to them. Participants were then given seven days to consider participation. Written informed consent was obtained, following which questionnaires were issued to patients by staff immediately pre and post exercise. The exercise sessions consisted of 45 minutes of moderate intensity aerobic exercise (intensity was self-reported). Participant anonymity was ensured through the use of ID numbers.

Participants met the inclusion criteria if they were: 1) a patient at the mental health hospital; 2) taking part in an exercise group at the hospital; 3) well enough on the day to complete the questionnaire; 4) over 18 years of age. Participants were informed that the questionnaire would take 10 - 15 minutes to complete pre-exercise and up to 5 minutes post exercise. Participants were able to withdraw from the study at any point. If participants requested support in filling out the questionnaire, this was provided by hospital staff. A private room was available for those completing the questionnaire. Analysis was undertaken on data collected as part of a service evaluation by the hospital. Ethical approval was granted for the analysis by Staffordshire University Faculty of Health Sciences Ethics Board; NHS ethics were informed, but as this was a service evaluation NHS ethics approval were not necessary.

3. Results. Due to incorrectly completed questionnaires 11 participants were removed from the study. As such analysis was undertaken on 54 participants.

Figure A6.1 highlights pre and post changes in mood and self-esteem. It can be observed that negative mood states all decrease, with the exception of fatigue. Vigour and self-esteem, which are positive moods state increase.

The data set was screened for parametric assumptions and was found to lack normal distribution. As such, non-parametric tests were applied. A Wilcoxon signed rank test for matched pairs was undertaken, using SPSS 17.

A significant difference was identified between pre and post scores for depression ($T = 0.5$, $p = 0.000$, $N = 54$, $r = 0.678$), anger ($T = 14.5$, $p = 0.000$, $N = 54$, $r = 0.530$) confusion ($T = 113.0$, $p = 0.008$, $N = 54$, $r = 0.364$), anxious tension ($T = 52.5$, $p = 0.000$, $N = 54$, $r = 0.575$) and vigour ($T = 342.0$, $p = 0.012$, $N = 54$, $r = 0.344$). There was no significant difference identified between fatigue scores. A significant difference was identified between the pre and post self-esteem scores ($T = 203.5$, $p = 0.000$, $N = 54$, $r = 0.505$).

Further post-hoc analysis was then undertaken to investigate any difference in scores regarding mental health diagnosis. A Kruskal-Wallis one way ANOVA by ranks was carried out for all five diagnoses, for each variable (*i.e.*, depression and post depression) and found

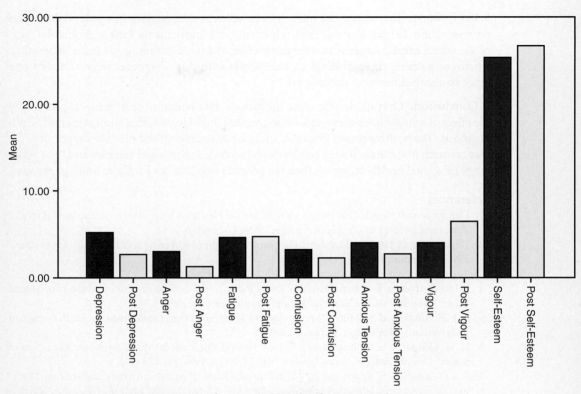

FIGURE A6.1 Graphical representation of mean mood and self-esteem results.

no significant difference between scores regarding mental health diagnosis. A significant difference was also not noted if those diagnoses with less than five participants were removed (*i.e.* analysis only on anxiety n = 28; and depression n = 17). Suggesting mental health diagnosis does not affect the pre-post relationship.

4. Discussion. This study was designed to assess the effect of a single, hospital based exercise session on mood and self-esteem in individuals with a clinical mental health diagnosis. The results suggest a significant improvement in six mood states; depression, anxious tension, anger, confusion and vigour and self-esteem.

The results replicate those of healthy populations suggesting that a single bout of exercise significantly influence mood states [12-15]. The findings also support the two previous studies in participants with a clinical diagnosis of depression [24,25].

The only mood state that did not show a significant difference was that of fatigue. However, this could be due to a misinterpretation regarding definition, with participants confusing mental fatigue with physical fatigue, thus this result should be taken with caution [24].

Previous research into the effect of a single bout of exercise on psychological outcomes, for individuals with a mental health diagnosis, has focused on depression [24,25]. The present study aimed to collect data from participants with a range of mental health diagnosis. A significant difference was recorded over time when participants were treated as a single cohort. Further analysis into mental health diagnosis noted no significant difference between diagnoses and psychological characteristics over time. Though due to low sample sizes (when separated by diagnosis) this is not surprising and warrants further investigation.

In comparison to previous research, the sample size used in this pilot study was larger [24,25], but this research used participants with a range of diagnosis. As such, if further research was to be undertaken it would be beneficial to collect a larger sample size to fully investigate the effect of a single bout of exercise on a range of clinical diagnosis.

5. Limitations. The measure of intensity was self reported, leading to a potential for miss representation. Sample size was relatively small when participants were separated by diagnosis, which caused issues with intergroup comparisons. Caution needs to be undertaken when generalising these findings as individuals with duel diagnosis were excluded and other co-morbidities were unreported.

6. Conclusion. Overall, despite some limitations, this remains the first investigation into the effect of a single bout of exercise on aggregated individuals with a clinical mental health diagnosis. The positive results from this study are encouraging and provide support for further research in the area. If such results can be recreated with larger samples and for a wider range of mental health diagnoses then the possible implications for these findings are vast.

References

1. Department of Health, "No Health without Mental Health: A Cross-Government Mental Health Outcomes Strategy for People of All Ages," HMSO, London, 2011.
2. Department of Health, "Making It Happen: A Guide to Delivering Mental Health Promotion," HMSO, London, 2001.
3. The Office of national Statistics, Cenus, 2001. www.ons.gov.uk
4. Sainsbury Centre for Mental Health, "Policy Paper 3: The Economic and Social Costs of Mental Illness," The Sainsbury Centre for Mental Health, London, 2001.
5. S. J. H. Biddle and N. Mutrie, "Psychology of Physical Activity: Determinants, Well-Being and Interventions," Routledge, Abingdon, 2008.
6. K. H. Cooper, J. S. Gallman and J. L. J. McDonald, "Role of Aerobic Exercise in Reduction of Stress," *Dental Clinics of North America*, Vol. 30, No. 4, 1986, pp. 133–142.
7. P. J. O'Connor, J. S. Raglin and E. W. Martinsen, "Physical Activity, Anxiety and Anxiety Disorders," *International Journal of Sport Psychology*, Vol. 31, No. 2, 2000, pp. 136–155.
8. L. L. Craft, "Exercise and Clinical Depression: Examining Two Psychological Mechanisms," *Psychology of Sport and Exercise*, Vol. 6, No. 2, 2005, pp. 151–171. doi:10.1016/j.psychsport.2003.11.003
9. P. C. Dinas, Y. Koutedakis and A. D. Flouris, "Effects of Exercise and Physical Activity on Depression," *Irish Journal of Medical Science*, Vol. 180, No. 2, 2011, pp. 319–325. doi:10.1007/s11845-010-0633-9
10. K. R. Fox, "The Influence of Physical Activity on Mental Well-Being," *Public Health Nutrition*, Vol. 2, Suppl. 3, 1999, pp. 411–418. doi:10.1017/S1368980099000567
11. D. Scully, J. Kremer, M. Meade, R. Grahma and K. Dudgeon, "Physical Exercise and Psychological Well Being: A Critical Review," *British Journal of Sports Medicine*, Vol. 32, No. 2, 1998, pp. 111–120. doi:10.1136/bjsm.32.2.111
12. P. Ekkekakis, E. E. Hall, L. M. Van Landuyt and S. J. Petruzello, "Walking in (Affective) Circles: Can Short Walks Enhance Affect?" *Journal of Behavioural Medicine*, Vol. 23, No. 3, 2000, pp. 245–275. doi:10.1023/A:1005558025163
13. T. C. North, P. McCullagh and Z. V. Tran, "Effect of Exercise on Depression," *Exercise and Sport Science Review*, Vol. 18, 1990, pp. 379–412. doi:10.1249/00003677-199001000-00016
14. A. Szabo, "Acute Psychological Benefits of Exercise Performed at Self-Selected Workloads: Implications for Theory and Practice," *Journal of Sports Science and Medicine*, Vol. 2, 2003, pp. 77–87.
15. R. R. Yeung, "The Acute Effects of Exercise on Mood State," *Journal of Psychosomatic Research*, Vol. 40, No. 2, 1996, pp. 123–141. doi:10.1016/0022-3999(95)00554-4
16. P. M. Dubbert, J. D. White, K. B. Grothe, J. O. Jile and K. A. Kirchner, "Physical Activity in Patients Who Are Severely Mentally Ill: Feasibility of Assessment for Clinical and Research Applications," *Archives of Psychiatric Nursing*, Vol. 20, No. 5, 2006, pp. 205–209. doi:10.1016/j.apnu.2006.04.002
17. K. A. Barbour, T. M. Edenfield and J. A. Blumrnthal, "Exercise as a Treatment for Depression and Other Psychiatric Disorders: A Review," *Journal of Cardiopul-monary Rehabilitation & Prevention*, Vol. 27, 2007, pp. 359–367.
18. D. Carless and K. Douglas, "The Role of Sport and Exercise in Recovery from Serious Mental Illness: Two Case Studies," *International Journal of Men's Health*, Vol. 7, No. 2, 2008, pp. 137–156. doi:10.3149/jmh.0702.137
19. D. S. Hutchinson, "Structured Exercise for Persons with Serious Psychiatric Disabilities," *Psychiatric Services*, Vol. 56, No. 3, 2005, pp. 353–354. doi:10.1176/appi.ps.56.3.353

20. F. J. Penedo and J. R. Dahn, "Exercise and Well-Being: A Review of Mental and Physical Health Benefits Associated with Physical Activity," *Current Opinion in Psychiatry*, Vol. 18, No. 2, 2005, pp. 189–193. doi:10.1097/00001504-200503000-00013

21. B. M. Wipfli, C. D. Rethorst and D. M. Landers, "The Anxiolytic Effects of Exercise: A Meta-Analysis of Randomized Trials and Dose-Response Analysis," *Journal of Sport & Exercise Psychology*, Vol. 30, No. 4, 2008, pp. 392–410.

22. C. D. Rethorst, B. M. Wipfli and D. M. Landers, "The Anti-Depressive Effects of Exercise: A Meta-Analysis of Randomized Trials," *Sports Medicine*, Vol. 39, No. 6, 2009, pp. 491–511. doi:10.2165/00007256-200939060-00004

23. N., Ellis, D. Crone, R. Davey and S. Grogan, "Exercise Interventions as an Adjunct Therapy for Psychosis: A Critical Review," *British Journal of Clinical Psychology*, Vol. 46, No. 1, 2007, pp. 95–111. doi:10.1348/014466506X122995

24. J. B. Bartholomew, D. Morrison and J. T. Ciccolo, "Effects of Acute Exercise on Mood and Well-Being in Patients with Major Depressive Disorder," *Medicine and Science in Sports and Exercise*, Vol. 37, No. 12, 2005, pp. 2032–2037. doi:10.1249/01.mss.0000178101.78322.dd

25. A. A. Weinstein, P. A. Deuster, P. L. Francis, C. Beadling and W. J. Kop, "The Role of Depression in Short-Term Mood and Fatigue Responses to Acute Exercise," *International Journal of Behavioral Medicine*, Vol. 17, No. 1, 2010, pp. 51–57. doi:10.1007/s12529-009-9046-4

26. R. R. Yeung and D. R. Hemsley, "Effects of Personality and Acute Exercise on Mood States," *Personality and Individual's Difference*, Vol. 20, No. 5, 1996, pp. 545–550. doi:10.1016/0191-8869(95)00222-7

27. D. Clark-Carter, "Quantitative Psychological Research," Third Edition, Psychology Press, New York, 2010.

28. K. Milton, F. C. Bull and A. Bauman, "Reliability and Validity Testing of a Single-Item Physical Activity Measure," *British Journal of Sports Medicine*, Vol. 6, 2010, pp. 348–352.

29. N. Ellis, C. Gidlow and R. Davey, "Exploring Mental Health Benefits of Physical Activity Using a Social Marketing Approach in Community Settings," *Care Service Improvement Partnership Document*, 2009.

30. T. Andrade, C. Arce, J. Torrado, J. Garrido, C. De Fancisco and I. Arce, "Factor Structure and Invariance of The Poms Mood State Questionnaire in Spanish," *Spanish Journal of Psychology*, Vol. 13, No. 1, 2010, pp. 444–452. doi:10.1017/S1138741600003991

31. D. M. McNaire, M. Lorr and L. F. Droppleman, "Manual for the Profile of Mood States," Education and Industrial Testing Service, San Diego, 1971.

32. P. C. Terry, A. M. Lane and G. J. Fogarty, "Construct Validity of the Profile of Mood States—Adolescents for the Use with Adults," *Psychology of Sport and Exercise*, Vol. 4, No. 2, 2003, pp. 125–139. doi:10.1016/S1469-0292(01)00035-8

33. P. C. Terry, A. M. Lane, H. J. Lane and L. Keohane, "Development and Validation of a Mood Measure for Adolescents," *Journal of Sport Sciences*, Vol. 17, No. 22, 1999, pp. 861–872. doi:10.1080/026404199365425

34. M. Rosenberg, "Society and the Adolescent Self-Image," Princeton University Press, Princeton, 1965.

35. W. C. Torrey, K. T. Mueser, G. H. McHugo and R. E. Drake, "Self-Esteem as an Outcome Measure in Studies of Vocational Rehabilitation for Adults with Severe Mental Illness," *Psychiatric Services*, Vol. 51, No. 2, 2000, pp. 229–233. doi:10.1176/appi.ps.51.2.229

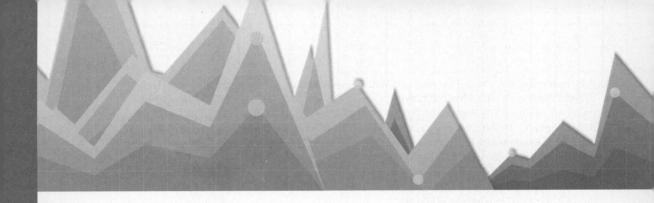

Appendix A-7

Clinical Study
The Use of Postoperative Restraints in Children After Cleft Lip or Cleft Palate Repair: A Preliminary Report

Jennifer Huth,[1] J. Dayne Petersen,[2] and James A. Lehman[1,3]

Received 13 November 2012; Accepted 3 December 2012
Academic Editors: A. Ferri and İ. Özyazgan

Hindawi Publishing Corporation
ISRN Plastic Surgery
Volume 2013, Article ID 540717, 3 pages
http://dx.doi.org/10.5402/2013/540717

Purpose: *This study examines whether the use of elbow restraints after cleft lip/palate repair has a relationship to postoperative complications. Methods. A comparative descriptive design was used to study a convenience sample of children undergoing repair of cleft lip/palate at Akron Children's Hospital with Institutional Review Board approval. The children were randomized into intervention or control groups with use of elbow restraints considered the intervention. The study consists of two arms; one examined children after cleft lip repair, the second examined children after cleft palate repair. Repairs were performed by a single surgeon. Data collected included age, comorbidities, patient discomfort measured by pain score, frequency and duration of pain medications, use of pacifier or finger/thumb sucking, and postoperative complications including disruption of the suture line. Results. With 47 post palate repair patients and 47 post cleft repair patients, there is no significant difference (P > 0.05) in the occurrence of postoperative complications. Conclusions. Study results provide prospective evidence to support postoperative observation of children by surgery staff and family following*

[1] Akron Craniofacial Center, Akron Children's Hospital, Akron, OH 44308, USA
[2] University of Oklahoma Section of Plastic Surgery and The Children's Hospital of Oklahoma, Norman, OK 73104, USA
[3] Faculty of Plastic Surgery, Northeast Ohio Medical University, Rootstown, OH 44274, USA

cleft lip or cleft palate repair without the use of elbow restraints. Clinicians should reevaluate the use of elbow restraints after cleft lip/palate repair based on the belief restraints prevent postoperative complications.

1. Introduction. The question of whether children require elbow restraints following cleft lip and palate repair is unresolved. The theory is that arm restraints prevent children from putting their fingers or objects into their mouth where they could disrupt the suture line. In a survey of plastic surgeons in the United Kingdom in 1993, 93% of plastic surgeons reported the use of arm restraints after repair [1]. Other reports also support the use of splints [2, 3].

In the United States, the use of arm restraints remains a part of the dogma. A survey of Cleft Palate Teams by Petersen [4] in 2008, showed 95% of respondents advocated postoperative arm restraints. A publications by Katzel et al. [5] in 2009, on current surgical practices in cleft care stated that 85% of cleft surgeons recommended the use of elbow restraints after surgery.

This approach has been generally accepted as good practice; however, Jiginni et al. [1] in 1993 found no statistically significant difference between the use or nonuse of arm restraints in the development of postoperative complications. This is the only evidence-based evaluation in the medical literature. With family centered care practiced in the majority of pediatric hospitals parents should be given evidence-based medical results in order to be able to make informed decision on the use of restraints for their child postoperatively

On this basis we conducted a prospective clinical trial to bridge the gap that still remains between practice and evidence based medicine in the use of arm restraints to prevent postoperative complications following cleft lip and palate repair.

2. Method

2.1 Participants. A comparative descriptive design was used to study a prospective sample of children undergoing repair of cleft lip/palate at our pediatric teaching hospital by a single surgeon. The study consisted of two arms. One arm examined children after cleft lip repair; the second arm examined children after repair of cleft palate. All cleft lip patients had a Millard rotation advancement repair, and all cleft palate patients had an intravelar veloplasty repair. All parents of children under the age of 2 who were scheduled for repair of their cleft lip or cleft palate by the study author were invited to give consent to enter their child in the study. Children who required transfer to the critical care setting were excluded from the study. The study received IRB approval.

Because the use of arm restraints is thought to protect the incision from damage infants can cause by placing their fingers/thumb in or at their mouth, we included children whose parents reported them to be finger, thumb, or pacifier suckers in both the cleft lip and the cleft palate repair groups.

2.2 Instrument. The data collected included the child's age, gender, type of cleft repair (lip or palate), preoperative thumb, finger, or pacifier sucking, and the existence of any comorbidity. During hospitalization in the post operative phase, antibiotic therapy, frequency of pain medications, premedication fiacc pain scores, length of hospital stay in days, and an every four hour assessment of the operative site for excessive bleeding or indication of infection were recorded. Phone calls to the parents were made at one week postcleft lip or palate repair. Parents were asked to identify any disruption of the suture line such as a broken stitch or separation of the wound, excessive bleeding from the mouth or nose, signs of infection including redness, edema, drainage, or fever, and the child's discomfort reported as the average flacc pain score and frequency of pain medicationsat one week postoperatively. These questions were also asked of the parents at the followup office visit where standardized photographs were taken of the surgical site, and documentation of any disruption of the suture line was noted by the surgeon.

2.3 Procedure. Participants were divided into a control group, which used restraints, or into the intervention group, with no use of arm restraints. This assignment occurred as they entered the PACU following repair and after receiving parental consent. Assignment to the intervention or control group was alternated every other child. The study procedures were reviewed with parents/guardians in the postanesthesia care unit. This included the deviations from usual care which included the absence of arm restraints in the intervention group and a followup phone call to the home of all participants. Other than the use of restraints, each group received the same standard of care. After signing the consent, parents were given a copy of the study procedures and researchers' contact information. Data collection continued on the nursing care units with assessments of the surgical site recorded every four hours. Educational materials on the study protocol were presented to nursing staff and maintained on each unit to facilitate competency among nurse data collectors. A copy of the fiacc pain scale (Merkel et al, 1997)[6] was reviewed with parents in the PACU and included in the home going instruction packet to parents. This aided parents in communicating a pain score assessment and use of pain medications with the nurse during the one-week postoperative phone call. Assessment of the surgical site and any complications were noted by the surgeon and office staff at the postoperative office visit.

3. Results. A total of 47 children were enrolled in the cleft lip repair arm of the study, and 47 children were enrolled in the cleft palate repair group (Table A7.1). Twenty one of the children enrolled in the control group of the cleft lip repair arm had good ($n = 5$) to excellent ($n = 16$) postoperative healing of the surgical site. Twenty-six children enrolled in the intervention or no arm restraint group of the cleft lip repair arm demonstrated good ($n = 4$) to excellent ($n = 20$) repair. Families of 2 children in the intervention group did not return for followup evaluation.

The surgical outcome in cleft lip repair was initially evaluated by our surgical nurse and the surgeon. Postoperative photos at 6 months were then used as a final evaluation. Excellent results had no off set of the vermilion and no elevation of the lip on the cleft side. Good results had minor vermilion offset (<2 mm) and minimal (<2 mm) elevation of the lip on the cleft side.

In the palatal repair arm, 2 of 22 (9%) developed postoperative fistulae in the intervention group, and 2 of 25 children (8%) developed postoperative fistulae in the control group. Lehman [7] reported a fistula rate of 16.1% in 136 consecutive palate repairs. When examining the use of arm restraints after the repair of a child's cleft lip or cleft palate, the results show no significant difference in the occurrence of postoperative complications ($P > 0.05$).

The preoperative habit of finger, thumb, or pacifier sucking did not exclude a child from participating in the study. 79% of parents of children undergoing repair of their cleft lip reported the children placed their thumb/fingers in their mouths. 66% of the parents in the cleft palate repair group reported their children placed fingers, thumbs, or pacifiers in their mouths frequently (Table A7.1). The history of finger, thumb, or pacifier sucking did

TABLE A7.1	Demographics of patients.				
STUDY GROUP	MALE	FEMALE	AGE IN MONTHS	USE OF PACIFIER OR THUMB	TYPE OF CLEFT
Lip repair splints	61.9% ($n = 13$)	38.1% ($n = 8$)	M = 5.05 mo, SD = 4.22 mo	90.5% ($n = 19$)	CL-9 BCLP-3 UCLP-9
Lip repair no splints	61.5% ($n = 16$)	38.5% ($n = 10$)	M = 4.0 mo, SD = 2.36 mo	69.2% ($n = 18$)	CL-12 BCLP-3 UCLP-11
Palate repair splints	52% ($n = 13$)	48% ($n = 12$)	M = 11.76 mo, SD = 3.53 mo	60% ($n = 15$)	CP-14 BCLP-5 UCLP-6
Palate repair no splints	63.6% ($n = 14$)	36.4% ($n = 8$)	M = 13.86, SD = 4.05 mo	72.7% ($n = 16$)	CP-9 BCLP-14 UCLP-9

not add any significance to the results. In the intervention group, there was 1 fistula in the thumb sucking group and one in the nonthumb sucking group. In the control or arm restraint group both fistulas occurred in nonthumb sucking group (Table A7.1).

Our goal was to have two equal groups of patients (*n*) with equal numbers in both the control and intervention subgroups. This did not occur, but we believe that the numbers are adequate to make a strong statement regarding the use of postoperative splints.

4. Discussion. The literature does not answer the questions of whether the use of elbow restraints following the repair of the cleft lip/plate provides any evidence-based benefit. Our study which was a prospective study was stimulated by this long standing controversy to provide evidence-based information for surgeons, parents, and healthcare providers.

We also included patients who had a history of finger, thumb, or pacifier sucking.

The traditional use of postoperative arm restraints following the repair of a child's cleft lip or cleft palate remains common. Two surveys of cleft surgeons by Jiginni [1] and Petersen [4] show continued support for the use of splints, and recent articles reinforce the postoperative use of arm splints. There is a cadre of other authors who have pointed out that they have had "no untoward effects" after abandoning the use of arm restraints [1, 8-10].

Two other publications add information to support not using restraints. Oxley [11] in 2001, in a small survey found that 53% of parents if given a choice would choose not to use restraints for their child postoperatively. Tokioka et al. [12] in 2009, observed no manipulating, scratching, or other harmful movements when eight infants were videotaped after repair of their cleft lip and/or palate without restraints.

Seventy-nine percent of parents of children undergoing lip repair and 66% of patients in the cleft palate repair group reported finger, thumb, or pacifier sucking. Because this is one of the major reasons surgeons advocate for splint use we felt this was important to include this subset of patients in our study. Interestingly, 3 of the 4 fistula occurred in the nonthumb sucking group.

The final results of our study showed there was no significant difference ($P > 0.05$) in the occurrence of postoperative complication in the group without elbow restraints. The question remains whether presenting restraint use after cleft repair with no evidence to support their use reflects adherence to the concept of family centered care [13].

5. Summary. We have presented a prospective study that demonstrates no statistical significant benefit to the use of arm restraints in children having cleft lip and palate surgery.

As healthcare professionals, we must provide evidence based information to parents, so that they can make informed decisions in the care of their child. We hope this study adds to the body of knowledge in the discussion of whether arm restraints are necessary after cleft lip/palate repair. We also believe a large multicenter study would enhance confirmation of our results.

References

1. V. Jiginni, T. Kangesu, and B. C. Sommerlad, "Do babies require arm splints after cleft palate repair?" *British Journal of Plastic Surgery, Vol. 46,* no. 8, pp. 681–685, 1993.
2. M. Hosnuter, E. Kargi, and A. Işikdemir, 'Another practical method for arm restraint in children with cleft lip/palate," *Plastic and Reconstructive Surgery, Vol. 110,* no. 4, pp. 1185–1186, 2002.
3. M. Muraoka, T. Taniguchi, and T. Harada, "A restraining device of elbow flexion made from flowerpot bottle net," *Plastic and Reconstructive Surgery, Vol. 110,* no. 1, p. 711, 2002.
4. D. Petersen, *Poster Presentation,* ACPA Meeting, Philadelphia, Pa, USA, 2008.
5. E. B. Katzel, P. Basile, P. F. Koltz, J. R. Marcus, and J. A. Girotto, "Current surgical practices in cleft care: cleft palate repair techniques and postoperative care," *Plastic and Reconstructive Surgery,* Vol. 124, no. 3, pp. 899–900, 2009.
6. S. I. Merkel, T. Voepel-Lewis, J. R. Shayevitz, and S. Malviya, "The FLACC: a behavioral scale for scoring postoperative pain in young children," *Pediatric Nursing, Vol. 23,* no. 3, pp. 293–297, 1997.

7. J. A. Lehman, "Cleft palate repair for the 1990's," *Problems in Plastic Surgery, Vol. 2*, no. l, pp. 1–17, 1992, 16.1% fistula rate in 136 consecutive patients.

8. P. J. Skoll and D. A. Lazarus, "Arm restraint in children with cleft lip and palate," *Plastic and Reconstructive Surgery, Vol. 113*, no. 5, p. 1523, 2004.

9. B. C. Sommerlad, T. Kangesu, O. Babuccu et al., "Arm restraint in children with cleft lip/palate," *Plastic and Reconstructive Surgery, Vol. 112*, no. 1, pp. 331–332, 2003.

10. S. O'Riain, "Cleft lip surgery without postoperative restraints," *British Journal of Plastic Surgery, Vol. 30*, no. 2, pp. 140–141, 1977.

11. J. Oxley, "Are arm splints required following cleft lip/palate repair?" *Paediatric Nursing, Vol. 13*, no. 1, pp. 27–30, 2001.

12. K. Tokioka, S. Park, Y. Sugawara, and T. Nakatsuka, "Video recording study of infants undergoing primary cheiloplasty: are arm restraints really needed?" *Cleft Palate-Craniofacial Journal, Vol. 46*, no. 5, pp. 494–497, 2009.

13. "What are the core concepts of patient- and family-centered care?" Institute for Family Centered Care, 2010, http://www.ipfcc.org/faq.html.

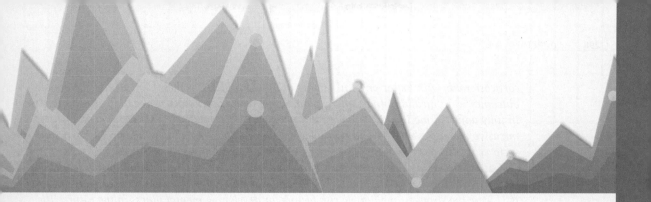

Appendix A-8

Investigating Risk Factors for Psychological Morbidity Three Months After Intensive Care: a Prospective Cohort Study

Dorothy M Wade[1,2]; David C Howell[2]; John A Weinman[3]; Rebecca J Hardy[4];
Michael G Mythen[5]; Chris R Brewin[6]; Susana Borja-Boluda[2]; Claire F Matejowsky[2]
and Rosalind A Raine[1]

Abstract

Introduction: *There is growing evidence of poor mental health and quality of life among survivors of intensive care. However, it is not yet clear to what extent the trauma of life-threatening illness, associated drugs and treatments, or patients' psychological reactions during intensive care contribute to poor psychosocial outcomes. Our aim was to investigate the relative contributions of a broader set of risk factors and outcomes than had previously been considered in a single study.*

Methods: *A prospective cohort study of 157 mixed-diagnosis highest acuity patients was conducted in a large general intensive care unit (ICU). Data on four groups of risk factors (clinical, acute psychological, socio-demographic and chronic health) were collected during ICU admissions. Post-traumatic stress disorder (PTSD), depression, anxiety and quality of life were assessed using validated questionnaires at three months (n = 100). Multivariable analysis was used.*

Results: *At follow-up, 55% of patients had psychological morbidity: 27.1% (95% CI: 18.3%, 35.9%) had probable PTSD; 46.3% (95% CI: 36.5%, 56.1%) probable depression, and 44.4% (95% CI: 34.6%, 54.2%) anxiety. The strongest clinical risk factor for PTSD was longer duration of sedation (regression coefficient = 0.69 points (95% CI: 0.12, 1.27) per day, scale = 0 to 51). There was a strong association between depression at three months and receiving benzodiazepines in the ICU (mean difference between groups = 6.73 points (95% CI: 1.42, 12.06), scale = 0 to 60). Use of inotropes or vasopressors was correlated with anxiety, and*

[1]Department of Applied Health Research, University College London (UCL), 1-19 Torrington Place, WC1E 7HB, UK
Full list of author information is available at the end of the article

Wade *et al. Critical Care 2012,* **16**:R192
http://ccforum.com/content/16/5/R192

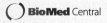

corticosteroids with better physical quality of life. The effects of these clinical risk factors on outcomes were mediated (partially explained) by acute psychological reactions in the ICU. In fully adjusted models, the strongest independent risk factors for PTSD were mood in ICU, intrusive memories in ICU and psychological history. ICU mood, psychological history and socio-economic position were the strongest risk factors for depression.

Conclusions: Strikingly high rates of psychological morbidity were found in this cohort of intensive care survivors. The study's key finding was that acute psychological reactions in the ICU were the strongest modifiable risk factors for developing mental illness in the future. The observation that use of different ICU drugs correlated with different psychological outcomes merits further investigation. These findings suggest that psychological interventions, along with pharmacological modifications, could help reduce poor outcomes, including PTSD, after intensive care.

Introduction. The mental health of intensive care survivors may be poor. Patients may suffer from post-traumatic stress disorder (PTSD), depression or anxiety with poor quality of life in the months following intensive care [1-3]. It is not clear whether poor psychological outcomes are associated with the traumatic effects of critical illness, intensive care treatment and drugs (clinical risk factors), or mood and stress reactions in intensive care (acute psychological factors). Outcomes might be better explained by chronic physical conditions and psychological history (chronic health factors) or socio-demographic factors, such as low socio-economic position [4]. There is an urgent need to explore the relative effects of a broader set of risk factors than has previously been investigated on different psychosocial outcomes, within a fully-powered single study of mixed-diagnosis, general intensive care patients.

Psychological outcomes after intensive care include PTSD, an "anxiety disorder that often follows exposure to an extreme stressor that causes injury, threatens life or physical integrity" [5]. The person's immediate response involves intense fear, helplessness or horror. The disorder is characterised by three clusters of symptoms: re-experiencing, avoidance and hyper-arousal, that persist for more than a month and cause distress or impaired functioning. Another outcome of interest, depression, is characterised by low mood or loss of interest for more than two weeks, with a range of other symptoms. Anxiety is a normal emotion that may become persistent and inappropriate. In systematic reviews, the median point prevalence of PTSD among intensive care survivors was 22% [1] with 28% prevalence of depression [2]. Rates of anxiety after intensive care vary from 5% to 43% [3]. In a meta-analysis of quality of life, physical functioning was 20 points (0 to 100) and mental health 10 points below UK norms [3].

Patients are exposed to many stressors in the intensive care unit (ICU), including illness, pain, sleep deprivation, thirst, hunger, dyspnea, unnatural noise and light, inability to communicate, isolation and fear of dying; and they may show extreme emotional reactions in response [6-8]. Interventions, such as mechanical ventilation (MV) or invasive monitoring for cardiovascular support, may be difficult for patients to tolerate. Furthermore, the onset of delirium, including frightening psychotic symptoms, such as hallucinations and paranoid delusions, is common in intensive care [9,10]. Delirium is associated with the pathophysiology of critical illness as well as drugs used in intensive care [11,12]. The question is whether exposure to stressors, such as MV, or acute psychological reactions, such as stress, mood and hallucinations, are direct risk factors for PTSD and other adverse outcomes. It may be that patients' emotional reactions to stress in intensive care are early signs of psychological morbidity.

Consistent risk factors for post-ICU psychological morbidity have not been definitively established [13,14], with associations mostly detected in very few studies. Socio-demographic risk factors for post-ICU PTSD include age [15,16,18], sex [17,18] and unemployment [19]. Psychological history is a known chronic health risk factor [12,15]. Acute psychological risk symptoms (extreme fear and agitation in the ICU) were found to be associated with PTSD in only one study to our knowledge [17]. Factual recall and memory of pain were associated with PTSD in one study [19], whereas delusional memories (of psychotic symptoms) following ICU discharge were more important in others [12,20]. Clinical risk factors include aspects of sedation [12,17,18,21] and duration of mechanical ventilation [15]. Two studies that found no association with mechanical ventilation and PTSD were small, with 41 [18] and 37 [22] participants. As mechanical ventilation is the most common intensive care intervention, replication of the positive result [15] is urgently needed.

The few risk factors identified for post-ICU depression and anxiety were mainly found in single or small studies or sub-groups of patients. Hypoglycemia [23] and benzo-diazepine dosage [24] were associated with post-ICU depression in patients with acute lung injury. Pessimism was associated with subsequent depression and anxiety in one study [19]. A more consistent group of risk factors (age, illness severity, ICU length of stay and prior health) were identified in studies of post-ICU quality of life [3].

The aim of our study was to investigate a broader set of clinical, acute psychological, socio-demographic and chronic health risk factors than had previously been tested, for different psychosocial outcomes within a single study of mixed general ICU patients. We used multi-variable analysis to determine relative contributions of risk factors in different domains. Furthermore, we aimed to identify modifiable clinical and acute psychological risk factors that might inform the development and evaluation of preventative interventions in intensive care.

Materials and methods

Study Design. This was a prospective cohort study with four groups of potential risk factors (clinical, acute psychological, socio-demographic and chronic health). Probable PTSD at three months was the primary outcome while depression, anxiety, and mental and physical quality of life at three months were secondary outcomes.

Participants. The sample consisted of consecutive, highest acuity adult patients who received level three care in a large general ICU at University College Hospital, London, England between November 2008 and September 2009. In the UK, level three patients are those receiving mechanical ventilation for more than 24 hours or patients with two or more organs supported. Patients were recruited in the ICU when physicians determined they were showing signs of recovery; when they had capacity to give informed consent, and were awake, alert and able to communicate. They were not recruited on a specific day of their ICU stay, as patients woke up and became alert at different times. They were excluded if they were not English-speaking; had dementia or remained confused or had a low GCS (Glasgow Coma Scale) until their discharge from ICU; were unable to communicate until their discharge from ICU; had severe sensory impairment; or were deemed terminally ill (for example, were receiving palliative care).

Ethics. The study was approved by the Joint University College London/University College London Hospitals Committee on the Ethics of Human Research.

Procedure. ICU patient lists were checked daily to identify eligible participants who had received level three care during their stay. After being assessed for capacity by a health psychologist (the first author), and giving informed consent, patients completed a psychological questionnaire. Patients found to have current confusion or inability to communicate were recruited later in their stay, if and when these problems had resolved. Clinical and socio-demographic data were collected from electronic patient notes held in the ICU. Three months after discharge from the ICU, patients were sent a postal questionnaire, which included measures of PTSD, depression, anxiety, Health-Related Quality of Life (HRQL) and socio-economic circumstances.

Data Collection. Socio-demographic data recorded include age, gender, ethnicity and socio-economic position, measured using the National Statistics Socio-Economic Classification [25].

The NS-SEC is a measure of employment relations and conditions of occupations, and is the most widely used measure of socio-economic positions in official UK statistics. The self-coded version of the NS-SEC used in this study has five classes of occupation: managerial and professional; intermediate; small employers and own account workers; lower supervisory and technical; semi-routine and routine. A sixth unclassified category was added.

Clinical data include: type of admission (elective surgical, emergency surgical, non-surgical), source of admission (theatre, ward, Accident & Emergency, other), acute physiology and chronic health evaluation II score (APACHE II) [26], length of stay (days), days of organ support, type of organ support, an infection biomarker (C-reactive protein) and highest therapeutic intervention (Therapeutic Intervention Scoring System, TISS) score during the admission [27]. The TISS score reflects the type and number of intensive care interventions received, with points added for each intensive care activity. Data on drugs administered included exposure to sleep medications (mainly zopiclone), benzodiazepines, anaesthetic agents (mainly propofol), antipsychotics, inotropes and vasopressors, systemically-administered corticosteroids, and opioids; number of psychoactive drug groups received (0 to 7); and the number of days patients were sedated.

Information on "chronic health" factors (chronic physical conditions, psychological history and alcohol use) was obtained from electronic medical records held in the ICU.

Psychological Measures. All acute psychological reactions were assessed once a patient was able to respond to questions. Mood in intensive care was measured with 15 items (on anger, anxiety, depression, positive mood and confusion) from the validated Profile of Mood States [28]. Stress reactions were assessed using a newly developed 18-item intensive care stress reactions scale (ICUSS) as validated stress questionnaires did not contain items relevant to the ICU context. The ICUSS has four subscales: "physical stress" (difficulty breathing, pain, discomfort from tubes, anxiety about breathing), "delirious symptoms" (hallucinations, nightmares, disorientation, agitation), control (communication, control, confidence, information) and support (dignity, emotional support).

Memory items, (on being admitted to the ICU, the ICU stay, and presence and content of early intrusive memories in the ICU), were developed with guidance from Professor Brewin, an expert in intrusive memories and stress. The content of intrusive memories was qualitatively assessed as "factual" (real experiences in the ICU) or "unreal" (hallucinations or delusions experienced in the ICU). The validated Brief Illness Perception Questionnaire (BIPQ) [29] was used to measure patients' subjective illness perceptions including "timeline" (how long they believed their illness would last).

Outcome Measures. Three months later, PTSD symptoms were assessed using the Post-traumatic Stress Diagnostic Scale (PDS), a well-validated instrument including a 17-item severity scale [30]. We selected the PDS as it conforms to diagnostic criteria for PTSD [5] and has high diagnostic agreement with the gold-standard Structured Clinical Interview for PTSD. Using a cut-point of 18 (on a scale of 0 to 51), shown to be a highly efficient scoring method [31], the PDS severity scale has sensitivity of 0.86, specificity of 0.87 and an overall efficiency of 0.87. Participants were asked to answer questions in relation to a specific trauma (in this case, admission to intensive care) according to PDS authors' instructions. Symptoms of depression were measured with the 20-item Center for Epidemiologic Studies Depression Scale (CES-D) [32], the most widely used measure of depression in epidemiological studies, validated for intensive care patients [33] and many other populations. We used a cut-point of 19 (on a scale of 0 to 60) rather than the usual 16, as recommended to deal with the effect of somatic items in patients with medical illness [34].

We assessed anxiety at three months using a validated short form of the State-Trait Anxiety Inventory (STAI) [35], a widely used questionnaire in many populations and health conditions. We used a cut-point of 44 (range of scores 0 to 80) as recommended for studies of medically ill patients [36]. The SF-12, extensively evaluated to establish reliability and validity, was used to measure quality of life. It yields mental and physical summary scales, transformed to have a mean of 50 and SD of 10 [37]. The follow-up questionnaire included an item about current or past psychological issues but few patients answered it, so we relied on electronic medical records to obtain details of psychological history. Three months was deemed a suitable time-point to measure outcomes, including acute PTSD [5], and to examine relationships between ICU clinical and stress factors and psychological outcomes.

Power. To obtain an initial estimate of the sample size required, a clinically significant difference in PTSD scores between two groups, defined by a binary risk factor (for example, sex), was deemed to be 10 points on the PDS [30]. For this effect size, 80% power and 5% significance, 34 patients were required in each of the two groups. As the analyses were to be carried out using multiple regression, with both continuous and categorical risk factors, the sample size needed to be inflated. With the initial sample size of 68, a correlation coefficient of 0.3 between a continuous risk factor and outcome could be detected [38]. To detect the same correlation coefficient (0.3) between a risk factor and outcome in a multiple regression model where all other variables in the model explained 30% of the total variation in outcome, calculations indicated that the sample size needed to be inflated by 40% [38]. This yielded a total sample size of 95 patients. A drop-out rate of approximately 30% was estimated on the basis of previous experience, raising the recruitment required to approximately 140 patients. During the study, the drop-out rate was higher than expected (36%) and 17 extra patients were recruited to ensure that the study retained power.

Statistical Analysis. All statistical analyses were conducted using SPSS for Windows (version 14) (SPSS Inc., Chicago, Illinois, USA).

Distributions of risk factors were assessed with frequency histograms and statistical tests for normality. Ordinary least squares regression models were used with PTSD and other outcomes treated as continuous variables. Model building was carried out in stages so that highly correlated variables (which confounded each other) were not included in the same model and to ensure parsimony of the final model. To facilitate this, four groups of risk factors (clinical, acute psychological, socio-demographic and chronic health) were predefined.

(i) *Univariable analysis.* In this stage of analysis, each risk factor was related to each outcome to estimate unadjusted associations. Correlations, t-tests and one-way analysis of variance were used with, respectively, continuous, binary and categorical risk factors. Spearman's rank correlation coefficients were used if continuous risk factors were not normally distributed.

(ii) *Multivariable analysis.* In recognition of the number of potential variables being tested in these analyses and the associated implications for sample size, a two-stage multivariable process was used.

Stage one: Separate multivariable models were built for each outcome from risk factors within each of the four groups (clinical, acute psychological, socio-demographic and chronic health) to identify the "strongest" risk factors from each group. Risk factors included in this first stage of multivariable analysis were those that showed significant unadjusted associations $(P < 0.05)$ with outcomes in univariable analysis. This first stage of multivariable analysis was not carried out for a group where two or fewer significant risk factors were identified in the univariable analysis. No more than eight variables were entered into a regression in this stage of multivariable analysis due to the sample size of 100 (a rule of thumb is to have 10 to 15 times more observations than variables).

Stage two: The strongest risk factors from each group identified in the first stage of multivariable analysis (based on an adjusted significance level of $P < 0.01$), were entered in a final series of multiple regressions to assess whether factors from different groups were independent of each other (also based on a significance level of $P < 0.01$). Factors were entered in the following order: socio-demographic, clinical, chronic physical, acute psychological and psychological history (at this stage of analysis, chronic factors were split up into chronic physical and psychological history). Residuals were found to be normally distributed in all multivariable models with no evidence of multicollinearity.

Results. A total of 157 level three patients were assessed before discharge from the ICU, and 100 patients (64%) were followed up at three months (see Figure A8.1). Most patients were mechanically ventilated for more than 24 hours, and most were sedated with benzodiazepines or anaesthetic agents (Table A8.1). Patients had elevated mean scores for mood disturbance and stress reactions in ICU (Table A8.2). Some 65 to 75% had hallucinations, agitation and nightmares. Memory impairment, including amnesia for time spent in ICU or unwanted intrusive memories of intensive care, were common.

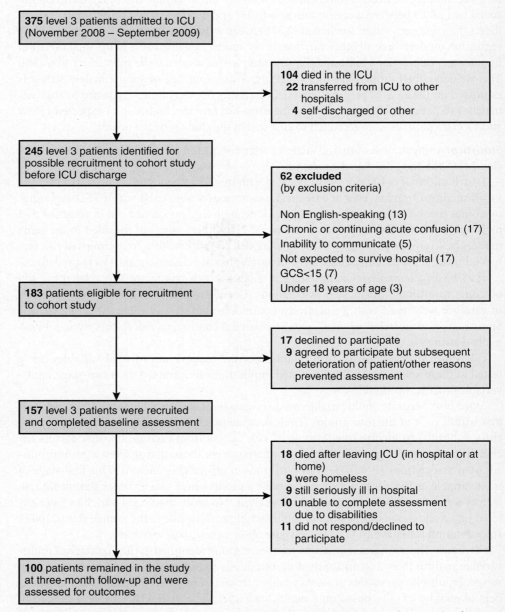

FIGURE A8.1 Flow diagram of patient recruitment and participation in a cohort study of psychological outcomes of intensive care survivors.

TABLE A8.1 Participants' Socio-Demographic and Clinical Characteristics

CHARACTERISTIC	FOLLOWED UP (N = 100)	LOST TO FOLLOW-UP/ DIED (N = 57)	P-VALUE
Age - years Mean (SD)	57.26 (17.40)	57.19 (15.62)	0.98
Male sex, No. (%)	52 (52%)	38 (66.7%)	0.07
White ethnicity, No. (%)	83 (85.6%)	49 (86%)	0.63
Occupation (by NS-SEC)*, No. (%)			
1. Professions/managerial	33 (33%)	No data	
2. Intermediate professions	10 (10%)		
3. Self-employed	21 (21%)		
4. Technical/craft	7 (7%)		
5. Semi-routine/routine	20 (20%)		
6. Unclassified	9 (9%)		
Type admission, No. (%)			
Elective surgical	23 (23%)	14 (24.6%)	0.63
Emergency surgical	14 (14%)	5 (8.8%)	
Non-surgical	63 (63 %)	38 (66.7%)	
Apache II score† Mean (SD)	22.01 (7.19)	22.44 (9.07)	0.76
Hospital length of stay - days Median (range)	27 (239)	27 (173)	0.81
ICU length of stay - days Median (range)	8 (85)	10 (37)	0.62
TISS score‡ Mean (SD)	24.61 (5.05)	24.37 (5.86)	0.79
Number of organs supported, Mean (SD)	4 (7)	5 (7)	<0.05
Number (%) receiving mechanical ventilation	79 (79%)	49 (88%)	0.43
Duration of MV in days, Median (range)	3 (80)	4 (28)	
Number (%) receiving cardiovascular support	52 (52%)	36 (63%)	0.24
Duration of CV support in days, Median (range)	1 (16)	1 (20)	
Duration of sedation - days Median (range)	2 (24)	2 (21)	0.18
Benzodiazepines in ICU (yes/no), No. (%)	60 (60%)	40 (70.2%)	0.19
Anaesthetic agents in ICU (yes/no), No. (%)	66 (66%)	39 (68.4%)	0.76
Antipsychotics in ICU (yes/no), No. (%)rows from here down have less space than rows above	39 (39%)	27 (47.4%)	0.70
Inotropes/vasopressors in ICU (yes/no), No.(%)	47 (47%)	35 (61.4%)	0.08
Steroids in ICU (yes/no), No. (%)	33 (33%)	20 (35.1%)	0.79
Opioids in ICU (yes/no), No. (%)	93 (93%)	53 (93%)	0.99
Highest C-reactive protein in ICU, Mean (SD)	212.72 (126.79)	No data	
Post-hospital destination**			<0.01
Primary body system††			0.63

*NS-SEC, National Statistics Socio-economic Classification (UK) [25]

†Scores for the Acute Physiology, Age, and Chronic Health Evaluation (APACHE II) [26] range from 0 to 71; higher scores indicate more severe illness

‡In the Therapeutic Intervention Scoring System [27] points are added for each new ICU activity

**Categories of post-hospital destination were 1. Home 2. Transfer to other hospital 3. Care or rehab centre 4. Died in hospital 5. Readmission since discharge home 6. Still in hospital at three months (not yet discharged). Numbers in each category are not reported here due to lack of space

††Primary body system had 11 categories: respiratory, cardiovascular, gastro-intestinal, neurological, trauma, poisoning, genito-urinary, endocrine, haematological, musculo-skeletal and dermatological. Numbers in each category are not reported here due to lack of space.

Subsequently, the incidence of probable PTSD at three months was 27.1% (95%CI: 18.3%, 35.9%). Prevalence of probable depression was 46.3% (95% CI: 36.5%, 56.1%) and anxiety 44.4% (95% CI: 34.6%, 54.2%). In all, 55% of patients had psychological morbidity at three months. There were 16% of patients with prior history of psychological morbidity (depression in all cases). Mean mental quality of life was 43.9 (95% CI: 41.6, 46.3), six points below the population norm (50). Mean physical quality of life was 34.4 (95% CI: 32.3, 36.6), 16 points below the norm.

All psychological measures used had reliability (internal consistency), using Cronbach's alpha (0.91 for Profile of Mood States (POMS); 0.93 for PDS; O.91 for CES-D; and 0.88 for STAI). After principal components analysis, the ICU stress reactions scale was found to

TABLE A8.2 Acute Psychological Responses in the Intensive Care Unit (ICU)

		FOLLOWED UP (N = 100)	DIED/LOST TO FOLLOW-UP (N = 57)	P-VALUE - DIFFERENCE
(i) Total ICU mood Mean (SD) disturbance		29.00 (13.60) Scale 0 to 60	27.18 (13.58)	P = 0.42
ii) Total ICU stress Mean (SD) reactions		32.89 (12.81) Scale 0 to 72	31.62 (11.98)	P = 0.54
a) Physical stress (subscale of ICU stress)		8.61 (4.46) Scale 0 to 16	7.57 (4.34)	P = 0.72
b) Delirious symptoms (subscale of ICU stress)		8.17 (5.04) Scale 0 to 20	7.86 (5.49)	P = 0.16
iii) Illness perceptions, Mean (SD)		Range 0 to 10	6.44 (2.93)	P = 0.69
a) Timeline - how long you think condition will last		6.64 (2.77)		
b) Concern about condition		7.34 (2.8)	7.09 (3.2)	P = 0.61
c) Control over condition		4 .00 (2.97)	4.62 (3.31)	P = 0.25
d) Understanding condition		7.06 (2.97)	7.41 (3.23)	P = 0.5
e) Emotional representation of condition		5.92 (3.4)	6.24 (3.75)	P = 0.59
iv) Memory No. (%)	Yes	34 (34.3%)	21(37.5%)	P = 0.69
a) Memory of initial admission to ICU	No	65 (65.7%)	35 (62.5%)	
b) Memory for whole ICU stay	Little	45 (45.5%)	21 (37.5%)	P = 0.19
	Some	29 (29.3%)	13 (23.2%)	
	Most	25 (25.3%)	22 (39.3%)	
c) Presence of early intrusive memories of ICU	Yes	49 (49.5%)	24 (42.8%)	P = 0.73
	No	50 (50.5%)	32 (57.1%)	
d) Content of early intrusive memories, if experienced	Factual	22.6%	No data	
	Delusional	20%		
	Both/other*	6.9%		

(i) Total mood disturbance was measured using the Profile of Mood States [28]
(ii) Total ICU stress, a) physical stress and b) delirious symptoms were measured with the ICU stress reactions scale
(iii) Illness perceptions were measured using the BIPQ [29]
*Patients had both factual and delusional memories, or did not describe the content of memories

have four factors: physical stress, delirious symptoms, personal control and support. The total scale and three subscales were reliable (Cronbach's alphas: 0.83 (total); 0.78 (personal control); 0.74 (delirious symptoms); 0.75 (physical stress)). ICU stress reactions scores were highly correlated with POMS [28] scores ($r = 0.73$, $P < 0.01$), suggesting concurrent validity. ICU stress reaction scores were also highly correlated with PTSD, depression and anxiety at three months, suggesting predictive validity.

PTSD. Because of the number of risk factors and outcomes investigated, the full three-stage statistical analysis is reported for PTSD only in the main paper. However, the same process was used for each outcome (see Tables A8.3 and A8.4 for univariable analyses of secondary outcomes, and Additional file 1 for further multivariable analyses tables).

Univariable Analysis - PTSD. Clinical risk factors significantly associated with PTSD were higher TISS scores, number of organs supported, days of mechanical ventilation, days of advanced cardiovascular support, days of sedation, number of drug groups and C-reactive protein during admission; and use of benzodiazepines, inotropes/vasopressors and antipsychotics (see Table A8.3). Significant acute psychological risk factors for PTSD were total mood disturbance in ICU, ICU stress reactions (including delirious symptoms), loss of memory in ICU, early intrusive memories in ICU and three illness perceptions (Table A8.4). Patients with ICU memory loss were more likely to have early intrusive memories (62% vs 39%, $P < 0.05$). No socio-demographic factors were significantly associated with PTSD. Psychological history and alcohol use were significant "chronic health" risk factors.

TABLE A8.3 Unadjusted Associations Between Clinical Factors and Psycho-Social Outcomes Three Months after Intensive Care

	POST-TRAUMATIC STRESS DISORDER*	DEPRESSION	ANXIETY	MENTAL QUALITY OF LIFE	PHYSICAL QUALITY OF LIFE
TISS (Therapeutic intervention scoring)	0.25, P = 0.01	0.08, P = 0.44	0.07, P = 0.52	−0.06, P = 0.62	0.04, P = 0.74
Number of organs supported	0.26, P < 0.01	0.12, P = 0.23	0.06, P = 0.57	−0.08, P = 0.47	0.08, P = 0.49
Duration of sedation	0.27, P < 0.01	0.19, P = 0.07	0.17, P = 0.09	−0.20, P = 0.06	0.03, P = 0.82
Number of drug groups	0.28, P < 0.01	0.10, P = 0.32	0.10, P = 0.31	−0.10, P = 0.47	−0.20, P = 0.07
Length of stay in ICU	0.11, P = 0.29	−0.05, P = 0.66	−0.06, P = 0.58	−0.02, P = 0.87	0.02, P = 0.87
Length of hospital stay	0.15, P = 0.15	0.21, P < 0.05	0.09, P = 0.39	−0.18, P = 0.12	−0.07, P = 0.56
Type of admission†	P = 0.81	P = 0.50	P = 0.12	P = 0.81	P = 0.53
Post-hospital destination	P = 0.38	P < 0.05	P = 0.23	P = 0.22	P = 0.90
Primary body system	P = 0.20	P = 0.03	P = 0.25	P = 0.30	P = 0.17
Duration of mechanical ventilation	0.20, P < 0.05	0.09, P = 0.39	0.06, P = 0.57	−0.013, P = 0.91	−0.014, P = 0.90
Duration of cardiovascular support	0.25, P < 0.05	0.14, P = 0.17	0.13, P = 0.22	−0.20, P = 0.06	−0.03, P = 0.79
Benzodiazepines ‡	6.96 (2.36, 11.57), P < 0.01	7.44 (1.81, 13.07), P = 0.01	5.95 (0.03, 11.87), P < 0.05	−4.08 (−8.73, .56), P = 0.08	−.27 (−4.67, 4.12), P = 0.90
Anaesthetics	1.64 (−3.35, 6.65), P = 0.51	−2.35 (−8.50, 3.80), P = 0.45	−2.61 (−8.88, 3.65), P = 0.41	2.02 (−2.9, 6.93), P = 0.42	4.45 (−0.04, 8.94), P = 0.05
Inotropes or vasopressors	4.84 (0.1, 9.57), P < 0.05	3.70 (1.99, 9.40), P = 0.20	7.63 (0.89, 13.37), P = 0.01	−4.51 (−9.08, .06), P = 0.05	0.06 (−4.29, 4.41), P = 0.98
Antipsychotics	5.81 (0.8, 10.81), P < 0.05	1.59 (−4.31, 7.39), P = 0.59	1.18 (−4.87, 7.25), P = 0.70	−1.58 (−6.28, 3.12), P = 0.51	4.14 (−0.15, 8.43), P = 0.06
Opioids	−0.55 (−10.42, 9.32), P = 0.91	−7.12 (−18, 3.77), P = 0.20	−7.79 (−19.25, 3.66), P = 0.18	7.42 (−0.96, 15.8), P = 0.08	0.29 (−7.65, 8.23), P = 0.94
Steroids	−0.28 (−5.33, 4.77), P = 0.91	−1.08 (−7.25, 5.08), P = 0.73	−1.57 (−7.85, 4.71), P = 0.62	−.59 (−5.48, 4.31), P = 0.81	5.57 (1.18, 9.96), P < 0.05
Highest C-reactive protein in ICU	0.22, P < 0.05	0.10, P = 0.32	0.08, P = 0.44	No data	No data

Effect sizes presented in the table are Pearson's r for normally distributed exposure variables, Spearman's rho for skewed variables, and mean difference with 95% CI for binary variables.

*Range of scores for outcome measures: PTSD 0-51 (PDS); depression 0 to 60 (CES-D); anxiety 0 to 80 (STAI); mental quality of life 0 to 100 (SF-12 mental component summary score); physical quality of life 0 to 100 (SF-12 physical component summary score)

†For type of admission, post-hospital destination and primary body system (categorical variables) the P-values of the F statistic are presented.

‡For all drug variables, the mean score of patients who did not receive the drug group was subtracted from the mean score of patients who did receive the drug.

TABLE A8.4 Unadjusted Associations between Socio-Demographic Variables, Acute Psychological Reactions in ICU, and Three Month Outcomes

	PTSD*	DEPRESSION	ANXIETY	MENTAL QUALITY OF LIFE	PHYSICAL QUALITY OF LIFE
Age	−0.18 $P = 0.07$	0.17 $P = 0.11$	−0.03 $P = 0.79$	0.10 $P = 0.38$	−0.10 $P = 0.38$
Sex (female - male)	4.30 (−0.44, 9.04) $P = 0.08$	4.01 (1.68, 9.69) $P = 0.17$	−3.39 $P = 0.26$	4.20 (−0.39, 8.79) $P = 0.07$	−0.81 (−5.16, 3.54) $P = 0.71$
Ethnicity (white/other)	$P = 0.60$	$P = 0.05$	$P = 0.49$	$P = 0.20$	$P = 0.15$
Socio-economic position	$P = 0.25$	$P < 0.01$	$P < 0.05$	$P < 0.05$	$P = 0.69$
1. Professions/managerial	11.77 (9.10)	14.46 (10.68)	39.27 (11.69)	48.47 (9.53)	35.86 (9.66)
2. Intermediate profession	15.61 (7.25)	30.33 (12.51)	53.00 (13.19)	39.58 (10.73)	31.16 (6.95)
3. Self-employed	13.12 (12.46)	22.71 (14.21)	43.33 (13.89)	45.55 (10.79)	34.13 (10.81)
4. Technical/craft	8.04 (4.79)	13.64 (8.59)	36.19 (11.45)	43.53 (8.75)	38.21 (10.77)
5. Semi-routine/routine	18.19 (13.77)	24.75 (15.65)	46.33 (16.11)	38.43 (9.48)	35.40 (11.32)
6. Unclassified	18.56 (18.66)	24.98 (21.30)	50.52 (21.30)	37.98 (12.97)	34.57 (11.45)
ICU mood† disturbance	0.50 $P < 0.01$	0.42 $P < 0.01$	0.38 $P < 0.01$	−0.47 $P < 0.01$	−0.01 $P = 0.92$
ICU stress reactions	0.60 $P < 0.01$	0.36 $P < 0.01$	0.32 $P < 0.01$	−0.37 $P < 0.01$	−0.90 $P = 0.41$
ICU delirious symptoms	0.40 $P < 0.01$	0.25 $P = 0.01$	0.20 $P = 0.05$	−0.27 $P = 0.01$	0.00 $P = 0.99$
ICU memory‡ (little memory - some/most memory)	6.30 (1.56, 10.98) $P = 0.01$	6.05 (0.37, 11.73) $P < 0.05$	3.06 (−2.91, 9.03) $P = 0.31$	−2.01 (−6.71, 2.68) $P = 0.40$	0.54 (−3.85, 4.95,) $P = 0.81$
ICU Intrusive memories (some - none)	9.39 (4.92, 13.85) $P < 0.01$	7.10 (1.47, 12.71) $P = 0.01$	5.85 (−0.02, 11.02) $P = 0.05$	−3.38 (−8.03, 1.27) $P = 0.15$	1.86 (−2.52, 6.23) $P = 0.40$
Illness perceptions Timeline§	0.28, $P < 0.01$	0.22, $P = 0.04$	0.23, $P = 0.03$	−0.16, $P = 0.16$	−0.39, $P < 0.01$
Concern	0.28 $P < 0.01$	0.32 $P < 0.01$	0.22 $P < 0.05$	−0.2 $P = 0.07$	−0.26 $P < 0.05$
Emotional representation	0.29 $P < 0.01$	0.31 $P < 0.01$	0.29 $P < 0.01$	−0.28 $P < 0.01$	−0.18 $P = 0.11$

Could these be fitted under the table like other tables? Effect sizes presented in the table are Pearson's 'r' or Spearman's 'rho' for continuous exposure variables, or mean differences + 95% CI for binary variables.

Range of scores (outcomes): PTSD 0 to 51 (PDS); depression 0 to 60 (CES-D); anxiety 0 to 80 (STAI); mental quality of life 0 to 100 (SF-12 mental component summary score); physical quality of life 0 to 100 (SF-12 physical component summary score)

*There were significant differences in depression scores between National Statistics Socio-economic Classification (NS-SEC) classes 1 and 2. There were no significant differences in anxiety between classes, although there was an overall effect of class. There was a significant difference of mean mental HRQL between NS-SEC classes 1 and 5.

†Range of scores (risk factors): mood 0 to 60 (POMS); stress 0 to 72 (ICUSS); delirious symptoms 0 to 20 (ICUSS).

‡ICU memory was used as a binary variable (little memory or some/most memory of ICU). Patients who had little memory of ICU had higher PTSD, depression and anxiety scores (more psychological morbidity) than patients with some/most memory of ICU. ICU intrusive memories (had or did not have intrusive memories) was also a binary variable. Patients with intrusive memories had higher PTSD, depression and anxiety scores (more psychological morbidity) than patients with intrusive memories.

§BIPQ, Brief illness perception questionnaire. BIPQ Timeline represents how long a person believes their condition will last.

Multivariable Analysis (Stage One) - PTSD. All significant factors identified by univariable analysis were now entered into three separate regressions, according to group (there was no socio-demographic group for PTSD). Within the clinical group, the strongest risk factors for PTSD were days of sedation, use of benzodiazepines, use of antipsychotics and use of inotropes or vasopressors (see Additional file 1, Table S1). Within the acute psychological group, the strongest risk factors were total ICU mood, intrusive memories and perceived illness timeline (Additional file 1, Table S2). Within the chronic health group, psychological history and alcohol use remained significant (Additional file 1, Table S3).

TABLE A8.5	Final Multiple Regression Models of Strongest* Risk Factors for Post-ICU PTSD at Three Months					
	R² CUMULATIVE VARIANCE	CLINICAL FACTORS† (COLUMN 1)		CLINICAL AND ACUTE PSYCHO-LOGICAL FACTORS (COLUMN 2)		CLINICAL, ACUTE PSYCHOLOGICAL AND CHRONIC PSYCHOLOGICAL FACTORS (COLUMN 3)
		Unstandardised coefficients (95% CI)	p	Unstandardised coefficients (95% CI)	p	Unstandardised coefficients (95% CI)	p
Duration of sedation - days		0.69 (0.12, 1.27)		0.35 (−0.17, 0.87)	0.18	0.33 (−0.18, 0.84)	
Benzodiazepines (yes/no)		3.98 (−1.01, 8.97)		1.26 (−3.22, 5.73)	0.58	0.352 (−4.01, 4.72)	0.87
Antipsychotics (yes/no)		3.32 (−1.61, 8.24)		1.88 (−2.47, 6.24)	0.39	1.06 (−3.18, 5.29)	0.62
	0.18 (18%)						
ICU Mood				0.31 (0.14, 0.47)	<0.01	0.25 (0.09, 0.42)	<0.01
BIPQ (timeline)				0.79 (0.05, 1.52)	<0.05	0.71 (−0.003, 1.43)	<0.05
Intrusions (yes/no)				5.21 (0.91, 9.51)	<0.05	5.83 (1.65, 10.02)	<0.01
	0.39 (39%)						
Psychological history (yes/no)						6.55 (0.99, 12.10)	<0.05
Alcohol use (yes/no)						4.63 (−1.51, 10.77)	0.14
	0.45 (45%)						

PTSD scores range from 0 to 51 on the post-traumatic stress diagnostic scale (PDS).

*Strongest risk factors were identified in a previous univariable analysis and separate multivariable analyses of each group of risk factors (clinical, acute psychological, chronic health)

†Factors were entered in this final multiple regression in the following order: 1. Clinical, 2. acute psychological, 3. chronic psychological. There are no socio-demographic factors or chronic physical conditions in this table as neither S-D factors nor chronic physical conditions had significant associations with PTSD in the univariable analysis.

BIPQ, Brief Illness Perception Questionnaire

Multivariable Analysis (Stage Two) - PTSD. The strongest risk factors from the groups identified by stage one multivariable analysis were now entered together in a final multiple regression (Table A8.5). As there were nine variables, the weakest of the four clinical factors (ino-tropes) was not included in this regression. Increasing duration of sedation was shown to be the strongest clinical risk factor for PTSD (Table A8.5, column 1). Overall, the strongest independent risk factors for PTSD were three acute psychological factors (ICU mood, intrusive memories and perceived illness timeline) and a chronic factor, psychological history (Table A8.5, column 3).

Depression and Anxiety. For secondary outcomes, depression and anxiety, only stage two of multivariable analysis is reported here. See Additional file 1, Tables S4-S6 for stage one multivariable analyses carried out for depression and anxiety.

Stage Two Multivariable Analysis - Depression. Receiving benzodiazepines in intensive care was the strongest clinical risk factor for depression (Table A8.6, column 1) after adjusting for socio-demographic factors. ICU mood, socio-economic position and psychological history were the strongest independent risk factors for depression in the fully adjusted model (Table A8.6, column 3).

Stage Two Multivariable Analyses - Anxiety. Receiving inotropes or vasopressors was the strongest clinical risk factor for higher anxiety (Table A8.7, column 1). Socio-economic

	R² CUMULATIVE VARIANCE	SOCIO-DEMOGRAPHIC (S-D), CLINICAL AND CHRONIC PHYSICAL FACTORS[†] (COLUMN 1)	P	S-D, CLINICAL, CHRONIC PHYSICAL AND ACUTE PSYCHOLOGICAL FACTORS (COLUMN 2)	P	S-D, CLINICAL, CHRONIC PHYSICAL, ACUTE PSYCHOLOGICAL AND CHRONIC PSYCHOLOGICAL (COLUMN 3)	P
		Unstandardised coefficients (95% CI)		Unstandardised coefficients (95% CI)		Unstandardised coefficients (95% CI)	
Ethnicity (white/ other)		5.34 (−1.40, 12.07)	0.12	3.78 (−2.66, 10.21)	0.25	5.15 (−1.17, 11.47)	0.11
SEC2[‡]		14.59 (4.71, 24.46)	<0.01	10.42 (0.76, 20.08)	<0.05	11.39 (2.04, 20.75)	<0.05
SEC3		7.86 (0.61, 15.12)	<0.05	8.40 (1.53, 15.26)	<0.05	7.61 (0.95, 14.27)	<0.05
SEC4		−1.75 (−12.14, 8.64)	0.74	−1.68 (−11.51, 8.14)	0.74	−0.38	0.94
SEC5		9.08 (1.93, 16.23)	<0.05	10.74 (3.90, 17.57)	<0.01	10.55 (3.95, 17.14)	<0.01
SEC6		7.64 (−2.08, 17.36)	0.12	7.67 (−1.52, 16.86)	0.10	7.40 (−1.46 16.26)	0.11
Benzodiazepines (yes/no)		6.73 (1.42, 12.05)	<0.05	4.54 (−0.65, 9.73)	0.09	3.80 (−1.24, 8.85)	0.14
Chronic physical health (yes/no)		5.05 (−0.20, 10.31)	0.06	2.82 (−2.32, 7.96)	0.28	3.10 (−1.86, 8.06)	0.22
	0.27 (27%)						
ICU Mood				0.35 (0.14, 0.55)	<0.01	0.28 (0.07, 0.48)	<0.01
	0.36 (36%)						
Psychological history (yes/no)						7.67 (0.86, 14.48)	<0.05
	0.39(39%)						

Depression was measured using the Center for Epidemiologic Studies Depression Scale (CES-D, range of scores 0 to 60).
*Strongest risk factors were identified in a previous univariable analysis, followed by multivariable analyses of each group of risk factors (socio-demographic, clinical, acute psychological, chronic health).
†Factors were entered in this final multiple regression in the following blocks: 1. Socio-demographic 2. Clinical 3. Chronic physical conditions 4. Acute psychological; 5. Chronic psychological (each stage is not shown in a separate column for space reasons).
‡Variables SEC2-SEC6 are dummy variables representing differences between occupational categories within the National Statistics Socio-economic classification (NS-SEC). In each dummy variable the numbered category is compared with the baseline of category 1. (NS-SEC categories are as follows: 1. Professions/ managerial 2. Intermediate professions 3. Self-employed 4. Technical/craft 5. Semi-routine/routine 6. Unclassified)

position, chronic physical health, ICU mood and psychological history were the strongest independent risk factors for anxiety in the final model (Table A8.7, column 3).

Multivariable Analyses - Quality of Life (Mental Component). As relatively few risk factors were identified for quality of life in univariable analyses, only one stage of multivariable analysis was necessary (Additional file 1, Table S7). Use of inotropes or vasopressors was the strongest clinical risk factor for worse mental quality of life (mean difference = −4.21 points on the SF-12 mental summary scale (95% CI: −8.45, 0.03)). ICU mood, chronic physical health and socio-economic position were the strongest independent risk factors for mental quality of life in the fully adjusted model.

Multivariable Analysis - Quality of Life (Physical Component). Better physical quality of life was most strongly associated with ICU steroid usage (mean difference = 4.81 points on the SF-12 physical summary scale, (95% CI: 1.66, 9.27) $P < 0.05$). Steroids confounded the effect of chronic physical conditions on physical quality of life. Use of anaesthetic agents

	R^2 CUMULATIVE VARIANCE EXPLAINED	SOCIO-DEMOGRAPHIC, CLINICAL AND CHRONIC PHYSICAL FACTORS[†] (COLUMN 1) Unstandardised coefficients (95% CI)	P	SOCIO-DEMOGRAPHIC, CLINICAL, CHRONIC PHYSICAL AND ACUTE PSYCHO-LOGICAL FACTORS (COLUMN 2) Unstandardised coefficients (95% CI)	P	SOCIO-DEMOGRAPHIC, CLINICAL, CHRONIC HEALTH, ACUTE PSYCHOLOGICAL AND PSYCHO-LOGICAL HISTORY (COLUMN 3) Unstandardised coefficients (95% CI)	P
SEC2[‡]		11.52 (1.50, 21.55)	<0.05	7.82 (−2.47, 18.10)	0.13	9.35 (−0.81, 19.52)	0.07
SEC3		5.87 (−2.06, 13.80)	0.15	5.92 (−1.84, 13.68)	0.13	4.73 (−2.94, 12.41)	0.22
SEC4		−2.17 (−13.37, 9.03)	0.70	−2.45 (−13.41, 8.51)	0.66	−1.37 (−12.15, 9.40)	0.80
SEC5		7.81 (−0.08, 15.7)	<0.05	8.14 (0.223, 16.05)	<0.05	7.99 (0.24, 15.73)	<0.05
SEC6		10.66 (0.37, 20.94)	<0.05	9.57 (−0.69, 19.82)	0.07	9.76 (−0.29, 19.80)	0.06
Inotropes or vasopressors (yes/no)		6.60 (0.67, 12.53)	<0.05	5.48 (−0.46, 11.42)	0.07	4.64 (−1.23, 10.50)	0.12
Benzodiazepines (yes/no)		4.06 (−1.87, 9.99)	0.18	2.59 (−3.34, 8.52)	0.39	2.08 (−3.74, 7.90)	0.48
Chronic physical health (yes/no)		6.57 (0.95, 12.12)	<0.05	4.62 (−1.14, 10.37)	0.1	5.16 (−0.50, 10.81)	0.07
	0.25 (25%)						
Mood				0.26 (0.04, 0.49)	<0.05	0.20 (−0.03, 0.428)	0.09
Timeline (BIPQ)				0.36 (−0.70, 1.43)	0.50	0.18 (−0.87, 1.24)	0.73
	0.30 (30%)						
Psychological history (yes/no)						8.37 (0.67, 16.08)	<0.05
	0.34 (34%)						

TABLE A8.7   Final Multiple Regression Models of Strongest*Risk Factors for Post-ICU Anxiety at Three Months

Anxiety was measured using the State-trait anxiety inventory (STAI), range of scores 0 to 80
*Strongest risk factors were identified in a previous univariable analysis, followed by multivariable analysis of each group of risk factors (socio-demographic, clinical, acute psychological, chronic health).
[†]Factors were entered in this final multiple regression in the following order: 1. Socio-demographic 2. Clinical 3. Chronic physical conditions 4. Acute psychological 5. Psychological history (each stage is not shown in a separate column for space reasons)
[‡]Variables SEC2-SEC6 are dummy variables representing differences between occupational categories within the National Statistics Socio-economic classification (NS-SEC). In each dummy variable the numbered category is compared with the baseline of category 1. (NS-SEC categories are: 1. Professions/managerial 2. Intermediate professions 3. Self-employed 4. Technical/craft 5. Semi-routine/routine 6. Unclassified

and the illness perception "timeline" were also independent predictors of better physical quality of life (see Additional file 1, Table S8).

Relative Contributions of Risk Factors. In the final regression models for PTSD, depression, anxiety (see Tables A8.5, A8.6, A8.7) and mental quality of life (Additional file 1, Table S7), the strongest clinical risk factors became weaker (effect sizes or unstandardised coefficients were reduced by up to a half) and were nonsignificant when acute psychological factors were added. This suggests that acute psychological reactions partially explained (or mediated) the effects of clinical risk factors on psychological outcomes. Additional mediational analyses carried out, but not reported here, confirmed that most associations between clinical risk factors and outcomes were mediated by acute psychological risk factors. Background factors, such as socio-economic position and chronic health (physical and psychological), were also strong, independent risk factors of psycho-social outcomes but did not confound the effects of acute psychological reactions in intensive care.

Discussion. In this prospective study, we found that level three patients with mixed diagnoses suffer considerable psychological distress both during and following a general ICU admission. Three months after being discharged, 27% had probable PTSD symptoms, 46% had probable depression and 44% had anxiety. Our PTSD estimate is broadly consistent with a systematic review in which median point prevalence of PTSD was 22% [1] and the expectation that 25 to 30% of people develop PTSD after a trauma [39]. Post-ICU depression and anxiety rates were high in this study, compared to 28% depression reported in a systematic review [2] and anxiety rates varying from 5 to 43% [3]. The varying rates of morbidity may be explained by differences in populations, admission criteria, and methods and timing of assessments. We believe our prevalence estimates are credible due to the high quality of questionnaires used to measure psychological morbidity and the representativeness of our level three samples.

Patients had high mean scores for mood disturbance and stress (see Table A8.2) in response to sleep deprivation, difficulty breathing, pain, inability to communicate, low control, hallucinations and nightmares. These stress reactions were measured during their ICU admission. Previous studies measured stress in ICU retrospectively [17] or in sub-groups, such as chronically critically ill [6] or terminally ill [8] patients. The presence of delirium has been well documented in intensive care patients [9,40]. In this study, we were interested in measuring specific delirium symptoms, such as hallucinations, nightmares and agitation, which we found to be at high levels.

Acute psychological risk factors for PTSD, identified in univariable analysis, include higher intensive care stress and delirious symptom scores (measured using the ICUSS). Associations were also found between ICU stress and delirious symptoms, and subsequent depression. However, in spite of moderate to large effect sizes, ICU stress and delirious symptoms were confounded by the variable ICU mood in the first stage of multivariable analysis. ICU mood and stress may have been overlapping variables [41] with mood showing slightly larger effect sizes. As one sub-scale in the ICU stress reactions scale was found unreliable and did not correlate with outcomes, omitting this sub-scale might increase the scale's utility in future.

The strongest acute psychological risk factors for PTSD identified in multivariable analysis were mood in the ICU, the perceived timeline of illness and early intrusive memories of intensive care. The strongest acute psychological risk factor for depression was also mood in the ICU. This mood variable was composed of symptoms, such as anger, nervousness, low mood and confusion. The first three are common stress reactions while the latter is arguably related to hypoxia, sedation or delirium. The identification of ICU mood as one of the strongest risk factors in the study suggests that emotional stress reactions in intensive care may be a trigger for, or early manifestation of, future psychological morbidity.

It was of interest that early intrusive memories in intensive care were associated with memory loss. Patients who remembered little of their ICU stay were more likely to have early intrusive memories than those who remembered more. It is known that periods of unconsciousness do not preclude the development of intrusive memories [42]. Other ICU studies emphasise the relationship between "delusional" memories and PTSD [12,20] but in our study there was no significant difference in outcomes between patients with factual or delusional intrusive memories. There is no consensus in the wider PTSD literature about the significance of early intrusive memories that immediately follow a trauma. Some studies predict successful recovery, but others predict a worse outcome [39].

Turning to clinical risk factors, it was of interest that many variables, such as TISS score [27], duration of mechanical ventilation and cardiovascular support, number of organs supported, drug groups given and length of sedation, were associated with PTSD in the univariable analysis. These results suggest that a level three admission, particularly when it involves multiple drugs and escalating invasive interventions, may be a traumatic stressor that can trigger PTSD symptoms if the patient survives.

During the first stage of multivariable analysis it emerged that the strongest clinical risk factors for PTSD were drug-related variables, particularly the number of days of sedation. In previous studies, PTSD was found to be associated with other aspects of sedation [12,17,18,21]. Our study also found strong associations in the first stage of multivariable analysis between other ICU drugs and psychological outcomes, including ben-zodiazepines and depression; inotropes/vasopressors and anxiety; and both steroids and anaesthetic agents (mainly propofol) with improved physical quality of life.

It has been hypothesised that benzodiazepines trigger depression by reducing central monoamine activity [43]. The association between benzodiazepine use in the ICU and delirium [11,12] also suggests pathways leading to long-term psychological morbidity. The association between inotropes and vasopressors in intensive care and subsequent anxiety has not previously been reported, although receiving noradrenaline or adrenaline was associated with short-term anxiety in medical patients [44]. These medications are known to enhance emotional memories [39], which are prominent in anxiety disorders. However, patients receiving inotropes and vasopressors are at risk for inadequate brain perfusion. Therefore, it should not be assumed the association is causal.

Regarding the association between corticosteroids and improved physical quality of life, it could be hypothesised that steroids offer protection by modifying the inflammatory response. In another study, patients receiving steroids in intensive care had a lower rate of PTSD [45]. However, caution is needed as the use of corticosteroids in intensive care has previously been associated with long-term physical impairments [46].

Few socio-demographic risk factors were identified in the analyses, perhaps suggesting that the stressful effects of intensive care transcend age or gender. However, lower socio-economic position was found to predict depression, anxiety and mental quality of life, although not PTSD. It may be that PTSD symptoms are directly triggered by traumatic experiences in intensive care, while depression and anxiety at three months are more affected by socio-economic factors. No previous studies of psychological outcomes after intensive care included a valid measure of socio-economic position, although this has been shown to predict mortality in ICU patients [4,47].

The most important finding in this study was that acute psychological reactions were among the strongest risk factors for post-ICU psychological morbidity. The second stage of multivariable analysis demonstrated that associations between clinical factors, such as duration of sedation, and outcomes, such as PTSD, were weakened when acute psychological factors were added to the regression. This suggests that the effects of clinical factors on outcomes were partially explained (or mediated) by acute psychological reactions. It is important to note that the effects of acute stress reactions in the ICU on outcomes were not confounded by psychological history. Thus, stress in the ICU was found to contribute to future psychological morbidity independently of preexisting psychological problems.

These results suggest that, as well as modifying clinical and sedation practices in the ICU, psychological interventions aiming to mitigate acute stress reactions in intensive care might have a positive impact on poor psycho-social outcomes.

The strengths of this study include the measurement of several important psychological outcomes with validated questionnaires, and of a comprehensive set of risk factors. The prospective design and participation of a representative sample of highest acuity "level three" general ICU patients, who are difficult to recruit, are also positive aspects of the study. The study was fully powered to detect associations between risk factors and outcomes using multiple regression models.

Limitations include the use of a single-centre. Another limitation was the necessary exclusion of patients who remained confused throughout the intensive care admission. Psychological questionnaires were used rather than clinician diagnosis of outcome. The ICU Stress Reactions Scale (ICUSS) was not validated before the study. However, this innovative instrument enables the measurement of ICU stress reactions in real time, not retrospectively, and preliminary validational data for the scale were collected. Records of patient's past medical history may not have been complete. The loss of 36% of participants to follow-up was due to death, homelessness, disability and hospitalisation. However, 90% of the patients who were able to participate in follow-up, completed the study.

Conclusions. This cohort study revealed that level three patients suffered considerable psychological morbidity after intensive care. We detected associations not found in previous studies: between inotropes/vasopressors and post-ICU anxiety; corticosteroids and better physical quality of life; and between delirious symptoms, early intrusive memories and memory loss with depression and PTSD. Our results lend weight to limited existing evidence that sedation is linked to depression and PTSD after intensive care. It was striking that different drug-related clinical risk factors were correlated with different outcomes, and further studies to assess mechanisms are warranted. The most important finding was that acute stress reactions in the ICU were stronger risk factors than clinical factors. This lends hope that modifying psychological as well as pharmacological risk factors may be possible, and preventative approaches to ICU stress could be developed and evaluated.

Key Messages
- High rates of psychological morbidity were found among level three patients three months after intensive care: PTSD (27%), depression (46%) and anxiety (44%).
- Strong acute psychological reactions in intensive care were among the risk factors most strongly associated with later psychological morbidity.
- Clinical risk factors for poor psychosocial outcomes included duration of sedation (PTSD); use of benzodiazepines (depression); inotropes and vaso-pressors (anxiety) and corticosteroids (better physical quality of life).
- The correlation of different clinical risk factors with different psychosocial outcomes suggests that investigations of psychobiological mechanisms are warranted.
- The risk factors identified suggest that psychological interventions, as well as pharmacological modifications, have the potential to reduce poor outcomes after intensive care.

Additional Material

Additional file 1: Tables showing full multivariable analyses. Tables showing the first stage of multivariable analyses for PTSD, depression and anxiety, and full multivariable analyses for physical and mental quality of life outcomes.

Abbreviations. APACHE: Acute Physiology and Chronic Health Evaluation; BIPQ: Brief Illness Perception Questionnaire; CES-D: Center for Epidemiologic Studies Depression Scale; DSM-IV: Diagnostic and Statistical Manual of Mental Disorders (4th Ed); GCS: Glasgow Coma Scale; HRQL: Health-Related Quality of Life; ICU: Intensive care unit; ICUSS: Intensive Care Stress Reactions Scale; MV: Mechanical ventilation; NS-SEC: National Statistics Socio-Economic Classification; PDS: Post-traumatic Stress Diagnostic Scale; PTSD: Post-traumatic stress disorder; POMS: Profile of Mood States; STAI: State-Trait Anxiety Inventory; TISS: Therapeutic Intervention Scoring System

Acknowledgements. We are extremely grateful to Dr. Robert Shulman, the intensive care pharmacist at UCLH, for sharing his expertise in relation to ICU drugs. We would like to thank Abu Bakarr Karim and Raksa Tupprasoot for their help with data collection. This study was funded by a Medical Research Council (MRC) PhD studentship awarded to Dorothy Wade. Rosalind Raine, David Howell and Michael Mythen receive a portion of their funding from the UCLH/UCL National Institute of Health Research Biomedical Research Centre. Rebecca Hardy is supported by the MRC.

Author Details. [1]Department of Applied Health Research, University College London (UCL), 1–19 Torrington Place, London, WC1E 7HB, UK. [2]Critical Care Unit, University College London Hospitals NHS Foundation Trust (UCLH), 235 Euston Rd, London, NW1 2BU, UK. [3]Psychology Department, Institute of Psychiatry, Kings College London, Guy's Campus, St. Thomas St, London, SE1 9RT, UK. [4]MRC Unit for Lifelong Health and Ageing, University College London, 33 Bedford Place, London, WC1B 5JU, UK. [5]UCLH/UCL NIHR Biomedical Research Centre, Maple House, 149 Tottenham Court Rd, London W1T 7DN, UK. [6]Psychology Department, University College London, Gower St, London, WC1E 6BT, UK.

Authors' Contributions. DW conducted the study under the academic supervision of RR, JW, RH and CB. RH led the design of the analysis plan. DH and MM contributed to study design, and provided clinical support and advice at every stage of the project. SB and CM advised on the inclusion of ICU clinical risk factors and helped DW with data collection. DW drafted the initial report and the other authors revised it. All authors read and approved the final version of the paper.

Competing Interests. The authors declare that they have no competing interests.

Received: 14 February 2012 Revised: 12 April 2012
Accepted: 18 July 2012 Published: 15 October 2012

References

1. Davydow DS, Gifford JM, Desai SV, Needham DM, Bienvenu OJ: **Posttraumatic stress disorder in general intensive care unit survivors: a systematic review**. *Gen Hosp Psychiat* 2008, **30**:421–443.
2. Davydow DS, Gifford JM, Desai SV, Bienvenu OJ, Needham DM: **Depression in general intensive care unit survivors: a systematic review**. *Intens Care Med* 2009, **35**:796–809.
3. Wade D, Raine R, Weinman J, Hardy R, Tupprasoot R, Mythen M, Howell DC: **What determines poor psychological outcomes after admission to the intensive care unit?** *The Intensive Care Society State of the Art meeting*. conference proceedings, December 2010 London: The Intensive Care Society; 2010.
4. Hutchings A, Raine R, Brady A, Wildman M, Rowan K: **Socioeconomic status and outcome from intensive care in England and Wales: a prospective cohort study**. *Med Care* 2004, **42**:943–951.
5. American Psychiatric Association: *Diagnostic and Statistical Manual of Mental Disorders*. 4 edition. Washington DC: American Psychiatric Association; 1994.
6. Nelson JE: **The symptom burden of chronic critical illness**. *Crit Care Med* 2004, **32**:1527–1534.
7. Novaes MA, Aronovich A, Ferraz MB, Knobel E: **Stressors in ICU: patients' evaluation**. *Intens Care Med* 1997, **23**:1282–1285.
8. Puntillo KA, Arai S, Cohen NH, Gropper MA, Neuhaus J, Paul SM, Miaskowski C: **Symptoms experienced by intensive care unit patients at high risk of dying**. *Crit Care Med* 2010, **38**:2155–2160.
9. Ely EW, Siegel MD, Inouye SK: **Delirium in the intensive care unit: an under-recognized syndrome of organ dysfunction**. *Semin Respir Crit Care Med* 2001, **22**:115–126.
10. Granberg A, Engberg IB, Lundberg D: **Acute confusion and unreal experiences in intensive care patients in relation to the ICU syndrome. Part II**. *Intens Crit Care Nurs* 1999, **15**:19–33.
11. Pandharipande P, Shintani A, Peterson J, Pun BT, Wilkinson GR, Dittus RS, Bernard GR, Ely EW: **Lorazepam is an independent risk factor for transitioning to delirium in intensive care unit patients**. *Anesthesiology* 2006, **104**:21–26.
12. Jones C, Backman C, Capuzzo M, Flaatten H, Rylander C, Griffiths RD: **Precipitants of posttraumatic stress disorder following intensive care: a hypothesis generating study of diversity in care**. *Intens Care Med* 2007, **33**:978–985.

13. Griffiths J, Fortune G, Barber V, Duncan Young J: **The prevalence of post traumatic stress disorder in survivors of ICU treatment: a systematic review.** Intens Care Med 2007, **33**: 1506–1518.

14. Hopkins RO, Key CW, Suchyta MR, Weaver LK, Orme JF Jr: **Risk factors for depression and anxiety in survivors of acute respiratory distress syndrome.** Gen Hosp Psychiat 2010, **32**: 147–155.

15. Cuthbertson BH, Hull A, Strachan M, Scott J: **Post-traumatic stress disorder after critical illness requiring general intensive care.** Intens Care Med 2004, **30**:450–455.

16. Scragg P, Jones A, Fauvel N: **Psychological problems following ICU treatment.** Anaesthesia 2001, **56**:9–14.

17. Samuelson KA: **Stressful memories and psychological distress in adult mechanically ventilated intensive care patients - a 2-month follow-up study.** Acta Anaesth Scand 2007, **51**:671–678.

18. Girard TD, Shintani AK, Jackson JC, Gordon SM, Pun BT, Henderson MS, Dittus RS, Bernard GR, Ely EW: **Risk factors for post-traumatic stress disorder symptoms following critical illness requiring mechanical ventilation: a prospective cohort study.** Crit Care 2007, **11**:R28.

19. Myhren H, Ekeberg O, Toien K, Karlsson S, Stokland O: **Posttraumatic stress, anxiety and depression symptoms in patients during the first year post intensive care unit discharge.** Crit Care 2010, **14**:R14.

20. Jones C, Griffiths RD, Humphris G, Skirrow PM: **Memory, delusions, and the development of acute posttraumatic stress disorder-related symptoms after intensive care.** Crit Care Med 2001, **29**:573–580.

21. Kress JP, Gehlbach B, Lacy M, Pliskin N, Pohlman AS, Hall JB: **The long-term psychological effects of daily sedative interruption on critically ill patients.** Am J Resp Critic Care Med 2003, **168**:1457–1461.

22. Richter JC, Waydhas C, Pajonk FG: **Incidence of posttraumatic stress disorder after prolonged surgical intensive care unit treatment.** Psychosomatics 2006, **47**:223–300.

23. Dowdy DW, Dinglas V, Mendez-Tellez PA, Bienvenu OJ, Sevransky J, Dennison CR, Shanholtz C, Needham DM: **Intensive care unit hypoglycemia predicts depression during early recovery from acute lung injury.** Crit Care Med 2008, **36**:2726–2733.

24. Dowdy DW, Bienvenu OJ, Dinglas VD, Sevransky J, Shanholtz C, Needham DM: **Are intensive care factors associated with depressive symptoms six months after acute lung injury?** Crit Care Med 2009, **37**:1702–1707.

25. National Statistics: **National Statistics Socio-economic Classification (NS-SEC).** London: National Statistics; 2010 [http://www.ons.gov.uk/ons/guide-method/ classifications/current-standard-classifications/soc2010/soc2010-volume-3-ns-sec–rebased-on-soc2010–user-manual/index.html].

26. Knaus WA, Zimmerman JE, Wagner DP, Draper EA, Lawrence DE: **APACHE -Acute Physiology and Chronic Health Evaluation: a physiologically based classification system.** Crit Care Med 1981, **9**:591–597.

27. Keene AR, Cullen DJ: **Therapeutic Intervention Scoring System: update.** Crit Care Med 1983, **11**:1–3.

28. McNair DM, Lorr M, Droppelman LF: Manual for the Profile of Mood States. San Diego, CA: Educational and Industrial Testing Service; 1971.

29. Broadbent E, Petrie KJ, Main J, Weinman J: **The Brief Illness Perception Questionnaire.** J Psychosom Res 2006, **60**:631–637.

30. Foa EB, Cashman L, Jaycox L, Perry K: **The validation of a self-report measure of posttraumatic stress disorder: the Posttraumatic Diagnostic Scale.** Psychol Assessment 1997, **9**:445–451.

31. Ehring T, Kleim B, Clark DM, Foa EB, Ehlers A: **Screening for posttraumatic stress disorder: what combination of symptoms predicts best?** J Nerv Ment Dis 2007, **195**:1004–1012.

32. Radloff LS: **The CES-D scale: a self-report depression scale for research in the general population.** Appl Psychol Meas 1977, **1**:385–401.

33. Weinert C, Meller W: **Epidemiology of depression and antidepressant therapy after Acute Respiratory Failure.** Psychosomatics 2006, **47**:399–407.

34. Covic T, Pallant JF, Conaghan PG, Tennant A: **A longitudinal evaluation of the Center for Epidemiologic Studies-Depression scale (CES-D) in a rheumatoid arthritis population using Rasch analysis.** Health Qual Life Outcomes 2007, **5**:41.

35. Spielberger CD, Gorsuch RL, Lushene R, Vagg PR, Jacobs GA: *Manual for the State-Trait Anxiety Inventory* Palo Alto, CA: Consulting Psychologists Press; 1983.

36. Kindler C, Harms C, Amsler F, Ihde-Scholl T, Scheidegger D: **The visual analog scale allows effective measurement of preoperative anxiety and detection of patients' anesthetic concerns.** *Anesthesia Anal* 2000, **90**:706–712.

37. Ware J, Kosinski M, Keller SD: **A 12-Item Short-Form Health Survey: construction of scales and preliminary tests of reliability and validity.** *Med Care* 1996, **34**:220–233.

38. Hsieh FY, Bloch DA, Larsen MD: **A simple method of sample size calculation for linear and logistic regression.** *Stat Med* 1998, **17**:1623–1634.

39. Brewin CR, Dalgleish T, Joseph S: **A dual representation theory of posttraumatic stress disorder.** *Psychol Rev* 1996, **103**:670–686.

40. Ely EW, Shintani A, Truman B, Speroff T, Gordon SM, Harrell FE Jr, Inouye SK, Bernard GR, Dittus RS: **Delirium as a predictor of mortality in mechanically ventilated patients in the intensive care unit.** *JAMA* 2004, **291**:1753–1762.

41. Kraemer HC, Stice E, Kazdin A, Offord D, Kupfer D: **How do risk factors work together? Mediators, moderators and independent, overlapping, and proxy risk factors.** *Am J Psychiat* 2001, **158**:848–856.

42. Harvey AG, Brewin CR, Jones C, Kopelman MD: **Coexistence of posttraumatic stress disorder and traumatic brain injury: towards a resolution of the paradox.** *J Int Neuropsychol Soc* 2003, **9**:663–676.

43. Longo LP, Johnson B: **Addiction: Part I. Benzodiazepines - side effects, abuse risk and alternatives.** *Am Fam Physician* 2000, **61**:2121–2128.

44. House A, Stark D: **Anxiety in medical patients.** *Br Med J* 2002, **325**:207–209.

45. Schelling G: **The effect of stress doses of hydrocortisone during septic shock on posttraumatic stress disorder in survivors.** *Biol Psychiat* 2001, **50**:978–985.

46. Herridge MS, Cheung AM, Tansey CM, Matte-Martyn A, Diaz-Granados N, Al-Saidi F, Cooper AB, Guest CB, Mazer CD, Mehta S, Stewart TE, Barr A, Cook D, Slutsky AS, for the Canadian Critical Trials Group: **One-year outcomes in survivors of the acute respiratory distress syndrome.** *N Eng J Med* 2003, **348**:683–933.

47. Welch CA, Harrison DA, Hutchings A, Rowan K: **The association between deprivation and hospital mortality for admissions to critical care units in England.** *J Crit Care* 2010, **25**:382–390.

doi:10.1186/cc11677

Cite this article as: Wade et al.: **Investigating risk factors for psychological morbidity three months after intensive care:** a prospective cohort study. *Critical Care* 2012 *16*:R192.

Submit your next manuscript to BioMed Central and take full advantage of:

- Convenient online submission
- Thorough peer review
- No space constraints or color figure charges
- Immediate publication on acceptance
- Inclusion in PubMed, CAS, Scopus and Google Scholar
- Research which is freely available for redistribution

Submit your manuscript at
www.biomedcentral.com/submit

( ) **BioMed** Central

Appendix A-9

Quality-of-Life Outcomes Between Mastectomy Alone and Breast Reconstruction: Comparison of Patient-Reported BREAST-Q and Other Health-Related Quality-of-Life Measures

Yassir Eltahir, M.D.; Lisanne L. C. H. Werners; Marieke M. Dreise;
Ingeborg A. Zeijlmans van Emmichoven, Ph.D.; Liesbeth Jansen, M.D., Ph.D.;
Paul M. N. Werker, M.D., Ph.D.; Geertruida H. de Bock, Ph.D.

Groningen, The Netherlands

Background: *Published data on quality of life in women after breast reconstruction are inconsistent. This cross-sectional study evaluated the quality of life of women after successful breast reconstruction in comparison with those who underwent mastectomy alone.*

Methods: *The quality of life was evaluated using two validated self-report questionnaires: the BREAST-Q and the RAND-36. Demographic information, patient anxiety, depression, and concerns about recurrences were measured by using standardized questionnaires. These questionnaires were sent to the participants. The quality of life of the mastectomy plus breast reconstruction group (n = 92) and the mastectomy-alone group (n = 45) were compared. Multiple regression analysis was used to evaluate the statistical signifcance of the authors' findings.*

Results: *Women with successful breast reconstruction were significantly more satisfied with the appearance of their chest/breasts (p = 0.003). They also fared better psychosocially (n = 0.008) and sexually (p = 0.007) than women with mastectomy alone. Furthermore, they functioned better physically (p = 0.012), experiencing less pain and fewer limitations (p = 0.007).*

Conclusions: *Successful breast reconstruction following mastectomy can greatly improve different aspects of the patient's life compared with women who do not undergo reconstructive surgery. These findings might be taken into consideration when the treating medical team and the patient study various treatment options. (Plast. Reconstr. Surg. 132: 201e, 2013.)*

CLINICAL QUESTION/LEVEL OF EVIDENCE: *Therapeutic, III.*

Disclosure: *The authors declare that they do not have any conflicts of interest financial, personal, or other that might affect the information, research, analysis, or interpretation of this article.*

From the University Medical Center Groningen.
Received for publication September 15, 2012; accepted February 6, 2013.

Breast cancer is recognized as the most common cancer in women worldwide and a leading cause of cancer-related mortality.[1] Despite improvements in screening and diagnosis and advances in treatment of breast cancer, mastectomy remains an important surgical option.[2] Prophylactic mastectomy is offered to decrease the risk of gene mutations,[3] most notably the risk associated with *BRCA1* or *BRCA2*.[4] However, mastectomy undoubtedly adds a traumatic burden to the lives of women diagnosed with breast cancer.[5] Psychological changes may often be detected.[6] Besides the obvious concerns over physiologic health, breast cancer sufferers are also apprehensive about their appearance following a disfiguring operation.[7] This perception may impact their social, personal, and sexual relationships.[8] Half of all women who undergo mastectomy perceive a negative self-image and experience negative changes in their sexuality.[9] For such women, particularly younger ones for whom physical appearance carries more signif-cance, breast reconstruction, in its various forms, should be considered as a possible solution.[10]

A retrospective study by Rowland et al.[11] concluded that there were no significant differences in quality of life of women who underwent either mastectomy alone, lumpectomy, or mastectomy with reconstruction. However, only one-third of the women replied to the self-reported questionnaire. Chen et al.[12] concluded that rigorous patient-reported outcomes data are essential and should be the focus of future research. A systematic review by Winters et al.[13] revealed that most of the studies were poorly designed, retrospective with significant limitations, and potentially biased. Furthermore, the studies were underpowered and they used generic quality-of-life instruments that were neither sensitive nor specific for breast reconstruction. We may conclude that published data on quality of life in women after breast reconstruction are inconsistent and point out various limitations.

The aim of this cross-sectional study was to determine whether successful breast reconstruction improves quality of life in women following mastectomy. For that, we performed a survey among women who underwent surgery for breast cancer at our university hospital and compared the quality of life in women with breast reconstruction to women with mastectomy alone. In addition to the RAND-36, we used the recently published BREAST-Q questionnaire to appraise the outcome of breast reconstruction as perceived by the patients themselves.[14] This is currently one of the few instruments in reconstructive breast surgery that meets international standards in terms of development and validation.[15] Naturally, we were also interested in learning of our patients' experiences. This knowledge would empower the future breast cancer sufferers and enable them to make a more informed decision. This decision would rely on an evidence-based protocol designed according to the patient's psychological and social needs.

Patients and Methods

Study Population. The study population consisted of women who had undergone mastectomy for either breast cancer or prophylaxis resulting from genetic predisposition. These patients were treated at the University Medical Center Groningen between 2006 and 2010. The patient selection procedure is shown in Figure A9.1. The study population consisted of two groups of women: mastectomy alone and mastectomy with successful breast reconstruction. We received approval from the medical ethics committee before conducting the study.

The inclusion criteria included female breast reconstruction patients, mastectomy patients (unilateral or bilateral), patients with a good understanding of the Dutch language, and signed consent. We excluded patients younger than 18 years, severely ill patients, women who were legally incompetent, and women who did not sign the consent form; also, 12 patients were excluded because of flap or prosthesis loss. In these patients, emotional trauma and disappointment were clear. We considered it unethical to ask women with failed reconstruction to answer questions about the new reconstructed breast.

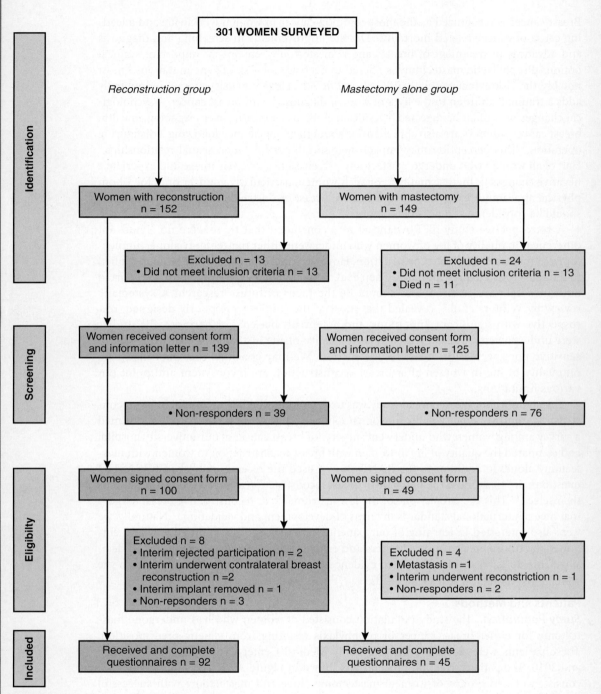

FIGURE A9.1 Patient selection flow diagram.

The initial number of patients considered for the study was 301. As depicted in the flow diagram, 264 of them were deemed eligible and thus approached to participate in the study. Of the 264 patients, 139 women had undergone mastectomy and a breast reconstruction, whereas 125 women had only mastectomy performed. We received signed informed consent from 149 subjects; nonetheless, 12 were still excluded as detailed in the flow diagram. Thus, a total of 137 patients with completed questionnaires and consent forms were included: 92 subjects with breast reconstruction and 45 in the mastectomy-alone group.

Methods. Clinical data were retrieved using digital patient recording by Poliplus software (Poliplus Software, Waterloo, Ontario, Canada). Where necessary, we turned to paper-based documentation. Demographic information (Table A9.1) such as employment, educational level, marital status, and the time interval since last treatment were obtained using the demographic questionnaire formerly used in the study by van den Beuken-van

TABLE A9.1	Characteristics of the Study Population Based on Treatment Indication			
CHARACTERISTICS	PROPHYLACTIC MASTECTOMY ALONE (%)	RECONSTRUCTION FOLLOWING PROPHYLACTIC MASTECTOMY (%)	THERAPEUTIC MASTECTOMY ALONE (%)	RECONSTRUCTION FOLLOWING THERAPEUTIC MASTECTOMY (%)
No.	2	26	43	66
Age at completion of questionnaires, yr				
Median	50.5	43.0	58.0	50.0
Range	50–51	26–57	40–76	26–78
Age at mastectomy, yr				
Median	47	40.5	57.0	45.5
Range	47–47	25–54	38–74	21–72
Comorbidity	1 (50.0)	3 (11.5)	11 (25.6)	14 (21.2)
BMI*				
Median	31.0	23.0	24.0	25.0
Range	31–31	20–34	19–35	18–33
BMI > 30*	2 (100)	2 (8.7)	2 (5.0)	10 (15.2)
Smoking	1 (50.0)	7 (26.9)	13 (31.0)	14 (21.9)
Chemotherapy	—	—	25 (58.1)	35 (53.8)
Radiotherapy	—	—	19 (46.3)	26 (40.0)
Bilateral mastectomy[†]	2 (100)	26 (100)	5 (11.6)	17 (25.8)
TNM staging[‡]				
Stage 0–IIB	—	—	33 (78.6)	46 (79.3)
Stage IIIA–IIIC	—	—	9 (21.4)	12 (20.7)
BRCA1 or *BRCA2* mutation	2 (100)	23 (88.5)	3 (7.0)	12 (18.2)
Time between the last operation and completing the questionnaires, mo				
Median	37.5	27.0	27.0	24.0
Range	28–47	5–48	11–45	4–52
Education				
Low	2 (100)	14 (56.0)	22 (52.4)	43 (65.2)
High	0	11 (44.0)	20 (47.6)	23 (34.8)
Family status[§]				
Single	1 (50.0)	2 (8.0)	8 (18.6)	12 (18.2)
Partner	1 (50.0)	23 (92.0)	35 (81.4)	54 (81.8)
HADS				
1: Anxiety	0 (0.0)	3 (11.5)	6 (14.0)	8 (12.1)
2: Depression	0 (0.0)	1 (3.8)	3 (7.0)	3 (4.5)
CARS				
1: General concerns	0 (0.0)	2 (7.7)	7 (16.3)	9 (13.6)
2: Concerns about health	0 (0.0)	5 (19.2)	7 (16.3)	18 (27.3)
3: Concerns about being a woman	0 (0.0)	0 (0.0)	1 (2.3)	5 (7.6)
4: Concerns about her role	0 (0.0)	0 (0.0)	0 (0.0)	2 (3.0)

HADS, Hospital Anxiety and Depression Scale; CARS, Dutch language version of the Concerns About Recurrence Scale.
*At the operation.
[†]Bilateral mastectomy: for therapeutic mastectomy alone, bilateral malignancy, $n = 2$, and for unilateral malignancy of one breast and prophylactic mastectomy of the other breast, $n = 3$. For therapeutic reconstruction, bilateral malignancy, $n = 3$, and for unilateral malignancy of one breast and prophylactic mastectomy of the other breast, $n = 14$.
[‡]Bilateral malignancy is classified as stage IIIA to IIIC; high education means (university of applied science and university) bachelor's degree and higher; low education is all degrees and levels below bachelor's degree.
[§]At completion of the questionnaires.

Everdingen et al.[16] In addition, all patients completed the Hospital Anxiety and Depression Scale[17,18] and a Dutch language version of the Concerns About Recurrence Scale.[19] The Hospital Anxiety and Depression Scale appears to be a good means of assessment of anxiety disorder (Cron-bach alpha, 0.68 to 0.93) and depression (Cron-bach alpha, 0.67 to 0.90).[18] The Dutch language version of the Concerns About Recurrence Scale measures the influence of fear of cancer recurrence on the quality of life in women with breast cancer.[19] Comorbidities noted included diabetes mellitus, fibromyalgia, hypertension, and psychological instability. American Society of Anesthesiologists classifcation was noted. In addition, we used tumor, node, metastasis staging. To further condense our population, we divided the tumors into two categories: stage 0 to IIB and stage III to IIIC. Two self-reported questionnaires were used to measure the quality of life in our patients: the BREAST-Q and the RAND-36.

BREAST-Q. The BREAST-Q patient-reported outcome instrument is designed to gauge the impact of mastectomy and breast reconstruction on quality of life and satisfaction, from the patient's perspective. The BREAST-Q reconstruction module (postoperative) consists of nine scales. The BREAST-Q mastectomy module (postoperative) consists of five scales. Each scale consists of three to five items. The score from each scale is transferred into a 100-point scale. Thus, each scale displays a score from 0 (very dissatisfied) to 100 (very satisfied). The BREAST-Q reconstruction module has good internal consistency (Cronbach alpha, 0.88 to 0.97).[20] The BREAST-Q mastectomy module was only recently released. However, we understand that this is similar to the reconstruction module. Before commencing the study, the questionnaires had a Dutch translation validated in accordance with the agreement with the MAPI Trust (http:// www.mapi-trust.org/). The translated version was approved by Pusic, the author of the BREAST-Q.

RAND 36-Item Health Survey. The RAND-36 questionnaire[21] consists of 36 items for assessing various topics related to health and quality of life concentrated under eight domains: physical functioning, physical role functioning, emotional role functioning, vitality, mental health, social role functioning, bodily pain, and general health. The Dutch translation has been validated.[22] The internal consistency of the domains is high (Cronbach alpha, 0.71 to 0.92).

Statistical Analysis. To present baseline characteristics, we distinguished the following groups of women: prophylactic mastectomy alone, reconstruction following prophylactic mastectomy, therapeutic mastectomy alone, and reconstruction following therapeutic mastectomy. We used the medians and ranges or proportions. Multivariate analysis made a distinction between mastectomy alone and reconstruction. The data on the BREAST-Q and the RAND-36 were presented by means and standard deviations. Differences on the BREAST-Q and the RAND-36 between mastectomy alone and reconstruction were tested by using linear regression modeling. For each dimension of the BREAST-Q and the RAND-36, we compared mastectomy alone versus reconstruction. To adjust for differences in baseline to each comparison, the covariates as measured at baseline were added, and in case of any significant effect, these covariates were included in the model. In these multiple models, the variables mastectomy and reconstruction were always included. The regression analyses were tested with a 95 percent confidence interval and a 5 percent significance level ($\alpha = 0.05$) (Table A9.2). The statistical analysis was performed using SPSS version 18.0 (SPSS, Inc., Chicago, Ill.). Lastly, we reviewed all recorded intraoperative and postoperative complications in both groups.

RESULTS. This cross-sectional study compared two cohorts in which 45 women underwent mastectomy alone and 92 women underwent successful breast reconstruction. The overall response rate was 56.44 percent (149 of 264). Only two women preferred to undergo mastectomy alone for preventive indications (Table A9.1). The median age was 50.5 years

TABLE A9.2 Results of the Multiple Linear Regression Analyses for the BREAST-Q and RAND-36 for Mastectomy Alone versus Reconstruction*

	Variables[†]	β	SE	95% CL FOR β Lower	95% CL FOR β Upper
BREAST-Q					
Satisfaction with breasts[‡]	None	10.12	3.33	3.53	16.72
Psychosocial well-being[‡]	None	8.89	3.29	2.39	15.40
Sexual well-being[‡]	None	11.59	4.26	3.17	20.02
Physical well-being: breast region	Unilateral or bilateral mastectomy; partner	4.55	2.88	−1.14	10.24
Satisfaction with the surgeon[‡]	Chemotherapy	11.34	3.02	5.36	17.32
Satisfaction with the medical team	Unilateral or bilateral mastectomy; education	1.99	3.56	−5.05	9.04
Satisfaction with the administration team	Age at completion of questionnaires; education	4.87	4.14	−3.33	13.06
RAND-36					
Physical functioning[‡]	Comorbidity	7.65	3.00	1.72	13.58
Social functioning	Comorbidity; partner	1.61	3.08	−4.49	7.71
Physical role problem	Time interval between the last operation and questionnaires completed; comorbidity; BRCA mutation	7.47	6.44	−5.28	20.21
Emotional role problem	Comorbidity; TNM staging	−0.07	7.45	−14.86	14.73
Mental health	Partner	2.86	2.53	-2.14	7.86
Vitality	Comorbidity	−1.82	3.11	−7.97	4.33
Pain[†]	BMI > 30	9.73	3.56	2.68	16.78
General health	Comorbidity	6.05	3.36	−0.60	12.69
Health change	None	−5.44	4.64	−14.61	3.73

β, coefficient for main effect (mastectomy alone)/reconstruction in the model; SE, standard error for β; CL, confidence limits; TNM, tumor, node, metastasis; BMI, body mass index.
*Coded as 0 for mastectomy alone and 1 for reconstruction.
[†]Variables are the variables included in the model except the main effect (mastectomy alone/reconstruction), age at mastectomy, age at breast reconstruction, age when quality of life reported, period between mastectomy and breast reconstruction in months, time between breast reconstruction and reporting quality of life, mastectomy indication, tumor/node/metastasis classification, comorbidity, body mass index, body mass index > 30, smoking, radiotherapy, chemotherapy, unilateral or bilateral mastectomy, unilateral or bilateral breast reconstruction, BRCA, primary/secondary breast reconstruction, education level, partner, nipple reconstruction, areola reconstruction, complications (asymmetry, scar, seroma, ptosis, wound healing), and secondary corrections.
[‡]Statistically significant.

at the time of completing the questionnaires. At the time of mastectomy, both subjects were aged 47 years. Both had *BRCA1* or *BRCA2* gene abnormality and both underwent bilateral mastectomy. However, 26 women underwent prophylactic mastectomy and reconstruction. The median age of the patients at the time of completing the questionnaire was 43 years (range, 26 to 57 years). The median age of the patients at the time of mastectomy was 40.5 years (range, 25 to 54 years). Existing comorbidity was noted in 11.5 percent of patients. The median body mass index at the time of reconstruction was 23 kg/m² (range, 20 to 34 kg/m²). All women had a bilateral mastectomy. *BRCA1* or *BRCA2* gene mutation was detected in 88.5 percent of the subjects in the said group.

Forty-three women had mastectomy alone for malignant disease (Table A9.1). Reconstruction following mastectomy for malignant indications was performed in 66 women. Patients undergoing only mastectomy had a significantly higher median age (58.0 years; range, 40 to 76 years) at the time of completing the questionnaire ($p < 0.001$) than subjects in the breast reconstruction group (50.0 years; range, 26 to 78 years). Also, the age at the time of mastectomy in the former group was significantly higher ($p < 0.001$) (57.0 years; range, 38 to 74 years) than in the reconstruction group (45.5 years; range, 21 to 72 years). Despite some differences in scores between mastectomy-alone and the reconstruction group, neither the Hospital Anxiety and Depression Scale nor the Dutch language version of the Concerns About Recurrence Scale produced any significant results. However, 73 percent of the mastectomy-alone group did not consider reconstruction.

No measured variables could explain the higher score of patients with reconstruction on satisfaction with breasts, psychosocial well-being, and sexual well-being (Table A9.2). Patients with mastectomy alone were less satisfied with their surgeon than breast reconstruction patients, regardless of whether the patients received chemotherapy or not. Breast reconstruction patients had a higher score on physical functioning, regardless of whether the patients had a comorbidity or not. Breast reconstruction patients reported less pain regardless of whether their body mass index was greater than 30 or not.

Table A9.3 details the score of both the BREAST-Q and RAND-36 questionnaires. The score for satisfaction with breasts was a mean of 60.3 in the mastectomy-alone group, whereas in the breast reconstruction group this value was statistically significantly higher (70.5; $p = 0.003$). Similarly, the score for psychosocial well-being was a mean of 66.6 in the former group. This value was again statistically significantly higher in the latter group (75.5; $p = 0.008$). Sexual wellness and satisfaction with surgeon also demonstrated statistically significantly higher values in the reconstruction group ($p = 0.007$ and $p < 0.001$, respectively). Other domains did not depict significant differences, as portrayed in Table A9.3. The scores for subgroups with therapeutic indications had similar significant differences in the same areas of the BREAST-Q, as in comparison between the mastectomy and the reconstruction groups. Comparing results from the RAND-36 questionnaire, two important domains showed a marked difference between the mastectomy and the reconstruction groups. Both physical functioning and pain domain scores were better with breast reconstruction. These results were statistically significant ($p = 0.012$ and $p = 0.007$, respectively). In other areas, striking differences were not observed between the two groups, as detailed in Table A9.3.

We looked at complications (e.g., bleeding, seroma formation, delayed wound healing) associated with mastectomy itself. The incidence of such complications was comparable between the two groups. However, as expected, additional complications were identified directly as a result of breast reconstruction. The most notable complications were related to the anastomosis, partial or total flap necrosis, and the loss of prosthesis.

TABLE A9.3   Mean BREAST-Q and RAND-36 Patient-Reported Scores

	MASTECTOMY ALONE (SD)	RECONSTRUCTION (SD)	P
BREAST-Q			
Satisfaction with breasts	60.33 (19.18)	70.46 (17.90)	0.003*
Satisfaction with the results	—	78.39 (19.07)	
Psychosocial well-being	66.62 (18.31)	75.52 (17.92)	0.008*
Sexual well-being	49.42 (19.44)	61.01 (22.39)	0.007*
Physical well-being			
Breast region	71.59 (13.93)	74.57 (16.27)	0.116
Abdomen	—	67.18 (34.96)	
Satisfaction with nipples	—	64.59 (30.34)	
Satisfaction with information	—	71.04 (15.11)	
Satisfaction with the surgeon	80.16 (19.67)	90.35 (15.28)	<0.001*
Satisfaction with the medical team	86.30 (18.24)	86.68 (20.08)	0.577
Satisfaction with the administration team	85.88 (20.70)	86.01 (19.24)	0.242
RAND-36			
Physical functioning	77.33 (21.86)	86.51 (15.34)	0.012*
Social functioning	83.06 (18.69)	85.48 (17.61)	0.603
Physical role problem	71.11 (40.23)	77.96 (34.15)	0.249
Emotional role problem	75.56 (40.45)	80.29 (35.52)	0.993
Mental health	75.11 (15.16)	77.81 (15.57)	0.259
Vitality	65.78 (15.59)	64.73 (18.01)	0.559
Pain	75.37 (21.64)	83.87 (17.28)	0.007*
General health	68.33 (21.40)	75.54 (17.75)	0.074
Health change	62.78 (25.91)	57.26 (25.16)	0.243

*Statistically signifcant.

In total, 12 patients (7.9 percent) were excluded because of flap loss (five patients) and implant loss (seven patients).

Discussion. Women with successful breast reconstruction were signifcantly more satisfied with the appearance of their chest/breasts ($p = 0.003$). They also fared better psychosocially ($p = 0.008$) and sexually ($p = 0.007$) than women with mastectomy alone. Furthermore, they functioned better physically ($p = 0.012$), experiencing less pain and fewer limitations ($p = 0.007$).

Mastectomy is potentially a very traumatic event. Besides immediate concerns over health and longevity associated with breast cancer, patients most likely agonize over their future appearance, social interactions, and sexual life. For these women, breast reconstruction is proposed as a possible solution. In this study, we investigated whether there was a difference in satisfaction and quality of life between women with mastectomy alone and women with mastectomy and successful breast reconstruction. Among the self-report questionnaires, the BREAST-Q in particular added extra strength to this study, as it is currently the only validated, condition-specific instrument for breast reconstruction surgery.

A previous systematic literature review by Lee et al.[23] could not find any evidence of disparity in satisfaction between patients with mastectomy alone and those undergoing breast reconstruction. However, they do point out the various limitations associated with most studies that make it very doubtful whether the above conclusion is justified. The results from our questionnaires do conclude that women with breast reconstruction are more satisfied with their appearance than women with only a mastectomy. They are also more content with their psychosocial and sexual well-being. Physical functioning in women following breast reconstruction was superior to that in patients with a mastectomy alone. Furthermore, they also experienced less pain and disability. These observations emphasize our proposition that breast reconstruction does facilitate breast cancer sufferers to better cope with various aspects of their lives following completion of their treatment.

In general, women with breast cancer surgery are content with the medical care they receive. However, in our study, breast reconstruction patients were more satisfied with their breast surgeon than were women with mastectomy alone. Nonetheless, this discrepancy may be because comparison is being drawn between possibly two different subspecialties and at different stages of treatment. The systematic review by Guyomard et al.[24] has reported high satisfaction rates with breast reconstruction, but the authors advised that more robust and evidence-based research is needed with validated quality-of-life measures.

Whether unilateral or bilateral breast reconstruction was undertaken also influenced the results in various domains of the BREAST-Q. This can be explained by the possible resultant asymmetry. Waljee et al.[25] drew a similar conclusion, emphasizing the importance of breast symmetry or the lack of it in psychosocial functioning of breast reconstruction recipients.

Educational level also correlated with satisfaction with the overall outcome. In our study, women with low educational background were more satisfied with the outcome than women with higher education. Similar findings were reported by Medina-Franco et al.[26] Perhaps patients with higher education have a higher expectation from breast reconstruction procedures.

We found that chemotherapy affected the BREAST-Q score. Although the comorbidity affected the RAND-36 scores, patients with reconstruction had a higher score on physical functioning. Patients who were overweight (body mass index > 30) and underwent reconstruction reported less pain. Lower quality of life is associated with the presence of other diseases. This may be explained by the fact that those parts of questionnaires focused on the overall picture of the patient's condition; they were not designed specifically for breast reconstruction surgery.

This study has some limitations. To begin with bias by indication, the reconstruction technique and study population were not randomized. However, randomization would have been difficult, because it is the patient who will make the decision on reconstruction.

We identified only two *BRCA*-positive patients, who chose to undergo mastectomy alone without reconstruction. Therefore, we decided to include prophylactic and therapeutic mastectomy patients in one group and performed multivariate regression analyses to control for differences in our population. The sample size was not sufficient to control for all biases. However, the power of the outcome "satisfaction with breasts" was 80 percent. A total of 115 women chose not to participate in this study. Their reasons and their characteristics were not clear. We cannot exclude that the nonparticipation might have influenced the findings in this study. The low response rate (56.44 percent) could be a potential selection bias. Furthermore, we excluded 12 patients who had flap or implant loss. However, features of failed breast reconstruction patients did not match the features of the breast reconstruction group. The BREAST-Q is a condition-specific instrument, and the reconstruction module measures satisfaction with questions about the breast (e.g., softness, size, implant). We found it inappropriate to ask women those questions after such a traumatic event. The quality-of-life study of Bellino et al.[26] excluded patients with cancer recurrences and subjects with breast reconstruction complications. Zhong et al.[27] reported a 20 percent rate of major postoperative complications, but no flap loss. After adjusting for complications, the gains in satisfaction with breast, psychosocial well-being, and sexual well-being remained significant.

The study reflects findings from a single institution treating a homogenous population. However, "homogenous population" can be considered as an advantage. In contrast, a multicenter study targeting various ethnic groups would add weight to our findings. Furthermore, we had little information on the emotional background of our patients. The median time between surgical intervention and completion of the questionnaires was 24 months (range, 4 to 52 months). The analysis showed that the time effect was not significant. The retrospective nature of our study could not possibly record the likely variations in perceived quality of life over time. Some women are still in the process of nipple reconstruction or nipple tattooing or are awaiting secondary correction. However, nipple reconstruction showed a positive effect on satisfaction. Previous studies have revealed that the time elapsed since surgery influences the quality of life in women with breast surgery.[28,29] Therefore, we currently are conducting a prospective study in which patients periodically complete a questionnaire. Nonetheless, to the best of the authors' knowledge, the BREAST-Q has never been used to evaluate satisfaction and quality of life in patients following mastectomy alone or combined with breast reconstruction. Furthermore, combining the validated BREAST-Q with the RAND-36, the Hospital Anxiety and Depression Scale, and the Dutch language version of the Concerns About Recurrence Scale in one study is also unique.

Conclusions. Breast reconstruction, in its various forms, has become an appropriate option offered to women diagnosed with breast cancer. Breast reconstruction may be accomplished in one sitting, but more often than not, it is a multistage process. As such, many months may lapse before the final intended aesthetic result is achieved. It may also be associated with additional surgical complications and higher costs. However, it is evident that patients do benefit from breast reconstruction following mastectomy. Of course, careful patient selection and ample patient education are important in empowering patients to make an informed decision in view of their treatment plan. Larger, more comprehensive studies are needed; nevertheless, results from this study will be helpful to both care providers and patients during that decision process.

Yassir Eltahir, M.D.
Department of Plastic Surgery
University Medical Center Groningen
University of Groningen
Hanzeplein 1, BB81
9700 RB Groningen, The Netherlands

References

1. Jemal A, Bray F, Center MM, Ferlay J, Ward E, Forman D. Global cancer statistics. *CA Cancer J Clin.* 2011;61:69–90.

2. De Vries J, van der Graaf WTA, Hollema H, Szabó BG, Bender W, Haagedoorn WML. Mammacarcinoom. In de Vries J, ed. *Oncologie voor de algemene praktijk.* Assen, The Netherlands: Van Gorcum; 2009:121–132.

3. Rebbeck TR, Friebel T, Lynch HT, et al. Bilateral prophylactic mastectomy reduces breast cancer risk in *BRCA1* and *BRCA2* mutation carriers: The PROSE Study Group. *J Clin Oncol.* 2004;22:1055–1062.

4. Hartmann LC, Sellers TA, Schaid DJ, et al. Efficacy of bilateral prophylactic mastectomy in *BRCA1* and *BRCA2* gene mutation carriers. *J Natl Cancer Inst.* 2001;93:1633–1637.

5. Ganz PA. Psychological and social aspects of breast cancer. *Oncology (Williston Park)* 2008;22:642–646, 650; discussion 650, 653.

6. Metcalfe KA, Semple J, Quan ML, et al. Changes in psychosocial functioning 1 year after mastectomy alone, delayed breast reconstruction, or immediate breast reconstruction. *Ann Surg Oncol.* 2012;19:233–241.

7. Helms RL, O'Hea EL, Corso M. Body image issues in women with breast cancer. *Psychol Health Med.* 2008;13:313–325.

8. Fobair P, Stewart SL, Chang S, D'Onofrio C, Banks PJ, Bloom JR. Body image and sexual problems in young women with breast cancer. *Psychooncology* 2006;15:579–594.

9. McGaughey A. Body image after bilateral prophylactic mastectomy: An integrative literature review. *J Midwifery Womens Health* 2006;51:e45–e49.

10. Lee C, Sunu C, Pignone M. Patient-reported outcomes of breast reconstruction after mastectomy: A systematic review. *J Am Coll Surg.* 2009;209:123–133.

11. Rowland JH, Desmond KA, Meyerowitz BE, Belin TR, Wyatt GE, Ganz PA. Role of breast reconstructive surgery in physical and emotional outcomes among breast cancer survivors. *J Natl Cancer Inst.* 2000;92:1422–1429.

12. Chen CM, Cano SJ, Klassen AF, et al. Measuring quality of life in oncologic breast surgery: A systematic review of patient-reported outcome measures. *Breast J.* 2010;16:587–597.

13. Winters ZE, Benson JR, Pusic AL. A systematic review of the clinical evidence to guide treatment recommendations in breast reconstruction based on patient- reported outcome measures and health-related quality of life. *Ann Surg.* 2010;252:929–942.

14. Pusic AL, Klassen AF, Scott AM, Klok JA, Cordeiro PG, Cano SJ. Development of a new patient-reported outcome measure for breast surgery: The BREAST-Q. *Plast Reconstr Surg.* 2009;124:345–353.

15. Pusic AL, Chen CM, Cano S, et al. Measuring quality of life in cosmetic and reconstructive breast surgery: A systematic review of patient-reported outcomes instruments. *Plast Reconstr Surg.* 2007;120:823–837; discussion 838.

16. van den Beuken-van Everdingen MH, Peters ML, de Rijke JM, Schouten HC, van Kleef M, Patijn J. Concerns of former breast cancer patients about disease recurrence: A validation and prevalence study. *Psychooncology* 2008;17:1137–1145.

17. Bjelland I, Dahl AA, Haug TT, Neckelmann D. The validity of the Hospital Anxiety and Depression Scale: An updated literature review. *J Psychosom Res.* 2002;52:69–77.

18. Spinhoven P, Ormel J, Sloekers PP, Kempen GI, Speckens AE, Van Hemert AM. A validation study of the Hospital Anxiety and Depression Scale (HADS) in different groups of Dutch subjects. *Psychol Med.* 1997;27:363–370.

19. Vickberg SM. The Concerns About Recurrence Scale (CARS): A systematic measure of women's fears about the possibility of breast cancer recurrence. *Ann Behav Med.* 2003;25:16–24.

20. Klassen AF, Pusic AL, Scott A, Klok J, Cano SJ. Satisfaction and quality of life in women who undergo breast surgery: A qualitative study. *BMC Womens Health* 2009;9:11.

21. Van der Zee KI, Sanderman R. *Het meten van de algemene gezondheidstoestand met de RAND-36: een handleiding.* Groningen, The Netherlands: Noordelijk Centrum voor Gezondheidsvraagstukken; 1993.

22. Aaronson NK, Muller M, Cohen PD, et al. Translation, validation, and norming of the Dutch language version of the SF-36 Health Survey in community and chronic disease populations. *J Clin Epidemiol.* 1998;51:1055–1068.

23. Lee C, Sunu C, Pignone M. Patient-reported outcomes of breast reconstruction after mastectomy: A systematic review. *J Am Coll Surg.* 2009;209:123–133.

24. Guyomard V, Leinster S, Wilkinson M. Systematic review of studies of patients' satisfaction with breast reconstruction after mastectomy. *Breast* 2007;16:547–567.

25. Waljee JF, Hu ES, Ubel PA, Smith DM, Newman LA, Alderman AK. Effect of esthetic outcome after breast-conserving surgery on psychosocial functioning and quality of life. *J Clin Oncol.* 2008;26:3331–3337.

26. Bellino S, Fenocchio M, Zizza M, Rocca G, Bogetti P, Bogetto F. Quality of life of patients who undergo breast reconstruction after mastectomy: Effects of personality characteristics. *Plast Reconstr Surg.* 2011;127:10–17.

27. Zhong T, McCarthy C, Min S, et al. Patient satisfaction and health-related quality of life after autologous tissue breast reconstruction: A prospective analysis of early postoperative outcomes. *Cancer* 2012;118:1701–1709.

28. Medina-Franco H, García-Alvarez MN, Rojas-García P, Trabanino C, Drucker-Zertuche M, Arcila D. Body image perception and quality of life in patients who underwent breast surgery. *Am Surg.* 2010;76:1000–1005.

29. Yueh JH, Slavin SA, Adesiyun T, et al. Patient satisfaction in postmastectomy breast reconstruction: A comparative evaluation of DIEP, TRAM, latissimus flap, and implant techniques. *Plast Reconstr Surg.* 2010;125:1585–1595.

Appendix A-10

Why People Living With HIV/AIDS Exclude Individuals From Their Chosen Families

Joan S Grant[1]; David E Vance[1]; Worawan White[2]; Norman L Keltner[1] and James L Raper[3]

Abstract: *Health professionals can gain a better understanding of key elements of social support by examining reasons why people living with human immunodeficiency virus/ acquired immunodeficiency syndrome (PLWH) exclude individuals from their chosen families (ie, families of choice). Our study identified reasons why PLWH excluded specific individuals from their chosen families. This mixed-method design was drawn from a larger study of 150 PLWH, in which 94 self-reported why they excluded individuals from their chosen families. Physical and emotional distance (n = 64; 68.1%); nonsupport, nonacceptance, and harm (n = 25; 26.6%); conditional caring and trust (n = 22; 23.4%); and no blood/familial relationship (n = 13; 13.8%) were the reasons PLWH excluded individuals from their chosen families. Demographic and personal characteristics were unrelated to these themes, supporting the conclusion that reasons for excluding family members are universal and not dependent on particular participant characteristics. For chosen family relationships to develop and exist, these findings emphasize the value of physical and emotional contact between individuals.*

Keywords: *families, stigma, social networks, human immunodeficiency virus, acquired immunodeficiency syndrome*

Introduction. Infection with the human immunodeficiency virus (HIV) is at epidemic levels and people living with HIV/acquired immunodeficiency syndrome (AIDS) (PLWH) may experience depression, stress, anger at their diagnosis, fear of disease progression, and worries about infecting others. Unfortunately, these factors are also associated with negative physiological and psychological outcomes, such as a decreased quality of life, nonadherence to care, faster disease progression, and increased mortality.[1-3] Unlike for people with many other chronic health conditions, PLWH are also faced with issues related to disclosure and potential stigma and discrimination.[4-6]

For some, their family is a major source of support. In fact, the family unit is the most important social unit in most countries of the world. Family life is important in the sense

[1]School of Nursing, University of Alabama at Birmingham, Birmingham, Alabama,
[2]Department of Nursing, Pensacola State College, Pensacola, Florida,
[3]School of Medicine, Department of Medicine, Division of Infectious Diseases, University of Alabama at Birmingham, Birmingham, Alabama, USA

Nursing: Research and Reviews 2013:3 33–42

that it gives individuals basic strength. Therefore, for PLWH, their family often influences how well they manage significant challenges associated with this disease. While family and friends can be significant sources of social support,[7] PLWH may also fear isolation and associated stigma and discrimination from them. Some feel betrayed, neglected, avoided, or shunned by those they expected to stand by them – their "family."[6,8]

Individuals who are marginalized due to stigma create alternative family structures for support and companionship in lieu of families related by blood or marriage. Therefore, many gay, lesbian, bisexual, and transgender individuals have chosen individuals other than those who are related by blood or marriage to provide them with social support. Therefore, in this paper, "family" is defined more broadly to include biologically related members and other social relationships, such as partners, friends, and relatives.[9–12]

A review of the literature failed to reveal any published empirical literature examining why PLWH exclude individuals from their chosen families. However, health professionals can gain a better understanding of key elements of social support by examining the reasons why PLWH exclude individuals from their chosen families (ie, families of choice). Our study identified reasons why PLWH excluded specific individuals from their chosen families.

While there was no available literature related to this specific topic, other studies regarding family structure, disclosure, and stigma added insight to this investigation. The chosen families of PLWH offer social support, love, and affection and are held together by inspiration, commitment, caring, and trust. Families also provide stability, structure, inspiration, mentorship, and encouragement to PLWH. Chosen families are sources of functional social support that offer emotional support by asking PLWH about their general well-being, giving general encouragement, and by talking with them about daily issues and challenges (but not necessarily about their HIV status). Instrumental support is provided through household and financial assistance (eg, food, shelter, monies).[13,14]

Grant et al offered further insight into why chosen family members are important to PLWH. Using a mixed-method design of a convenience sample of 150 PLWH aged 19-68 years old they reported reasons why PLWH included specific individuals in their chosen families.[11] Self-reported reasons for including specific individuals in their chosen families were love and acceptance (n = 135; 90.0%), support (n = 100; 66.7%), blood and family ties (n = 37; 24.7%), and commonality (n = 28; 18.7%). These findings emphasize the importance of relationships between PLWH and those who provide love and acceptance, support, blood/familial ties, and have common interests.

Further, Serovich et al examined reasons why 48 HIV-positive men who have sex with men (MSM) felt their families of origin (through blood, adoption, and marriage) were important.[15] Participants were recruited from a large Midwestern city in the USA. Family as a unique relationship was a significant reason why MSM felt their families of origin were important, emphasizing the value of biological ties. Contact and proximity were also an important factor. While participants had more consistent exchanges with their friends, they also had significant close relationships with biological families. Family closeness or the loving nature of the biological family was yet another reason why their families of origin were important to MSM and significantly influenced whether they disclosed their serostatus to their relatives. However, a quarter of the MSM also had a family of creation that was at least as important as, if not more important than, their biological family to them.

Because social support is important to both physical and mental health, Peterson examined social support challenges of women living with HIV.[8] A qualitative approach was used to interview 45 women living with HIV/AIDS. Participants were recruited from three cities in the US Midwest. These participants encountered numerous challenges in seeking and receiving social support. The women feared abandonment by family members and that their families would not keep their status private. Many were worried that telling their family would result in others knowing about their diagnosis. The women also recounted instances in which they were treated differently by their family (eg, separate eating utensils, a specific place to sit, and limited or no physical contact with children). The women also balanced their need for social support with overburdening their families. In disclosing to children, these participants often failed to share their HIV status for fear of worrying them or causing them sadness.

In examining disclosure to specific family members, Serovich et al examined 135 HIV-positive MSM.[16] These participants were drawn from a larger longitudinal study of HIV disclosure regarding mental and physical health, social support, disease progression, and sexual risk-taking behaviors. Of the 597 family members of participants, 50% had been informed of their HIV status. Participants disclosed their HIV status in greater proportion to their mother (77%) than to others: 47% to fathers, 50% to sisters, and 41% to brothers. After accounting for characteristics of participants and family members, there was no difference in the rate at which family members were told. In examining patterns of support in PLWH, Bor et al suggested that it was not the type of relationship that facilitated talking about HIV status, but, rather, other qualities such as openness and emotional closeness.[17] Further, knowing that a person was not prejudiced might simplify to whom MSM with HIV confide about their HIV status.

In another study, Paiva et al examined disclosure of HIV-positive serostatus by 250 heterosexual and bisexual men to sexual partners.[18] Fear of rejection led to isolation and distress, thus hindering disclosure to current and new partners. HIV/AIDS diagnosis was more commonly disclosed to steady partners, partners who were HIV-positive themselves, and female partners. These investigators suggested stigma management is an important element underlying personal motivation that must be considered while enhancing comprehensive care for HIV-positive men.

Gaskins et al[19] also examined reasons for disclosure and nondisclosure of HIV status among 40 rural African-American men in the Southern USA. From audiotaped interviews, the authors determined that the most common reasons this sample disclosed to other people were to relieve their stress, satisfy their need to tell, to help others, and to receive support. The most common reasons for not disclosing their status were a fear of negative reactions or stigma from others, worrying the disclosure recipient would tell others, a belief that there was no need to tell, not being ready to tell, and not wanting to burden others with their disclosure.

Latkin et al[20] also examined correlates of disclosure of MSM and seropositive HIV status to individuals in their social networks. Data for the study were drawn from a cohort of African-American MSM recruited for a pilot HIV risk-reduction intervention in Baltimore, Maryland. In these 187 African-American MSM, disclosure of MSM behavior to social network members was more common among participants who were younger, had a higher educational level, and were HIV infected. Participants were more likely to disclose their MSM behavior to people in their social networks who were HIV infected, gave them emotional support, socialized with them, and were not a female sex partner. Younger participants were more likely to disclose their positive HIV status to those who were older, HIV infected, provided emotional support, loaned them money, and were not a male sex partner.

In a review of the HIV disclosure literature, Obermeyer et al[21] also found that few people kept their status completely secret. Stigmatization increased the fear of disclosure and disclosure tended to be a gradual process, with more PLWH revealing their HIV status to those in their social networks over time. Disclosure also appeared to be higher in the USA and Europe. Sharing positive HIV status to partners varied greatly but appeared to be lower with casual partners than with steady partners. Further, disclosure to relatives appeared to be higher than to friends.

Their survey of people living with HIV[21] found that stigma in family settings – in particular, avoidance, exaggerated kindness, and being told to conceal one's status – was a significant predictor of psychological distress. This was believed to be due to the absence of unconditional love and support that families are expected to provide. Furthermore, people living with HIV are often worried about losing family and friends if they disclose their status.

Finally, Serovich et al[22] examined the prevalence of regret related to the disclosure of serostatus and sexual orientation to family members among HIV-positive MSM. They also explored participant, family member, and relationship characteristics that influenced the likelihood of experiencing regret over disclosure. Almost half of participants indicated no regret in disclosing either their HIV-positive serostatus or sexual orientation. Among those who did experience some regret, the prevalence of regret over disclosing to one or more family members was similar for HIV-positive serostatus (39.4%) and for sexual orientation (37.3%).

Parker and Aggleton[23] emphasized how stigma and discrimination, as social processes, strengthen and reproduce existing inequalities of gender, race, and social class. For example, in addition to stigma around HIV and homosexuality faced by PLWH, regional factors such as higher rates of poverty; racism that helps drive and fuel the problem; cultural conservatism that serves as a barrier to sensitization/education; stigma toward drug addiction, prostitution and promiscuity; and sexism play an important role in higher incident rates of HIV in the US South. In addition, religious or moral beliefs lead some people to believe that being infected with HIV is the result of moral fault (such as promiscuity or "deviant sex") that deserves to be punished.

Stigma arises and develops within the context of culture and power, and is used by individuals, communities, and others to produce and reproduce inequality. Parker and Aggleton[23] suggest new agendas for research and action, focusing on conceptual studies that examine social, cultural, political, and economic causes and consequences of stigmatization and discrimination. Further, these authors recommend developing our understanding of the social processes at work in HIV and the ways that these social processes influence HIV vulnerability.[23]

In summary, because of the isolation, rejection, and stigmatization that are usually associated with HIV/AIDS, some PLWH become distant from their traditional families. However, PLWH manage to create chosen families that include those they consider family. Proximity, support, love and acceptance, and biological ties appear to be important in defining the chosen families of PLWH. HIV disclosure appeared to a gradual process and more PLWH disclosed to those who provided emotional support and socialized with them.

Participants and Methods. This investigation was drawn from a larger study of 150 PLWH in the southeastern USA examining relationships of individuals who PLWH included in their chosen families as well as why PLWH either include or exclude specific individuals from their chosen families. Relationships of individuals who PLWH included in their chosen families and reasons why PLWH include these specific individuals in their chosen families are reported elsewhere.[7,11] In the present study, using a mixed-method design, content analysis was used to identify why PLWH exclude individuals from their chosen families and quantitative analysis was used to report their most common reasons. Of the larger sample, 94 out of the 150 PLWH gave reasons for excluding specific individuals from their chosen families. Demographic and personal characteristics were also examined to determine if these reasons were associated with identified themes for excluding an individual as a family member.

Participants. Study approval was obtained from The University of Alabama at Birmingham (Birmingham, AL, USA) institutional review board and study facilities; this included an approved written consent form for participants to sign. In this study, a convenience sample was recruited from two HIV outpatient clinics in the southeastern USA. Inclusion criteria included being a male or nonpregnant female with a self-reported diagnosis of HIV; 19 years of age or older; and able to speak, read, and write English. Further, participants also were cognitively unimpaired, as indicated by a score > 10 on the HIV Dementia Scale.[24]

Of this subsample (n = 94), participants ranged in age from 19 to 61 years old and were primarily male (81.9%) and African-American (70.2%). Participants' self-described sexual orientation was almost equally heterosexual (52.1%) and homosexual/bisexual/ other (47.9%).

Procedures. Posters and flyers describing the study were posted in each clinic to recruit study participants. Physicians and nurse practitioners in the clinics also shared basic information about the study with their patients. Interested potential participants subsequently contacted the investigators to learn more about the study. A trained research nurse interviewed potential participants to explain the study, verify eligibility, and secure informed consent prior to completing study questionnaires.

Eligible participants completed an investigator-developed questionnaire privately in a private room in one of the outpatient clinics where they sought care. Following questionnaire completion, participants were given US$10 for their time and participation. Questionnaire completion was assessed prior to participants leaving the clinic.

Measures

Cognitive Status. The HIV Dementia Scale[24] was used to screen PLWH' cognitive status to determine their eligibility to be enrolled in the study. Scores on this instrument range from 0 to 16, with a cut-off of 10 or less suggesting HIV-associated cognitive impairment or dementia. This scale has good internal consistency (Cronbach's alpha = 0.75).

Sociodemographic and Family Data Questionnaire. An investigator-developed questionnaire was used to assess sociodemographic characteristics, individuals PLWH included or did not include in their chosen families, and reasons why they included or excluded them from their families. The sociodemographic section of the questionnaire included questions concerning age, gender, race, education, sexual orientation, employment and income status, and HIV-related information (eg, duration of HIV infection, current viral load and HIV medications, emotional/mental problems, and recent opportunistic infections). The questionnaire contained a list of persons with whom participants could potentially have a relationship. This list included relatives by blood or marriage (eg, fathers, mothers, children, brothers and sisters, spouses, relatives, in-laws, and grandparents) as well as other individuals not related by blood or marriage (eg, friends, dates, partners, sexual partners [lovers]). Using this list of existing relationships, participants were asked to indicate individuals they included or did not include as a member of their family of choice and provide a rationale for this inclusion and exclusion. Participants checked "Does not apply" when a respective person was non-applicable (eg, death of a parent, grandparent). Data analyses for this article focus on individuals who PLWH did not include in their chosen families.

The appropriateness and clarity of the instrument items were evaluated by three experts who collectively had expertise in family dynamics, psychometrics, and HIV/AIDS. Using two rounds of a modified Delphi technique, all content experts agreed regarding the appropriateness and clarity of instrument items, supporting the instrument's content validity.

Data Analysis. Data were analyzed using SPSS (v 14.0; IBM, Armonk, NY). Measures of central tendency and variability, frequencies, and percentages were used to quantify reasons participants excluded individuals from their chosen families. Only participants with existing relationships were included in the analyses. Demographic and personal characteristics (ie, gender, race) were examined to determine if they were statistically related to excluding specific individuals from their chosen families.

Prior to analyzing the quantitative data, a conventional content analysis[25] was conducted. Similar codes were grouped together and aggregated under a single inclusive definition for the broader conceptual meaning of why PLWH excluded individuals from their chosen families. Two research team members with backgrounds in HIV, psychometrics, and family dynamics generated descriptive codes for emerging themes in the data and refined those codes until the team reached consensus that the terms were adequate for defining, explaining, and categorizing reasons why participants excluded specific individuals from their family of choice.

Once the coding scheme was determined, all transcripts were independently reviewed a second time and coded in their entirety according to the newly developed coding scheme. To ensure coding reliability, the research team met to discuss coding interpretations. Coding discrepancies were discussed until consensus about the appropriate code was obtained. Another team member randomly selected 10% of the transcripts and recoded them independently again in terms of the existing descriptive codes. In comparing the coding of participants' responses between this team member and the other investigators, the Cohen's kappa coefficient was 0.94. Validity was addressed by checking transcripts against themes and interpretations.

Results. Of the sample, 94 of the 150 PLWH identified specific persons they excluded from their chosen families and gave reasons for excluding them. Descriptive statistics regarding the 94 participants are presented in Table A10.1 and trends shown in this table reflect the

TABLE A10.1	Characteristics of Participants who Provided Reasons for Including/Excluding Individuals from their Chosen Families (N = 94)		
CHARACTERISTIC	MEAN (SD)	N	%[a]
Age (years)	40.4 (8.0)		
Gender			
Male		17	
Female		77	
Sexual orientation			
Heterosexual		49	52.1
Homosexual		34	36.2
Bisexual and/or other		11	11.7
Race			
Caucasian (non-Hispanic)		23	24.5
African-American		66	70.2
Other (eg, Asian, Hispanic)		5	5
Current marital status			
Single		63	67.0
Married		4	4.3
Live with partner		10	10.6
Divorced		5	5.3
Other		12	12.8
Current employment status			
Employed part-time		11	11.7
Employed full-time		10	10.6
Unemployed		24	25.5
On disability		48	51.1
Other			1.1
Highest education achieved (years)	12.4 (2.4)		
Less than high school		23	24.5
Completed high school		25	26.6
Some college		28	29.8
College graduate		7	7.4
Graduate degree			1.1
Others (eg, training certificates)		10	10.6
Annual income (USD)			
≤$10,000		71	75.5
$10,001–$29,999		19	20.2
≥$30,000		4	4.3

Note: [a]Sum of percentages may be > 100 due to rounding.
Abbreviation: SD, standard deviation.

larger overall sample of 150 participants. Participants' ages ranged from 19 to 61 years with a mean age of 40.4 years (standard deviation = 8.0). They were primarily single (n = 85; 90.4%), male (n = 77; 81.9%), and African-American (n = 66; 71.3%); had completed high school education or more (n = 46; 48.9%); were on disability (n = 48; 51.1%) and unemployed (n = 73; 77.7%); had an annual income of <US$10,000 (n= 71; 75.5%); and reported no current emotional/mental problems (n = 62; 66.0%). The number of participants identifying themselves as heterosexual (n = 49; 52.1%) was comparable to those identifying themselves as homosexual (n = 34; 36.2%). Further, eleven (11.7%) individuals specified an "other" (eg, bisexual) sexual preference.

Participants had an average 9.1 years (standard deviation = 5.5) of known HIV-positive status. Most self-reported they were prescribed at least one HIV medication (n = 73, 77.7%) and had had no opportunistic infections during the previous 3 months (n = 68; 72.3%). The average CD4+ lymphocyte count and viral load of the sample was 364.5 cells/mm^3 (SD = 258.1) and 56,529 copies/mL (SD = 141,442.0), respectively. However, approximately one-third (n = 29; 30.9%) of participants had an undetectable viral load (<50 copies/mL) and approximately one-third (n = 28; 29.8%) had AIDS (ie, a CD4+ lymphocyte count of ≤200 cells/mm^3). Most (n = 89; 94.7%) had revealed their HIV status to someone in their lives.

Themes. Physical and emotional distance (n = 64; 68.1 %); nonsupport, nonacceptance, and harm (n = 25; 26.6%); conditional caring and trust (n = 22; 23.4%); and no blood/familial relationship (n = 13; 13.8%) were the four reasons PLWH excluded individuals from their chosen families. While 65 (69.1%) participants voiced one of these reason themes, 28 (29.8%) participants voiced two themes and one participant (69.1%) voiced three themes.

Physical and Emotional Distance. The most frequent reason for PLWH excluding individuals from their chosen families was physical and emotional distance. PLWH excluded these individuals because of a limited or lack of tangible and affective closeness. Further, this reason was often given because the contact and sharing of specific information, such as their HIV-positive serostatus, was considered irrelevant to those individuals they excluded from their chosen families. Specific responses included:

- "We have no contact at all."
- "We are not and have never been close."
- "Disowned me growing up, didn't care what happened to me."
- "Don't see them. They don't know if I am dead or alive."
- "None of their business."
- "Don't want them to know my status […]."
- "Just don't need to know."
- "It isn't easy to talk about, not close so I don't tell them everything."

Nonsupport, Nonacceptance, and Harm. PLWH excluded individuals from their chosen families for providing them no support or not accepting their homosexuality and HIV-positive serostatus. A lack of understanding between PLWH and particular individuals, and rejection, was inherent in this exclusion. Further, there was dissonance or disagreement between PLWH and others regarding acceptance of their homosexuality and HIV-positive serostatus. Those excluded from their family of choice included both biological and nonbiological relations. Some participants cited physical and sexual harm to themselves in previous years as a reason for exclusion of specific individuals. Therefore, rejection of the participant as a person, their homosexuality, and HIV status was the major and underlying reason for excluding specific individuals as part of their chosen families. Specific responses included:

- "He is not good to me (raped me when I was young)."
- "One sister loved me but didn't like the color I was dating and my HIV status."

- "… they react differently to people with HIV."
- "They are not understanding at all."
- "Smothering, they both know, I have explained but they don't understand what HIV is."
- "Not gay friendly, they react to me differently b/c [because] of my being gay."
- "I don't include my brother because he's a snob."
- "Rejects and acts differently to me."

Conditional Caring and Trust. Whereas the previous theme was based on actual nonsupport, nonacceptance, and harm, participants also cited many reasons for excluding an individual from their chosen families because of tentative or conditional emotional closeness and trust. PLWH feared negative consequences, such as rejection or loss of a relationship or employment, if these individuals knew their HIV status. They also feared that others would be told of their HIV status if they made it known to specific individuals they excluded from their chosen families. Specific responses included:

- "Not open minded, doesn't know about my HIV, but wouldn't accept it."
- "They don't know about my HIV, afraid of them telling other people."
- "I don't trust them."
- "They have no knowledge; they might break up the friendship."
- "They don't know my status; they would reject me because they have no knowledge."
- "Afraid of being stereotyped and …"
- "They don't know, don't want to expect or experience a negative reaction."
- "She doesn't know and I haven't told her. I'm afraid she would not be able to take it and get disappointed."

No Blood/Familial Relationship. PLWH also excluded certain individuals from their chosen families because there was no blood or familial tie. Therefore, a lack of kinship was an important reason to exclude someone from their family. For example, some friends were excluded because they were not related by blood. Further, although participants had positive relationships with friends, participants sometimes excluded specific friends because of a lack of kinship. Individuals with whom PLWH had relationships that were at an early stage or were for sexual gratification were also not viewed by PLWH as members of their chosen families. Specific responses included:

- "They are not blood related."
- "They are friends, not blood related."
- "I care for them, but not like my family."
- "We only see each other once per week, pretty much just sex."
- "They are just friends, not a family."
- "Not blood related despite a good and close relationship."
- "They're friends, associates, not blood related …"
- "It is just a casual (superficial relationship)."

Themes Expressed by Groups. In follow-up analyses using the entire sample of 150 participants, demographic and personal characteristics were examined to determine if they were associated with excluding individuals from being chosen family members. In Table A10.2, the demographic and personal characteristics of the sample are compared, using chi-squares, according to whether they identified with any of the four themes. Only one demographic was related by theme: those who were employed were more likely to voice physical and emotional distance as a reason for excluding someone from being a member of their chosen family (χ^2 [N = 150] = 7.7, P = 0.005). However, using a Bonferroni correction (alpha of 0.05 divided by 40 tests = alpha correction of 0.00125), this relationship was no longer significant. Therefore, based upon the lack of significant findings between

TABLE A10.2	Themes Expressed by Grouping Variables (N = 150)			
GROUPING VARIABLE	PHYSICAL AND EMOTIONAL DISTANCE (n = 64)	NONSUPPORT, NONACCEPTANCE, AND HARM (n = 25)	CONDITIONAL CARING AND TRUST (n = 22)	NO BLOOD/ FAMILIAL RELATIONSHIP (n = 13)
Age[a] (years)				
<40 (n = 56)	24 (42.9%)	12 (21.4%)	10 (17.96%)	6 (10.7%)
≥40 (n = 94)	40 (42.6%)	13 (13.8%)	12 (12.8%)	7 (7.4%)
Gender				
Male (n = 118)	47 (39.8%)	24 (20.3%)	19 (16.1%)	11 (9.3%)
Female (n = 31)	17 (54.8%)	1 (3.2%)	3 (9.7%)	2 (6.5%)
Transgendered (n = 1)	0 (0%)	0 (0%)	0 (0%)	0 (0%)
Sexual orientation				
Heterosexual (n = 71)	34 (47.9%)	13 (18.3%)	14 (19.7%)	8 (11.3%)
Homosexual (n = 65)	24 (36.9%)	8 (12.3%)	7 (10.8%)	3 (4.6%)
Other (n = 14)	6 (42.9%)	4 (28.6%)	1 (7.1%)	2 (14.3%)
Race				
African-American (n = 105)	43 (41.0%)	15 (14.3%)	18 (17.1%)	10 (76.9%)
Caucasian (n = 39)	20 (51.3%)	8 (20.5%)	3 (7.7%)	2 (5.1%)
Other (n = 6)	1 (16.7%)	3 (33.3%)	1 (0.7%)	1 (16.7%)
Marital status				
Single (n = 132)	55 (41.7%)	23 (17.4%)	19 (14.4%)	13 (9.8%)
Coupled (n = 18)	9 (50.0%)	2 (11.1%)	3 (16.7%)	0 (0%)
Highest education				
High school or less (n = 81)	29 (35.8%)	13 (16.9%)	13 (16.0%)	8 (9.9%)
Higher than high school (n = 69)	35 (50.7%)	12 (17.4%)	9 (13.0%)	5 (7.2%)
Current employment status				
Employed (n = 27)	18 (66.7%)a	3 (11.1%)	5 (18.5%)	2 (7.4%)
Unemployed (n = 123)	46 (37.6%)	22 (17.9%)	17 (13.8%)	11 (8.9%)
Annual income (USD)				
<$10,000 (n = 116)	48 (41.4%)	18 (15.5%)	18 (15.5%)	13 (11.2%)
≥$10,000 (n = 34)	16 (47.1%)	7 (20.6%)	4 (11.8%)	0 (0%)
Current emotional/mental problems				
Yes (n = 51)	19 (37.3%)	8 (15.7%)	7 (13,7%)	6 (11.8%)
No (n = 99)	45 (45.5%)	17 (17.2%)	15 (15.2%)	7 (7.1%)
Disclose HIV status to someone				
Yes (n = 145)	63 (43.4%)	23 (15.9%)	21 (14.5%)	12 (8.3%)
No (n = 5)	1 (20.0%)	2 (40.0%)	1 (20.0%)	1 (20.0%)

Note: [a]Chi-square significant at $P < 0.05$.
Abbreviation: HIV, human immunodeficiency virus.

demographic and personal characteristics and expressed themes, the findings suggest that these themes may be universal to human behavior and not dependent on particular participant characteristics.

Discussion. The purpose of this study was to identify why PLWH exclude individuals from their chosen families. The most common reasons PLWH excluded individuals from their chosen families were physical and emotional distance; followed by nonsupport, non-acceptance, and harm; conditional caring and trust; and no blood/familial relationship. Demographic and personal characteristics (ie, gender, race) were not related to the exclusion of individuals from their chosen families. These themes emphasize that distance, both emotional and physical, and a lack of support, acceptance, caring, and trust are reasons why PLWH exclude other individuals from their chosen families. Further, a portion of this sample excluded individuals from their chosen family based upon whether they were related by blood or marriage, reinforcing the value of these ties.

These findings are similar to those cited by Gaskins et al for not disclosing HIV status, including fear of negative reactions, worrying that disclosure recipients would tell others, belief that there was no need to tell, and not wanting to burden others.[19] In contrast, our study findings also emphasize essential components for disclosing HIV-positive status to others. Similar to reasons suggested by Bor et al,[17] we found that PLWH need an open, emotionally close, and unprejudiced relationship with others to trust them enough to disclose their HIV status.

While these findings indicate reasons for excluding individuals from chosen families, they also have implications for health professionals in terms of appropriate behaviors when interacting with and providing care to PLWH. These findings emphasize the importance of health professionals demonstrating supportive behaviors that indicate they value and accept PLWH. Further, interactions should be frequent enough to build therapeutic relationships that are built upon caring and trust.

Moreover, basic counseling skills are essential to address the stigma experienced by PLWH. Stigma management programs are important tools in this respect, as they lessen negative attitudes and beliefs about HIV.[18] Given Peterson's[8] findings, who cited examples of how PLWH were treated differently by their family (ie, those related to them by blood or marriage) when they disclosed their status to them, the development of family counseling and support programs to improve the physical and psychological health of individuals living with HIV and their family is essential.

Balaji et al[26] concurred in their study of the role of familial, religious, and community influences on the experiences of young black MSM. Their results suggest that homosexuality remains highly stigmatized in the men's families, religious communities, and the African-American community. To manage stigma, many participants used "role flexing," in which they changed their behavior to adapt to a situation.[26] Thus, interventions should focus on social, political, and economic causes of stigma and stigmatization and concentrate on aggregates and communities rather than just on individuals. Further, priority should be given to intervention programs that focus on communities developing new models for advocacy and social change. These programs should be part of a multidimensional effort, with structural and environmental interventions directed at transforming the context in which both individuals and communities operate as they respond to HIV.[26,27]

Cahill et al also emphasized the necessity for other community-based HIV prevention interventions that combat prejudice against MSM and transgender women.[27] Community-based prevention intervention programs that assert the healthy formation of gay and transgender identities are necessary. These investigators also recognized the value of gay-affirming school-based interventions and resiliency-focused social-marketing campaigns that have already had a positive impact on health outcomes and should be implemented on a broader scale to address anti-gay stigma.[27] One might hold out hope that, given the broadening acceptance/tolerance of marriage equality, someday the burden of homosexual stigma may also be removed along with a social cascade of factors that relate to the negativity of being infected with HIV.

Peterson also emphasized the value of physical and emotional contact between individuals for relationships among chosen families to develop and exist.[8] Many individuals excluded biological family members because of distant relationships and a lack of tangible and affective closeness between themselves and others. In interacting with their chosen families, therapeutic and supportive communication between PLWH and others is important. If personal face-to-face contact is not possible, then contact by letter, email, and/or telephone may be feasible.

Our study has limitations, including the use of a cross-sectional design. Because participation was initiated by volunteers in response to study flyers and information provided by health care providers, the limitations of a self-selected sample must be recognized in this study. Considering these study findings have limited generalizability, future studies of other populations such as women would be valuable in examining why PLWH exclude individuals from their chosen families. Further, this study should be replicated in parts of the country other than the southeastern USA to examine the similarity of themes. Although this study did examine whether demographic and personal characteristics were related to certain themes, a more in-depth examination of such potential factors is important in future research.

Conclusion. Reasons for excluding individuals from their family of choice include a lack of physical and emotional contact; nonsupport and nonacceptance because of their HIV status as well as harm to themselves; tentative caring and trust between PLWH and others; and a lack of biological/familial ties. These study findings emphasize the potential and actual stigma and rejection PLWH face.

Health professionals have an essential role in reducing the stigma associated with HIV and improving the quality of life of PLWH by increasing awareness about this chronic disease, challenging prejudice, providing nonjudgmental care, teaching adaptive coping skills, and serving as role models.[28]

Disclosure. The authors report no conflicts of interest in this work. All authors made substantial contributions to this study in terms of (1) the conception and design, acquisition of data, or analysis and interpretation of data; (2) drafting the article or revising it critically for important intellectual content; and (3) giving final approval of the version to be published.

References

1. Freudenreich O, Goforth HW, Cozza KL, et al. Psychiatric treatment of persons with HIV/AIDS: an HIV-psychiatry consensus survey of current practices. *Psychosomatics*. 2010;*51*(6):480–488.
2. Horberg MA, Silverberg MJ, Hurley LB, et al. Effects of depression and selective serotonin reuptake inhibitor use on adherence to highly active antiretroviral therapy and on clinical outcomes in HIV-infected patients. *J Acquir Immune Defic Syndr*. 2008;*47*(3):384–390.
3. Leserman J. Role of depression, stress, and trauma in HIV disease progression. *Psychosom Med*. 2008;*70*(5):539–545.
4. Greene K, Banjeree SC. Disease-related stigma: comparing predictors of AIDS and cancer stigma. *J Homosex*. 2006;*50*(4):185–209.
5. Rao D, Kekwaletswe TC, Hosek S, Martinez J, Rodriguez F. Stigma and social barriers to medication adherence with urban youth living with HIV. *AIDS Care*. 2007;*19*(1):28–33.
6. Stutterheim SE, Bos AE, Pryor JB, Brands R, Liebregts M, Schaalma HP. Psychological and social correlates of HIV status disclosure: the significance of stigma visibility. *AIDS Educ Prev*. 2011;*23*(4):382–392.
7. Prachakul W, Grant JS, Pryor E, Keltner NL, Raper JL. Family relationships in people living with HIV in a city in the USA. *AIDS Care*. 2009;*21*(3):384–388.
8. Peterson JL. The challenges of seeking and receiving support for women living with HIV. *Health Comm*. 2010;*25*(5):470–479.
9. Butler SS. Gay, lesbian, bisexual and transgender (GLBT) elders: the challenges and resilience of this marginalized group. *J Hum Behav Soc Environ*. 2004;*9*(4):25–44.
10. de Vries B, Blando JA. The study of gay and lesbian aging: Lessons for social gerontology. In: Herdt G, de Vries B, editors. *Gay and Lesbian Aging: Research and Future Directions*. New York, NY: Springer;2004:3–28.
11. Grant JS, Vance DE, Keltner NL, White W, Raper JL. Reasons why persons living with HIV include individuals in their chosen families. *J Assoc Nurses AIDS Care*. 2013;*24*(1):50–60.
12. Wright F. The role of the family as a support system for people with AIDS. *Nurse Pract Forum*. 1991;*2*(2):134–136.
13. George S, Garth B, Wohl AR, Galvan FH, Garland W, Myers HF. Sources and types of social support that influence engagement in HIV care among Latinos and African Americans. *J Healthcare Poor Care Underserved*. 2009;*20*(4):1012–1035.

14. Poindexter C, Shippy RA. Networks of older New Yorkers with HIV: fragility, resilience, and transformation. *AIDS Patient Care STDS*. 2008;*22*(9):723–733.

15. Serovich JM, Grafsky EL, Craft SM. Does family matter to HIV-positive men who have sex with men? *J Marital Fam Ther*. 2011;*37*(3):290–298.

16. Serovich JM, Esbensen AJ, Mason TL. HIV disclosure by men who have sex with men to immediate family over time. *AIDS Patient Care STDs*. 2005;*19*(8):506–517.

17. Bor R, du Plessis P, Russell M. The impact of disclosure of HIV on the index patient's self-defined family. *J Fam Ther*. 2004;*26*(2):167–192.

18. Paiva V, Segurado AC, Filipe EM. Self-disclosure of HIV diagnosis to sexual partners by heterosexual and bisexual men: A challenge for HIV/ AIDS care and prevention. *Cad Saude Publica*. 2011;*27*:1699–1710.

19. Gaskins S, Payne Foster P, Sowell R, Lewis T, Gardner A, Parton J. Reasons for HIV disclosure and non-disclosure: an exploratory study of rural African American men. *Issues Ment Health Nurs*. 2011;*32*(6): 367–373.

20. Latkin C, Yang C, Tobin K, Roebuck G, Spikes P, Patterson J. Social network predictors of disclosure of MSM behavior and HIV-positive serostatus among African American MSM in Baltimore, Maryland. *AIDS Behav*. 2012;*16*(3):535–542.

21. Obermeyer CM, Baijal P, Pegurri E. Facilitating HIV disclosure across diverse settings: a review. *Am J Public Health*. 2011;*101*(6): 1011–1023.

22. Serovich JM, Grafsky EL, Reed S. Comparing regret of disclosing HIV versus sexual orientation information by MSM. *AIDS Care*. 2010;*22*(9):1052–1059.

23. Parker R, Aggleton P. HIV and AIDS-related stigma and discrimination: a conceptual framework and implications for action. *Soc Sci Med*. 2003;*57*(1):13–24.

24. Power C, Selnes OA, Grim JA, McArthur JC. HIV Dementia Scale: a rapid screening test. *J Acquir Immune Defic Syndr Hum Retrovirol*. 1995;*8*(3):273–278.

25. Hsieh HF, Shannon SE. Three approaches to qualitative content analysis. *Qual Health Res*. 2005;*15*(9):1277–1288.

26. Balaji AB, Oster AM, Viall AH, Heffelfinger JD, Mena LA, Toledo CA. Role flexing: how community, religion, and family shape the experiences of young black men who have sex with men. *AIDS Patient Care STDS*. 2012;*26*(12):730–737.

27. Cahill S, Valadéz R, Ibarrola S. Community-based HIV prevention interventions that combat anti-gay stigma for men who have sex with men and for transgender women. *J Public Health Policy*. 2013;*34*(1):69–81.

28. Lewis R. Stamping out stigma in HIV. *Nurs Times*. 2011;*107*(11): 16–17.

Nursing: Reasearch and Reviews   Dovepress

Publish your work in this journal

Nursing: Reasearch and Reviews is an ininternational, peer-reviewed, open access journal publishing original research, reports, reviews and commentaries on all aspects of nursing and patient care. These include patient education and counselling, ethics, management and organizational issues, diagnostics and prescribing, economics and resource management, health outcomes, and improving patient safety in all settings. The manuscript management system is completely online and includes a very quick and fair peer-review system. Visit http://www.dovepress.com/testimonials.php to read real quotes from published authors.

Submit your manuscript here: http://www.dovepress.com/nursing-research-and-reviews-journal

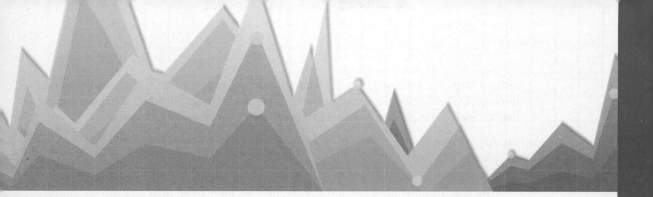

Appendix B

Demographic Characteristics as Predictors of Nursing Students' Choice of Type of Clinical Practice

Abstract

This descriptive study examined predictors of nursing students' choice of field of clinical practice using a convenience sample of 30 baccalaureate students in a Midwestern university. Students voluntarily completed a written questionnaire and responded to a subjective question about experiences influencing their choice of field. Students favored acute settings such as intensive care and emergency rooms over less acute settings, and their age and self-rating of health were related to these choices. Three types of experiences were described as meaningful contributors to choice of field of practice.

The nursing shortage is of grave concern to the public and to the profession of nursing itself, and nursing workforce planning is a priority. Nursing workforce planning needs to address the number of nurses prepared and the level of nursing preparation (Institute of Medicine, 2010). In considering nursing workforce needs, one needs to consider not just the numbers of nurses but also the choice of clinical practice of those nurses. While declining enrollments in schools of nursing affect the availability of nurses in all settings, settings that are less "popular" among new graduates will be even harder hit by this shortage. This includes long-term health care settings and primary care settings. The needs for nurses in these types of settings vary from country to country. For example, in South Africa, the number of nursing positions in hospitals is much smaller than those in primary health clinics. In contrast, in the United States, the aging population makes needs in long-term care facilities greater than those in primary care.

BACKGROUND. In the United States, the general public's image of nursing continues to be the dedicated individual providing bedside nursing for acute health problems. Often the only image nursing students have of the field as they begin their education comes from television shows such as *House ER* or *Grey's Anatomy*. These portrayals usually project an image of nurses as either oversexed or always in the midst of life-threatening crises. The impact of such portrayals of nurses is reflected in the common situation when students, who think they may be interested in primary care or public health nursing "someday," often plan to do "real nursing" in a hospital first. As long-term planning for the nursing workforce continues, it will be important to be able to predict which students are more likely to fill gaps in the different and varied fields of nursing practice. This will allow nursing programs to target student recruitment toward those students most likely to move into clinical practice

339

settings with the greatest need. Therefore, this study examined the relationships among nursing students' demographic characteristics and their choice for practice following graduation. Specifically, the study addressed the following three questions:

1. Are age, gender, race, and marital status associated with choice of first clinical practice after graduation?

2. Do older students and those with higher levels of perceived well-being select primary care settings for clinical practice after graduation more often than do younger students and those with lower levels of well-being?

3. What student experiences bring meaning to their choices of field of nursing practice?

METHODS

Sample. This study used a convenience sample of undergraduate baccalaureate nursing students in the second semester of their junior year of their program. The students were completing a required research course. The NLN-accredited nursing program located in a large Midwestern university enrolls 120 undergraduate students each year. The university draws students from throughout the Midwest and reports a generally diverse student body, including representative numbers of Latino and black students. Programs to earn a bachelor's degree in nursing include a traditional 4-year program, an RN to BSN program, and an LPN to BSN program. Students in all three of these programs take the research course that provided the sample for this study. Participation in the study was voluntary, and completion of the questionnaire was anonymous. A total of 30 out of 33 students participated.

Procedure. An independent faculty member who was not teaching the course administered the questionnaires, and the subjects placed the questionnaires in a sealed box themselves. Subjects were told that the questionnaire was part of the nursing department's efforts to plan future programs. In order to avoid any overt breach in confidentiality, all students remained in the classroom while the questionnaires were being completed, and all students placed questionnaires in the box, whether or not they had completed the questionnaire.

Measures. The entire questionnaire consisted of three sections. The first section asked about demographic characteristics, the second section asked about postsecondary education, perceived well-being, and planned choice of career, and the last section asked about subjects' preferences of automobiles. The last section was included to be used as a class exercise for the research course itself. Each section is described below.

Demographic characteristics included in this study were age, gender, and marital status. Each of these variables could reflect selected life experiences of students that might influence their choice of practice site after graduation.

The section asking about postsecondary education, well-being, and planned career choice included items asking about completion of previous technical programs, or associate or undergraduate degrees. Subjects were asked whether they were currently licensed to practice as either an LPN or RN and to give the total number of years of postsecondary education they had completed. Well-being was measured on a 4-point scale rating that perceived health as excellent, good, fair, and poor (Kaplan & Camacho, 1983). This single self-report item has been used in a number of studies, including the Human Population Laboratory Studies in Alameda County, CA (Kaplan & Camacho, 1983). The item has demonstrated reliability and validity. It has been shown to be strongly related to a persons' baseline physical health status and to be significantly related to different mortality rates for both men and women of all ages who perceived their health as excellent versus poor (Kaplan & Camacho, 1983).

The last questions in the second section of the questionnaire asked subjects about their anticipated choice of field of nursing immediately post graduation and long-term.

Responses were selected from a list of nursing career options, eliminating the need to code individual responses. Subjects also were asked a single open-ended qualitative question, "What experiences in your life have led to your anticipated choice for field of nursing practice?" Subjects were provided with a single page of lined paper for this response.

The third section of the questionnaire regarding automobile preferences included questions about ownership of an automobile, and a rating on a 10-point scale of the condition of that automobile or how much they want an automobile if they do not own one. Subjects were asked to rank their color preferences for automobiles and to answer a series of dichotomous questions about their use of various forms of transportation.

The questionnaire was reviewed for face validity by three undergraduate faculty members of nursing. It was then pilot-tested with a sample of five graduate student nurses in their research course in order to assure clarity and relevancy. Only very minor changes in language resulted from this pilot test.

Analysis. Only the results from the first two sections of the questionnaire are reported here. Objective data from the questionnaires were analyzed using SPSS (Statistical Package for the Social Sciences) software program. Written subjective responses were directly transcribed and were analyzed using common phenomenological methods (Boyd & Munhall, 1993). Analysis included data reduction, identification of common themes, and conclusion drawing and was aided by use of QRS NUD.IST (Non-Numerical Unstructured Data Indexing Searching and Theory-building Multi-Functional) software program.

RESULTS. The sample included 30 undergraduate baccalaureate nursing students, 25 female and 5 male. Ninety percent were single ($n = 27$) and the average age of subjects was 23 ($SD = 2$).

The majority of the subjects (60%) were traditional 4-year baccalaureate students; however, subjects did represent all of the different programs offered. Many subjects had completed more than 3 years of postsecondary education ($M = 3.5$, $SD = 1$). Only 20% of subjects rated their own health as "fair or poor." Students' choices of field of nursing immediately post graduation and for a long-term career are reported in Table B.l. In both cases, the majority of students selected acute care settings, with an emphasis on intensive care and emergency department care as their anticipated field of nursing.

Choice of field or setting was dichotomized for acute setting versus nonacute setting for additional analysis. There was a significant difference in age of subjects who selected the two settings ($t = 2.4$, $p < .05$). with younger students selecting acute fields of practice. There also was a significant difference in rating of health ($t = 2.1$, $p < .05$), with subjects who rated their health higher choosing acute care fields of practice more than those with lower levels of self-rated health. Lastly, there was an association between type of nursing program

TABLE B.1	Students' Choices of Field of Nursing	
FIELD OF CHOICE	NUMBER (%) SELECTING FIELD IMMEDIATELY POST GRADUATION	NUMBER (%) SELECTING FIELD AS LONG-TERM GOAL
Intensive care (adult)	18 (60%)	9 (30%)
Neonatal or pediatric intensive care	3 (10%)	6 (20%)
Emergency department	3 (10%)	9 (30%)
Obstetrics	1 (3%)	0
Medical/Surgical	0	0
Pediatrics	2 (7%)	2 (7%)
Health department	0	0
Long-term care, nursing home	2 (7%)	0
Primary care clinic or health care provider office	1 (3%)	4 (13%)

and choice of field of study ($\chi^2_{[10, N = 30]} = 23, p < .05$). There was no significant association between race or gender and choice of field of study, and no differences in number of years of postsecondary education and field of study. Logistic regression indicated that only age of subject and rating of health statistically contributed to the odds of selecting a nonacute care field of study when age, health rating, and type of nursing program were entered. One-way analysis of variance indicated that students who were older were more likely to be in the LPN to BSN program or the RN to BSN program.

Analysis of subjective findings yielded three distinct themes that represent the meaning of life experiences related to choice of field of nursing. The themes and selected quotes from subjects are included in Table B.2. The first theme was personal life experiences such as illness or death of a loved one, or their own acute illness. Subjects described experiences with nurses in the emergency room and the hospital and how these gave unique meaning to the health crisis being faced.

The second theme was direct experiences with family or close friends who provided nursing care in the field chosen by the subject. Subjects described love and respect and a desire to follow in the footsteps of these role models who had influenced their plans for the field of nursing.

The last theme was experiences with fictional media including novels, movies, and television shows. These subjects described being moved and excited by descriptions or scenes showing nurses providing care in the fields they expected to choose post graduation.

DISCUSSION. Overall, students in this study identified that their choice of nursing field was intensive care and emergency room care. Maternity care and care of children were the second most commonly identified fields, with public health, primary care, and long-term care being the least frequently chosen. Objectively, the major demographic characteristic that was associated with choice of acute care field of practice was age, with younger nursing

TABLE B.2	Definitions of Themes and Examples that Represent Meaning of Experiences in Relation to Choice of Nursing Field
THEMES	EXAMPLES OF EXPERIENCES
Personal life experience: direct interactions with health care providers and the health care system surrounding student's own health or that of others	"Seeing how those nurses took care of my mother as she lay there unconscious with so many tubes and machines hooked to her made me decide right then and there that this was what I wanted to do." "It was the nurse holding my hand as the doctor in the emergency room told me about my brother that made it possible for me to keep going. I want to be like that nurse and help others in such terrible times of life." "After I got home from the hospital a nurse came to visit and change my dressing. She was so caring and kind and gentle. Taking nursing into people's homes is what I want to do."
Experiences with nursing role models: direct interactions with significant others who are nurses	"My aunt was a nurse. She always was so strong and sure of herself—I wanted to be just like her and work in the emergency department." "In our town Mrs. Timms was the person everyone went to with a question or for help. It seemed like her being a nurse just made her able to help everyone. Mrs. Timms worked in the Health Department Clinic so that seems to me to be a good place to practice nursing."
Experiences with fictional media: vicarious experiences of providing nursing care in certain settings as described or depicted in books, television, and the movies	"Watching the nurses in *ER*; they always knew what was going on and were really there for the patients—that is why I want to practice in the emergency room."

students more frequently choosing acute fields compared with older students. Students who were older were more likely to be in the RN to BSN program or the LPN to BSN program, and therefore, the type of baccalaureate program was also related to choice of field. Lastly, self-rating of health was related to choice of field of practice, with students who rated themselves in better health being more likely to choose acute care fields.

Subjectively, students described experiences in their personal lives, with role models and with fictional characters as meaningful in their decisions about choice of field. Age of students may very well relate to these types of experiences, since one would expect that older students would be more likely to have a range of personal life experiences with various fields of nursing. Younger students are more likely to have primarily experienced health care in the acute setting, if at all, and may well depend on role models and fictional characters more than older students. Certainly, the fictional characters available to these students would create an emphasis on acute settings. The differences in self-rating of health further support this idea, since students who are in poor health are more likely to have personal experiences with a variety of health care fields, not just acute care. The subjective transcribed data was not connected to the objective demographic data, so it was not possible to explore these possibilities more completely.

Given the changes in health care in this country and throughout the world and the increased emphasis on primary health care and early discharge from hospitals, it is clear that not all graduates who wish to practice in intensive care and emergency rooms will be able to do so. Nursing programs that are particularly concerned about shortages in nonacute settings may be able to expand this workforce by focusing their recruitment efforts on older students and by further developing or expanding RN to BSN and LPN to BSN programs. In addition, nursing needs to make fields of nursing other than acute care more visible to the public at large in order to widen the number of meaningful experiences nursing students might have that will affect their choice of field of practice.

References

Boyd, C. O., & Munhall, P. L. (1993). Qualitative research proposals and reports. *NLN Publications*, *19*(2535), 424–453.

Institute of Medicine. (2010). The future of nursing: Leading change, advancing health. Retrieved January 2014 from http://books.nap.edu/openbook.php?record_id=12956&page=R1

Kaplan, B. A., & Camacho, T. (1983). Perceived health and mortality: A nine-year follow-up of the Human Population Laboratory cohort. *American Journal of Epidemiology*, *111*, 292–304.

Appendix C

Sample In-Class Data Collection Tool

This questionnaire is for use in this research class only. Completing the questionnaire is entirely voluntary. If you do choose to fill out the questionnaire, please answer each question fully and thoughtfully.

DO NOT PUT YOUR NAME ON THIS FORM

<u>Section One</u>

What is your AGE in years? _____

Are you MALE FEMALE (circle one)

What is your MARITAL STATUS? (check one) _____ Single

_____ Married

_____ Divorced or Widowed

_____ Partnered

<u>Section Two</u>

How many YEARS school have you <u>completed</u> since finishing high school? _____

In general, how would you rate your OVERALL HEALTH? (circle one)

Excellent   Good   Fair   Poor

Below, you will find a list of possible fields for healthcare practice. Please check which one you want as your FIRST CHOICE for practice when you graduate from this nursing program.

CHECK ONLY ONE!

_____ Emergency Department

_____ Health Department

_____ Intensive Care Unit for Adults

_____ Long-Term Care, Nursing Home

_____ Medical/Surgical Unit

_____ Neonatal or Pediatric Intensive Care

_____ Obstetrics

_____ Pediatric Unit

_____ Primary Care Clinic or Health Care Provider Office

Below, you will find the same list of healthcare practice fields. This time, please check which one you want as your FIRST CHOICE for practice as a **long-term goal.**

_____ Emergency Department

_____ Health Department

_____ Intensive Care Unit for Adults

_____ Long-Term Care, Nursing Home

_____ Medical/Surgical Unit

_____ Neonatal or Pediatric Intensive Care

_____ Obstetrics

_____ Pediatric Unit

_____ Primary Care Clinic or Health Care Provider Office

On the back of this questionnaire, please describe <u>the one major experience</u> in your life that has led you to select the field of healthcare that you indicated above.

Section Three

Do you currently own a car? (check one) _____ YES _____ NO

- IF "YES," please answer the following questions about the car you own.
- If "NO," please answer the following questions for the car you expect to own in the immediate future.

Is the car (check one) _____ NEW _____ USED

Please **rate** the overall condition of the car you own or expect to own in the <u>immediate</u> future by circling ONE rating from the scale below.

1   2   3   4   5   6   7   8   9   10

Terrible   OK   Excellent

Please select your preferences for the CAR OF YOUR DREAMS:

Color (write in your primary color choice) _____

Type (such as SUV, sedan, convertible) _____

Transmission type (check one) _____ Automatic _____ Standard 5 speed

Engine cylinders (check one) _____ 4 cylinder _____ 6 cylinder _____ 8 cylinder _____ Unknown

From a range of 0% to 100%, how often do you wear seat belts while riding or driving in a vehicle? _____% of the time.

Thank you for completing this questionnaire, which we will use for practice in this class only.

Appendix D

In-Class Study Data for Practice Exercise in Chapter 5

CASE NUMBER	MARITAL STATUS	HEALTH RATING
1	Single	4
2	Married	3
3	Divorced/widowed	3
4	Married	2
5	Married	1
6	Single	3
7	Single	1
8	Single	4
9	Single	4
10	Divorced/widowed	3
11	Married	2
12	Single	3
13	Single	3
14	Single	2
15	Married	2
16	Married	3
17	Single	4
18	Single	3
19	Divorced/widowed	3
20	Single	4
21	Married	3
22	Married	2
23	Single	3
24	Single	2
25	Single	3
26	Divorced/widowed	4
27	Single	3
28	Single	3
29	Married	2
30	Married	3

Glossary

Abstract a summary or condensed version of the research report. Chapter 1, p. 21.

Aggregated data data that are reported for an entire group rather than for individuals in the group. Chapter 11, p. 226.

Analysis of variance (ANOVA) a statistical test for analyzing differences in the means in three or more groups. Chapter 5, p. 99.

Anonymous a participant in research is anonymous when no one, including the researcher, can link the study data from a particular individual to that individual. Chapter 7, p. 138.

Assent to agree or concur; in the case of research, assent reflects a lower level of understanding about the meaning of participation in a study than consent. Assent is often sought in studies that involve older children or individuals who have a level of impairment that limits their ability but does not preclude their understanding of some aspects of the study. Chapter 7, p. 143.

Assumptions ideas that are taken for granted or viewed as truth without conscious or explicit testing. Chapter 11, p. 220.

Audit trail written and/or computer notes used in qualitative research that describe the researcher's decisions regarding both the data analysis process and the collection process. Chapter 8, p. 155.

Beta (β) value a statistic derived from regression analysis that tells us the relative contribution or connection of each factor to the dependent variable. Chapter 5, p. 101.

Bias some unintended factor that confuses or changes the results of the study in a manner that can lead to incorrect conclusions; bias distorts or confounds the findings in a study, making it difficult to impossible to interpret the results. Chapter 6, p. 116.

Bivariate analysis statistical analysis involving only two variables. Chapter 4, p. 73.

Bridge Theory the Gersch & Rebar Evidence-Based Bridge Theory explains how individual healthcare professionals can use evidence-based information (EBI) in clinical practice. The premise of the theory: there is a gap that exists between available research (EBI) and the need for active application of this research (EBI) to enact positive growth and/or change within the individual's professional environment. Chapter 1, p. 5.

Categorization scheme an orderly combination of carefully defined groups where there is no overlap among the categories. Chapter 4, p. 74.

Central tendency a measure or statistic that indicates the center of a distribution or the center of the spread of the values for the variable. Chapter 4, p. 82.

Clinical trial a study that tests the effectiveness of a clinical treatment; some researchers would say that a clinical trial must be a true experiment. Chapter 9, p. 195.

Cluster sampling a process of sampling, in stages, starting with a larger element that relates to the population and moving downward into smaller and smaller elements that identify the population. Chapter 6, p. 119.

Codebook a record of the categorization, labeling, and manipulation of data for the variables in a quantitative study. Chapter 11, p. 224.

Coding reducing a large amount of data to numbers or conceptual groups (see data reduction) in qualitative research; giving individual datum numerical values in quantitative research. Chapter 4, p. 74–75.

Coercion the involvement of some element that controls or forces someone to do something. In the case of research, coercion occurs if a patient is forced to participate in a study to receive a particular test or service, or to receive or not to receive the best quality of care. Chapter 7, p. 139.

Comparison group a group of subjects that differs on a major independent variable from the study group, allowing comparison of the subjects in the two groups in terms of a dependent variable. Chapter 9, p. 188.

Conceptual framework an underlying structure for building and testing knowledge that is made up of concepts and the relationships among the concepts. Chapter 10, p. 203.

Conceptualization a process of creating a verbal picture of an abstract idea. Chapter 3, p. 60.

Conclusions the end of a research report that identifies the final decisions or determinations regarding the research problem. Chapter 2, p. 30.

Confidentiality assurance that neither the identities of participants in the research will be revealed to anyone else, nor will the information that participants provide individually be publicly divulged. Chapter 7, p. 138.

Confidence intervals the range of values for a variable, which would be found in 95 out of 100 samples; confidence intervals set the boundaries for a variable or test statistic. Chapter 5, p. 93.

Confirmation the verification of results from other studies. Chapter 3, p. 58.

Confirmability the ability to consistently repeat decision making about the data collection and analysis in qualitative research. Chapter 8, p. 154–155.

Construct validity the extent to which a scale or instrument measures what it is supposed to measure; the broadest type of validity that can encompass both content- and criterion-related validity. Chapter 8, p. 166.

Content analysis the process of understanding, interpreting, and conceptualizing the meanings imbedded in qualitative data. Chapter 4, p. 74.

Content validity validity that establishes that the items or questions on a scale are comprehensive and appropriately reflect the concept they are supposed to measure. Chapter 8, p. 165.

Control group a randomly assigned group of subjects that is not exposed to the independent variable of interest to be able to compare that group to a group that is exposed to the independent variable; inclusion of a control group is a hallmark of an experimental design. Chapter 9, p. 188.

Convenience sample a sample that includes members of the population who can be readily found and recruited. Chapter 6, p. 114.

Correlation the statistical test used to examine how much two variables covary; a measure of the relationship between two variables. Chapter 5, p. 97.

Correlational studies studies that describe interrelationships among variables as accurately as possible. Chapter 9, p. 188.

Covary when changes in one variable lead to consistent changes in another variable; if two variables covary, then they are connected to each other in some way. Chapter 5, p. 97.

Credibility the confidence that the researcher and user of the research can have in the truth of the findings of the study. Chapter 8, p. 156.

Criteria for participation factors that determine how individuals are selected for a study; they describe the common characteristics that define the target population for a study. Chapter 6, p. 112.

Criterion-related validity the extent to which the results of one measure match those of another measure that is also supposed to reflect the variable under study. Chapter 8, p. 165–166.

Cross-sectional a research design that includes the collection of all data at one point in time. Chapter 9, p. 187.

Data the information collected in a study that is specifically related to the research problem. Chapter 2, p. 32.

Data analysis a process that pulls information together or examines connections between pieces of information to make a clearer picture of all the information collected. Chapter 2, p. 32.

Data reduction organizing large amounts of data, usually in the form of words, so that it is broken down (or reduced) and labeled (or coded) to identify to which category it belongs. Chapter 4, p. 74–75.

Data saturation the point at which all new information collected is redundant of information already collected. Chapter 4, p. 75.

Deductive knowledge a process of taking a general theory and seeking specific observations or facts to support that theory. Chapter 10, p. 202.

Demographics descriptive information about the characteristics of the people studied. Chapter 4, p. 84.

Dependent variable the outcome variable of interest; it is the variable that depends on other variables in the study. Chapter 4, p. 77.

Descriptive design research design that functions to portray as accurately as possible some phenomenon of interest. Chapter 9, p. 183.

Descriptive results a summary of results from a study without comparing the results with other information. Chapter 2, p. 33.

Directional hypothesis a research hypothesis that predicts both a connection between two or more variables and the nature of that connection. Chapter 10, p. 209.

Discussion the section of a research report that summarizes, compares, and speculates about the results of the study. Chapter 3, p. 57–58.

Distribution the spread among the values for a variable. Chapter 4, p. 80.

Dissemination the spreading or sharing of knowledge; communication of new knowledge from research so that it is adopted in practice. Chapter 11, p. 225.

Electronic databases categorized lists of articles from a wide range of journals, organized by topic, author, and journal source available on CDs or online. Chapter 1, p. 20.

Error the difference between what is true and the answer we obtained from our data collection. Chapter 8, p. 150.

Ethnography qualitative research methods used to participate or immerse oneself in a culture in order to describe it. Chapter 9, p. 184.

Evidence-based information (EBI) evidence or findings in a research study that addresses a research question related to clinical practice. Chapter 1, p. 5.

Evidence-based practice (EBP) the process that nurses use to make clinical decisions and to answer clinical questions about delivery of care to patients. Chapter 1, p. 3.

Evidence-based practice (EBP) model framework that provides structures or guidelines for use in practice and contains specific steps in validating EBI and applying EBI to practice (EBP). Chapter 1, p. 6.

Exempt a category of research that is free from some of the constraints that are normally imposed upon research involving human subjects (United States Department of Health & Human Services, 2007). Chapter 7, p. 143.

Experimental designs quantitative research designs that include manipulation of an independent variable, a control group, and random assignment to groups. Chapter 9, p. 176.

Experimenter effects a threat to external validity that occurs when some characteristic of the researchers or data collectors themselves influence the results of the study. Chapter 9, p. 181.

External validity the extent to which the results of a study can be applied to other groups or situations; how accurate the study is in providing knowledge that can be applied outside of or external to the study itself. Chapter 9, p. 178.

Factor analysis a statistical procedure to help identify underlying structures or factors in a measure; it identifies discrete groups of statements that are more closely connected to each other than to all the other statements. Chapter 5, p. 101.

Field notes documentation of the participant's tone, expressions, and associated actions, and what is going on in the setting at the same time; they are a record of the researcher's observations about the overall setting and experience of the data collection process while in that setting or field itself; field notes are used to enrich and build a set of data that are thick and dense. Chapter 8, p. 152.

Five human rights in research rights that have been identified by the American Nurses Association guidelines for nurses working with patient information that may require interpretation; they include the right to self-determination, the right to privacy and dignity, the right to anonymity and confidentiality, the right to fair treatment, and the right to protection from discomfort and harm (ANA, 1985). Chapter 7, p. 136.

Frequency distribution a presentation of data that indicates the spread of how often values for a variable occurred. Chapter 4, p. 80.

Generalizability the ability to say that the findings from a particular sample can be applied to a more general population; *see* Generalization. Chapter 6, p. 122.

Generalization the ability to say that the findings from a particular study can be interpreted to apply to a more general population. Chapter 3, p. 61.

Grounded theory a qualitative research method that is used to study interactions to understand and recognize linkages between ideas and concepts, or to put in different words, to develop theory; the term *grounded* refers to the idea that the theory that is developed is based on or grounded in participants' reality. Chapter 9, p. 184.

Group interviews the collection of data by interviewing more than one participant at a time. Chapter 8, p. 153.

Hawthorne effect a threat to external validity that occurs when subjects in a study change simply because they are being studied, no matter what intervention is applied; reactivity and the Hawthorne effect are the same concept. Chapter 9, p. 181.

Historical research method a qualitative research method used to answer questions about linkages in the past to understand the present or plan the future. Chapter 9, p. 185.

History a threat to internal validity that occurs because of some factor outside those examined in a study, affecting the study outcome or dependent variable. Chapter 9, p. 180.

Hypothesis a prediction regarding the relationships or effects of selected factors on other factors under study. Chapter 2, p. 40.

Independent variables those factors in a study that are used to explain or predict the outcome of interest; independent variables also are sometimes called *predictor variables* because they are used to predict the dependent variable. Chapter 4, p. 77.

Inductive knowledge a process of taking specific facts or observations together to create general theory. Chapter 10, p. 202.

Inferential statistics statistics that are most commonly used in quantitative studies allowing the researcher to draw conclusions based on evidence obtained from a sample population. Chapter 4, p. 71.

Inference the reasoning that goes into the process of drawing a conclusion based on evidence. Chapter 4, p. 71.

Informed consent the legal principle that an individual or his or her authorized representative is given all the relevant information needed to make a decision about participation in a research study and is given a reasonable amount of time to consider that decision. Chapter 7, p. 137.

Instrument a term used in research to refer to a device that specifies and objectifies the process of collecting data. Chapter 8, p. 158.

Instrumentation a threat to internal validity that refers to the changing of the measures used in a study from one time point to another. Chapter 9, p. 180.

Institutional review board (IRB) a group of members selected for the explicit purpose of reviewing any proposed research study to be implemented within an institution or by employees of an institution to ensure that the research project includes procedures to protect the rights of its subjects; the IRB is also charged to decide whether or not the research is basically sound in order to ensure potential participants' rights to protection from discomfort or harm. Chapter 7, p. 134.

Internal consistency reliability the extent to which responses to a scale is similar and related. Chapter 8, p. 164.

Internal validity the extent to which we can be sure of the accuracy or correctness of the findings of a study; how accurate the results are within the study itself or internally. Chapter 9, p. 178.

Inter-rater reliability consistency in measurement that is present when two or more independent data collectors agree in the results of their data collection process. Chapter 8, p. 163.

Items the questions or statements included on a scale used to measure a variable of interest. Chapter 8, p. 159.

Key words terms that describe the topic or nature of the information sought when searching a database or the Internet. Chapter 1, p. 20.

Knowledge information that furthers our understanding of a phenomenon or question. Chapter 1, p. 17.

Likert-type scale a response scale that asks for a rating of an item on a continuum that is anchored at either end by opposite responses. Chapter 8, p. 161.

Limitations the aspects of how the study was conducted that create uncertainty concerning the conclusion that can be derived from the study as well as the decisions that can be based on it. Chapter 2, p. 32.

Literature review a synthesis of existing published writings that describes what is known or has been studied regarding the particular research question or purpose. Chapter 2, p. 13; Chapter 10, p. 205.

Logistic regression a statistical procedure that looks at relationships between more than two factors and test whether those relationships are likely to occur by chance. Chapter 2, p. 35

Longitudinal research design a research design that includes the collection of data over time. Chapter 9, p. 187.

Matched sample the intentful selection of pairs of subjects that share certain important characteristics to prevent those characteristics from confusing what is being explained or understood within the study. Chapter 6, p. 117.

Maturation a threat to internal validity that refers to changes that occur in the dependent variable simply because of the passage of time, rather than because of some independent variable. Chapter 9, p. 180.

Mean the arithmetic average for a set of values. Chapter 4, p. 82.

Measurement effects a threat to external validity because various procedures used to collect data in the study changed the results of that study. Chapter 9, p. 181.

Measure of central tendency a measure that shows the common or typical values within a set of values; central tendency measures reflect the "center" of a distribution, or the center of the spread; the mean, the mode, and the median are the three most commonly used. Chapter 4, p. 82.

Measures the specific method(s) used to assign a number or numbers to an aspect or factor being studied. Chapter 2, p. 38.

Median a measure of central tendency that is the value in a set of numbers that falls in the exact middle of the distribution when the numbers are in order. Chapter 4, p. 82.

Member checks a process in qualitative research where the data and the findings from their analysis are brought back to the original participants to seek their input as to the accuracy, completeness, and interpretation of the data. Chapter 8, p. 156.

Meta-analysis a quantitative approach to knowledge by taking the numbers from different studies that addressed the same research problem and using statistics to summarize those numbers, looking for combined results that would not happen by chance alone. Chapter 2, p. 42.

Metasynthesis a report of a study of a group of single research studies using qualitative methods. Chapter 2, p. 42.

Methods the methods section of a research report describes the overall process of implementing the research study, including who was included in the study, how information was collected, and what interventions, if any, were tested. Chapter 2, p. 35.

Mixed methods some combination of research methods that differ in relation to the function of the design, the use of time in the design, or the control included in the design. Chapter 9, p. 193.

Mode the value for a variable that occurs most frequently. Chapter 4, p. 82.

Model the symbolic framework for a theory or a part of a theory. Chapter 9, p. 189.

Mortality a threat to internal validity that refers to the loss of subjects from a study due to a consistent factor that is related to the dependent variable. Chapter 9, p. 180.

Multifactorial a study that has a number of independent variables that are manipulated. Chapter 9, p. 190.

Multivariate more than two variables; multivariate studies examine three or more factors and the relationships among the different factors. Chapter 2, p. 34.

Nondirectional hypothesis a research hypothesis that predicts a connection between two or more variables but does not predict the nature of that connection. Chapter 10, p. 209.

Nonparametric a group of inferential statistical procedures that are used with numbers that do not have the bell-shaped distribution or that are categorical or ordinal variables. Chapter 5, p. 94.

Nonprobability sampling a sampling approach that does not necessarily assure that everyone in the population has an equal chance of being included in the study. Chapter 6, p. 116.

Normal curve a type of distribution for a variable that is shaped like a bell and is symmetrical. Chapter 4, p. 80.

Novelty effects a threat to external validity that occurs when the knowledge that what is being done is new and under study somehow affects the outcome, either favorably or unfavorably. Chapter 9, p. 181.

Null hypothesis a statistical hypothesis that predicts that there will be no relationship or difference in selected variables in a study. Chapter 5, p. 102.

Operational definition a variable that is defined in specific, concrete terms of measurement. Chapter 8, p. 149.

Outcomes research a type of research that evaluates the impact of healthcare on the health outcomes of patients and populations, including evaluation of economic impacts linked to health outcomes, such as cost effectiveness and cost utility (NLM, 2008). Chapter 1, p. 5.

Parametric Statistics a group of inferential statistical procedures that can be applied to variables that are (1) normally distributed and (2) interval or ratio numbers such as age or intelligence score. Chapter 5, p. 94.

Participant observation a qualitative method where the researcher intentionally imbeds himself or herself into the environment from which data will be collected and becomes a participant. Chapter 8, p. 153.

Peer review the critique of scholarly work by two or more individuals who have at least equivalent knowledge regarding the topic of the work as the author of that work. Chapter 10, p. 207.

Peer reviewed an article or journal that has been evaluated by other professionals in the same field, adding strength to the validity of the research findings. Chapter 1, p. 20.

Phenomenology a qualitative method used to increase understanding of experiences as perceived by those living the experience; assumes that lived experience can be interpreted or understood by distilling the essence of that experience. Chapter 9, p. 183.

Pilot study a small research study that is implemented for the purpose of developing and demonstrating the effectiveness of selected measures and methods. Chapter 11, p. 230.

Population the entire group of individuals about whom we are interested in gaining knowledge. Chapter 6, p. 110–111.

Power analysis a statistical procedure that allows the researcher to compute the size of a sample needed to detect a real relationship or difference, if it exists. Chapter 6, p. 123.

Practice actions that are planned and implemented exclusively for the enhancement of health and the improvement of the well-being of an individual. Chapter 7, p. 135.

Predictor variables those factors in a study that are expected to affect the dependent variable in a specified manner; predictor variables are also called *independent variables*. Chapter 4, p. 77.

Pretest–posttest a research design that includes an observation both before and after the intervention. Chapter 9, p. 190.

Primary sources use of sources of information as they were originally written or communicated. Chapter 10, p. 206.

Printed indexes written lists of professional articles that are organized and categorized by topic and author, covering the time period from 1956 forward. Chapter 1, p. 18–19.

Probability the percentage of the time that the results found would have happened by chance alone. Chapter 5, p. 93.

Probability sampling strategies to assure that every member of a population has an equal opportunity to be in the study. Chapter 6, p. 118.

Problem section of a research report that describes the gap in knowledge that will be addressed by the research study or a statement of the general gap in knowledge that will be addressed in a study. Chapter 2, p. 39.

Procedures specific actions taken by researchers to gather information about the problem or phenomenon being studied. Chapter 2, p. 37.

Process improvement a management system in which all participants involved strives to improve customer outcomes. Chapter 2, p. 44.

Prospective designs a research design that collects data about events or variables moving forward in time. Chapter 9, p. 187.

Purposive sample inclusion in a study of participants who are intentionally selected because they have certain characteristics that are related to the purpose of the research. Chapter 6, p. 114.

***p* value** a numerical statement of the percentage of the time the results reported would have happened by chance alone. For example, a *p* value of .05 means that in only 5 out of 100 times would one expect to get the results by chance alone. Chapter 2, p. 34.

Qualitative methods approaches to research that focus on understanding the complexity of humans within the context of their lives and tend to focus on building a whole or complete picture of a phenomenon of interest; qualitative methods involve the collection of information as it is expressed naturally by people within the normal context of their lives. Chapter 2, p. 35.

Quality improvement a process of evaluation of healthcare services to see whether they meet specified standards or outcomes of care. Chapter 2, p. 44.

Quality improvement study a study that evaluates whether or not certain expected clinical care was completed. Chapter 2, p. 44.

Quantitative methods approaches to research that focus on understanding and breaking down the different parts of a picture to see how they do or do not connect; quantitative methods involve the collection of information that is very specific and limited to the particular pieces of information being studied. Chapter 2, p. 35.

Quasi-experimental designs a research design that includes manipulation of an independent variable but will lack either a control group or random assignment. Chapter 9, p. 190.

Questionnaire a written measure that is used to collect specific data, usually offering closed or forced choices for answers to the questions. Chapter 8, p. 159.

Quota sampling selection of individuals from the population who have one or more characteristics that are important to the purpose of the study; these characteristics are used to establish limits or quotas on the number of subjects who will be included in the study. Chapter 6, p. 117.

Random assignment the process ensuring that all subjects in a study have an equal chance of being in any particular group within the study. The sample itself may be one of convenience or purposive, so there may be some bias influencing the results. But, since that bias is evenly distributed among the different groups to be studied, it will not unduly affect the outcomes of the study. Chapter 6, p. 121.

Random selection the process of creating a random sample; selection of a subset of the population where all the members of the population are identified, listed, and assigned a number and then some device, such as a random number table or a computer program, is used to select who actually will be in the study. Chapter 6, p. 118.

Reactivity effects threats in external validity that refer to subjects' responses to being studied. Chapter 9, p. 181.

Regression a statistical procedure that measures how much one or more independent variables explain the variation in a dependent variable. Chapter 5, p. 101.

Reliability the consistency with which a measure can be counted on to give the same result if the aspect being measured has not changed. Chapter 8, p. 163.

Repeated measures designs that repeat the same measurements at several points in time. Chapter 9, p. 187.

Replication a study that is an exact duplication of an earlier study; the major purpose of a replication study is confirmation. Chapter 3, p. 58–59.

Research design the overall plan for acquiring new knowledge or confirming existing knowledge; the plan for systematic collection of information in a manner that assures the answer(s) found will be as meaningful and accurate as possible. Chapter 9, p. 175.

Research hypothesis a prediction of the relationships or differences that will be found for selected variables in a study. Chapter 5, p. 97; Chapter 10, p. 208.

Research objectives clear statements of factors that will be measured in order to gain knowledge regarding a research problem; similar to the research purpose, specific aims, or research question. Chapter 10, p. 204–205.

Research problem a gap in existing knowledge that warrants filling and can be addressed through systematic study. Chapter 10, p. 201.

Research process a set of systematic processes that formalize the development of evidence. Chapter 1, p. 16.

Research purpose a clear statement of factors that are going to be studied in order to shed knowledge on the research problem. Chapter 10, p. 204.

Research questions statements in the form of questions that identify the specific factors that will be measured in a study and the types of relationships that will be examined to gain knowledge regarding a research problem; similar to the research objectives, purposes, and specific aims. Chapter 10, p. 208.

Research utilization the use of research in practice. Chapter 1, p. 3.

Response rate the proportion of individuals who actually participate in a study divided by the number who agreed to be in a study but did not end up participating in it. Chapter 6, p. 127.

Results a summary of the actual findings or information collected in a research study. Chapter 2, p. 32.

Retrospective designs quantitative designs that collect data about events or factors going back in time. Chapter 9, p. 187.

Rigor a strict process of data collection and analysis as well as a term that reflects the overall quality of that process in qualitative research; rigor is reflected in the consistency of data analysis and interpretation, the trustworthiness of the data collected, the transferability of the themes, and the credibility of the data. Chapter 8, p. 154.

Risk-to-benefit ratio a comparison of how much risk is present for human subjects compared with the level of benefit to the study. Chapter 7, p. 138.

Sample a subset of the total group of interest in a research study; the individuals in the sample are actually studied to learn about the total group. Chapter 2, p. 31; Chapter 6, p. 36.

Sampling frame the pool of all potential subjects for a study; that is, the pool of all individuals who meet the criteria for the study and, therefore, could be included in the sample. Chapter 6, p. 116.

Sampling unit the element of the population that will be selected for the study; the unit depends on the population of interest and could be individuals, families, communities, or outpatient prenatal care programs. Chapter 6, p. 122.

Saturation a point in qualitative research where all new information collected is redundant of information already collected; *see* Data saturation. Chapter 4, p. 70; Chapter 6, p. 115.

Scale a set of written questions or statements that in combination are intended to measure a specified variable. Chapter 8, p. 159.

Secondary sources someone else's description or interpretation of a primary source. Chapter 10, p. 206.

Selection bias when subjects have unique characteristics that in some manner relate to the dependent variable, raising a question as to whether the findings from the study were due to the independent variable or to the unique characteristics of the sample. Chapter 9, p. 180.

Selectivity the tendency of certain segments of a population agreeing to be in studies. Chapter 6, p. 126.

Semistructured questions questions asked in order to collect data that specifically targets objective factors of interest. Chapter 8, p. 158.

Simple random sampling a sample in which every member of the population has an equal probability of being included; considered the best type of sample because the only factors that should bias the sample will be present by chance alone, making it highly likely that the sample will be similar to the population of interest. An approach for acquiring the population of interest in which the researcher uses a device such as a random number table or computer program to randomly select subjects for a study. Chapter 6, p. 118.

Significance a statistical term indicating a low likelihood that any differences or relationships found in a study happened by chance alone. Chapter 2, p. 34.

Skew a distribution where the middle of the distribution is not in the exact center; the middle or peak of the distribution is to the left or right of center. Chapter 4, p. 82.

Snowball sampling a strategy for recruiting individuals in a study that starts with one participant or member of the population and then uses that member's contacts to identify other potential participants. Chapter 6, p. 114.

Specific aim clear statements of the factors to be measured and the relationships to be examined in a study to gain new knowledge about a research problem; similar to research purpose, objectives, or questions. Chapter 10, p. 204–205.

Speculation a process of reflecting on the results of a study and putting forward some explanation for them. Chapter 3, p. 59.

Standard deviation a statistic that is the square root of the variance; it is computed as the average differences in values for a variable from the mean value; a big standard deviation means that there was a wide range of values for the variable; a small standard deviation means that there was a narrow range of values for the variable. Chapter 4, p. 79.

Stratified random sampling an approach to selecting individuals from the population by dividing the population into two or more groups based on characteristics that are considered important to the purpose of the study and then randomly selecting members within each group. Chapter 6, p. 118.

Structured questions questions that establish what data are wanted ahead of the collection and do not allow the respondent flexibility in how to answer. Chapter 8, p. 158–159.

Study design the overall plan or organization of a study. Chapter 3, p. 63.

Systematic review the product of a process that includes asking clinical questions, doing a structured and organized search for theory-based information and research related to the question, reviewing and synthesizing the results from that search, and reaching conclusions about the implications for practice. Chapter 1, p. 17; Chapter 2, p. 42.

Systematic sampling an approach to the selection of individuals for a study where the members of the population are identified and listed and then members are selected at a fixed interval (such as every fifth or tenth individual) from the list. Chapter 6, p. 119.

Testing a threat to internal validity where there is a change in a dependent variable simply because it is being measured or due to the measure itself. Chapter 9, p. 180.

Test–retest reliability consistency in the results from a test when individuals fill out a questionnaire or scale at two or more time points that are close enough together that we would not expect the "real" answers to have changed. Chapter 8, p. 164.

Themes results in qualitative research that are ideas or concepts that are implicit in the data and are recurrent throughout the data; abstractions that reflect phrases, words, or ideas that appear repeatedly as a researcher analyzes what people have said about a particular experience, feeling, or situation. A theme summarizes and synthesizes discrete ideas or phrases to create a picture out of the words that were collected in the research study. Chapter 2, p. 27; Chapter 4, p. 75.

Theory an abstract explanation describing how different factors or phenomena relate. Chapter 2, p. 39–40.

Theoretical definition a conceptual description of a variable. Chapter 8, p. 149.

Theoretical framework an underlying structure that describes how abstract aspects of a research problem interrelate based on developed theories. Chapter 10, p. 203.

Transferability the extent to which the findings of a qualitative study are confirmed or seem applicable for a different group or in a different setting from where the data were collected. Chapter 8, p. 155.

Triangulation a process of using more than one source of data to include different views, or literally to look at the phenomenon from different angles. Chapter 8, p. 156.

Trustworthiness the honesty of the data collected from or about the participants. Chapter 8, p. 154.

t **test** a statistic that tests for differences in means on a variable between two groups. Chapter 5, p. 95.

Univariate analysis statistical analysis about only one variable. Chapter 4, p. 72–73.

Unstructured interviews questions asked in an informal open fashion without a previously established set of categories or assumed answers, used to gain understanding about a phenomenon or variable of interest. Chapter 8, p. 152.

Validity how accurately a measure actually yields information about the true or real variable being studied. Chapter 8, p. 164.

Variable some aspect of interest that differs among different people or situations; something that varies: it is not the same for everyone in every situation. Chapter 4, p. 72.

Variance the diversity in data for a single variable; a statistic that is the squared deviations of values from the mean value and reflects the distribution of values for the variable. Chapter 4, p. 79.

Visual analog a response scale that consists of a straight line of a specific length that has extremes of responses at either end but does not have any other responses noted at points along the line. Subjects are asked to mark the line to indicate where they fall between the two extreme points. Chapter 8, p. 161.

Withdrawal a right of human subjects to stop participating in a study at any time without penalty until the study is completed. Chapter 7, p. 139.

Index

Note: Page numbers followed by *f* indicate figures; those followed by *t* indicate tables; and those followed by *b* indicate boxed material.

A

Abstracts, 21
    example of, 23
    in journals, 21–22
    research reports, 21–23
Advances in Nursing Science, 4
Agency for Healthcare Research and Quality (AHRQ),
        5–6, 46
Aggregated data, 226
AHRQ (Agency for Healthcare Research and Quality),
        5–6, 46
Alpha coefficient, 164
American Nurses Association (ANA), 135
Anonymity, for research subjects, 136, 136*t*,
        138, 143*t*
ANOVA (analysis of variance) test, 95, 96*t*, 99–100
Arm restraint in children with cleft lip/palate repair,
        292–295
Assent, of research subjects, 143
Assumptions, identification of, 220–221
Attachment Theory, 202
Audit trail, 155
Autonomy, ethical principle, 135

B

Background section, 51*f*–52*f*, 202–205
    errors in, 212–213
    purpose of, 204
Belmont Report, 137
Beneficence, ethical principle, 135
Beta (β) value, 101
Bias
    in sampling, 116, 126, 127*t*, 180, 180*b*
    selection, 180, 180*b*
Bivariate analysis, 73
Bivariate correlation, 97–99
Bivariate tests, 95–102, 96*t*
Body mass index (BMI), 33
Body satisfaction in overweight adolescents, 237–240
Body Shape Satisfaction Scale, 33
Breast reconstruction and mastectomy, quality-of-life
        of, 316–324
Bridge theory, 5, 6*f*

British Medical Journal, 4
Brown University, 6
Brunel Universal Mood States (BRUMS)
        questionnaire, 288

C

Caring Climate Scale (CCS), 252
Categorization scheme, 74–75
Cementless total hip arthroplasty (THA), leg length
        discrepancy (LLD) in, 255–259
Center for Epidemiological Studies Depression Scale
        for Children, 33
Center for Evidence-based Medicine, 6
Central tendency, measure of, 77, 82–83, 83*f*
Cleft lip/palate, use of elbow restraints
        after repair of, 292–295
Clinical trials, 195
Cluster analysis, 102
Cluster sample, 119, 120*t*, 122*t*
Codebook, 224, 225
Coding reduction, 74–75
Coefficient, correlation, 97–99, 98*f*
Coercion, 139
Comparison group(s), 188
Computer software
    database, 18*t*–19*t*, 20–21
    data collection, 155, 225
Conceptual framework, for research problem,
        203–205
Conceptualization, 60
Conclusions, 30–32, 30*t*, 58*t*, 62–65, 170–171.
        See also Discussions; Results
    data collection and, 170–171
    descriptive results and, 84
    disagreement in, 64
    errors in, 65
    examples of, 65
    incomplete, 65
    inferential results and, 103–105
    insufficiently supported, 65
    irrelevant, 65
    limitations of, 62–63
    in meta-analysis, 42, 43*t*

methods in, 63
overinterpretation of, 65
practice implications of, 50–51, 64
in research reports, 30–32, 30*t*, 58*t*, 62–65
sampling and, 128–129
statistical significance and, 104–105
in systematic reviews, 42, 43*t*, 64–65
Concurrent validity, 166
Confidence intervals (CIs), 93–94, 94*t*
Confidentiality, of research subjects, 136,
136*t*, 138, 143*t*
Confirmability, 154–155, 156*t*
Confirmation, 58, 58*t*
Consent form, 140, 140*b*–141*b*, 141–142.
See also Informed consent
five rights of research subjects and,
136–140, 136*t*
Construct validity, 166, 167*t*
Content analysis, 74, 75, 76*f*
Content validity, 165, 167*t*
Continuous Quality Improvement (CQI), 46
Continuum, for data analysis, 91*f*
Control factors, in research design, 177, 177*f*, 182*f*,
186*f*, 187–188
Control group, 188, 189
Convenience sample, 114, 116, 120*t*, 121*t*
Correlation, 98*f*
bivariate, 97–99
coefficient, 97–99, 98*f*
designs, 188–189, 189*f*, 191*t*, 192
Pearson product–moment, 99
Correlational studies, 188–189
Covariance, 97–99, 98*f*
CQI (Continuous Quality Improvement), 46
Credibility, 156, 156*t*
Criteria for participation, 112, 139
Criterion-related validity, 165–166, 167*t*
Cronbach alpha coefficient, 164
Cross-sectional study, 187
Curve
normal, 80, 81*f*, 83*f*
skewed, 81*f*, 82, 83*f*

D

Data, 32, 72
aggregated, 226
coding, 74–75
confirmability of, 154–155, 156*t*
credibility of, 156, 156*t*
demographic, 84
diversity, 73–83
saturation of, 115
transferability of, 155–156, 156*t*
trustworthiness of, 154, 156*t*
Data analysis, 32, 34, 72–73, 224
bivariate, 73
content, 74, 75, 76*f*
continuum for, 91*f*
documentation of, 224
multivariate, 34, 72
in qualitative studies, 73–76, 75*f*

in quantitative studies, 76–83. *See also* Statistical
concepts
in research process, 47*f*, 48–49, 224–225
in research report, 39
rigor in, 154–156, 156*t*
univariate, 72–73, 83
Databases, electronic, 18*t*–19*t*, 20–21
Data collection, 72
conclusion and, 170–171
confirmability and, 154–155, 156*t*
credibility and, 156, 156*t*
documents and records in, 154
errors in, 154–156, 156*t*, 162–169, 167*t*
in implementation, 167–168
in qualitative research, 154–156, 156*t*
in quantitative research, 162–168, 167*t*
in reports, 168–169
examples of, 149, 170–171
field notes in, 152
free write in, 153
group interviews in, 153
instruments in, 158, 160*b*
journals in, 153
from medical records, 166
participant observation in, 153
physiologic measurements in, 157
in qualitative research, 152–156, 156*t*, 169
for quality improvement studies, 46
in quantitative research, 157–168, 167*t*
questionnaires in, 48, 159, 160*b*, 167–168
reliability in, 163–164, 167*t*
results and, 170–171
rigor in, 154–156, 156*t*
sampling and, 170–171
scales in, 159, 160*b*
software for, 155, 225
systematic observation in, 158
transferability and, 155–156, 156*t*
triangulation in, 156
trustworthiness and, 154, 156*t*
unstructured interviews in, 152
validity in, 164–167, 167*t*
Data entry, 224–225
Data reduction, 74–75
Data saturation, 75
Deductive knowledge, 202
Deming Cycle, steps in, 45–46
Demographic data, 84
Dependent variables, 73*t*, 76–77, 149
Descriptive design, 183, 188–189, 191*t*, 192
Descriptive results, 33, 70–86. *See also* Results
conclusions and, 84
confusing presentation of, 85
errors in reports, 84–85
incomplete, 84–85
vs. inferential results, 70–72, 91–92
in qualitative studies, 73–76
in quantitative studies, 76–83. *See also* Statistical
concepts
Descriptive statistics, 70–86
Dignity, of research subjects, 136*t*, 139–140, 143*t*
Directional hypothesis, 209

Discussions, 57–62, 58*t*. *See also* Conclusions
    comparison in, 58–59, 58*t*
    conclusion in, 57, 58*t*
    confirmation in, 58, 58*t*
    data collection and, 170–171
    examples of, 66
    incomplete, 65
    practice implications of, 61–62
    speculation in, 59–61
    summary in, 58, 58*t*
Dissemination, of research findings, 49, 225–227
Distribution, 80
    normal curve, 80, 81*f*, 83*f*
    of parametric/nonparametric statistics, 92–93,
        93*f*, 94–95
Documentation
    of data analysis, 224
    of observation, 223–224
    in research process, 224–225
Documents, 154
Duke Evidence-based Practice Center, 6

E

EBP (evidence-based practice), 3, 231
    approaches used in, 9–11
    critical reading results sections of research reports
        for use in, 85–86, 85*b*
    essential elements of, 10*f*, 10*t*
    healthcare research and, 4–5
    research synthesis study for, 195–196
    systematic reviews in, 23–25, 42–46, 43*t*,
        64–65, 191*t*
Effect(s)
    experimenter, 181
    Hawthorne, 181
    measurement, 181
    novelty, 181
    reactivity, 181
Electronic databases, 18*t*–19*t*, 20–21
Error(s)
    in conclusions, 65
    in data collection
        in implementation, 167–168
        in qualitative research, 154–156, 156*t*
        in quantitative research, 162–168, 167*t*
        in reports, 167–168
    in literature review, 212–213
    in measurement, 150
    in research reports
        in background section, 212–213
        in data collection section, 168–169
        in literature review section, 212–213
    translation, 168
    in variables, 150–151
Ethical issues, 133–145
    common errors in sampling for, 144
    five rights of research subjects and,
        136–140, 136*t*
    informed consent, 135–143, 136*t*
    IRB and, 136–140
    risk–benefit ratio, 138
Ethical principles, 135

Ethnographic method, 183*t*, 184, 191*t*
Ethnonursing, 183
Evidence-based bridge theory, 5, 6*f*
Evidence-based centers, 6
Evidence-based information (EBI), 5, 193
Evidence-based medicine (EBM) literature searching
        skills, teaching and reinforcing
    during preclinical and clinical years, 261–269
Evidence-based models, 5–8
Evidence-based nursing practice, 106–107,
    129–131
Evidence-based practice (EBP), 3, 231
    approaches used in, 9–11
    critical reading results sections of research reports
        for use in, 85–86, 85*b*
    essential elements of, 10*f*, 10*t*
    healthcare research and, 4–5
    research synthesis study for, 195–196
    systematic reviews in, 23–25, 42–46, 43*t*,
        64–65, 191*t*
Evidence for healthcare practice, 42–46
Exemption, research, 143–144
Experimental design, 189–191, 189*b*, 191*t*
Experimenter effects, 181
External checks, 155
External validity, 178–179, 178*f*, 179*t*
    generalizability and, 178
    threats to, 179*t*, 180–182

F

Face validity, 165
Factor analysis, 101–102
Fair treatment, of research subjects, 136*t*, 138, 143*t*
Field notes, 152
Financial support, for research, 229
Fisher exact test, 97
Five rights of research subjects, 136–140,
        136*t*, 143*t*
    informed consent and, 135–143, 136*t*, 143*t*
Foreign languages, translation errors and, 168
"*F* ratio" value, 100
Free write, 153
Frequency distribution, 80, 81*f*
Friedman test, 97, 100
Funding, research, 229

G

Generalizability, 122
    external validity, 178
Generalization, 61
Glasgow Coma Scale score, 98, 99, 105
Grounded theory, 183*t*, 184–185
Group interviews, 153

H

Harvard Medical Journal, 4
Hawthorne effect, 181
HCI (Health Care Improvement) project, 45
Healthcare decision making process *vs.* research
        process, 230–231, 231*t*
Health Care Improvement (HCI) project, 45

Healthcare research
  healthcare profession's role in, 3–4
  history of, 4–5
  systematic, 16, 23–25
Histogram, 77, 78f, 81f
Historical method, 183t, 185–186
History, 180
Hypothesis, 40
  defined, 102
  directional, 209
  nondirectional, 209
  null, 102, 209–210
  research, 102, 208, 209–210
  testing, 102–103

I

Independent (predictor) variables, 73t, 77, 149
  manipulation of, 189, 190
Indexes, printed, 18–20, 18t–19t
Inductive knowledge, 202
Inferential results, 70–72, 90–107. See also Results
  common errors in, 105–106
  conclusions and, 103–105
  confusing presentation of, 105
  vs. descriptive results, 70–72, 91–92
  example of, 91, 105
  for in-class study data, 103
  incomplete, 105
  purpose of, 90–92
Inferential statistics, 70–72, 90–107
Informants, in qualitative studies, 114. See also
    Sample/sampling
Informed consent, 135–143. See also Subject(s)
  vs. assent, 143
  definition of, 137
  ethical issues, 133–145, 136t
  five rights and, 136–140, 136t, 143t
  form for, 140, 140b–141b, 141–142
  participants, 135–143
Institutional Review Board (IRB), 134,
    136–140, 221, 223
Instrumentation, internal validity and, 179t, 180
Instruments. See also Measures; Scale(s)
  data collection, 158, 160b
  external factors affecting, 168
  reliability of, 163–164
  validity of, 164–167
Interlibrary loan, 21
Internal consistency reliability, 164, 167t
Internal validity, 178–180
  history and, 180, 180b
  testing and, 180, 180b
  threats to, 179–180, 180b
International Council of Nurses (ICN), 135
Internet, 18t–19t, 20
Interrater reliability, 163, 167t
Interviews
  group, 153
  transcription of, 224–225
  unstructured, 152
Introduction
  in meta-analysis, 42, 43t

  in research report, 28, 30t, 39, 43t, 48, 202–205,
    211–212
    errors in, 212–213
  in systematic review, 43t, 44
Intuition, 9, 15
Iowa model, of evidence-based practice, 6, 7f
Items, on scale, 159, 160, 160b

J

Joanna Briggs Institute model, of evidence-based
    practice, 6, 9f
Johns Hopkins University, 6
Journal of Medical Internet Research, 4
Journal of Nursing Scholarship, The, 21
Journals. See also Research reports
  abstracts in, 21–22
  for data collection, 153
  online, 21
  peer-reviewed, 207
  refereed, 207
  for research reports, 228
  research summaries in, 17, 22–23
Justice, ethical principle, 135

K

Keywords, 20
Knowledge, 17
  deductive, 202
  inductive, 202
Knowledge gaps, identification of, 47f, 48
Kruskal–Wallis one-way analysis of variance
    test, 95, 96t

L

Lancet Medical Journal, 4
Language, 29–30, 30t, 50
  foreign, translation errors and, 168
  of qualitative studies, 73–76, 74b
  of quantitative studies, 76–83
  of research design, 191
  of sampling, 113, 124t
Lazarus's theory of stress and coping, 40, 40f, 189, 189f
Lean Six Sigma process improvement model, 45
Leg length discrepancy (LLD), in cementless total hip
    arthroplasty (THA), 255–259
Likert-type response scale, 160b, 161, 161f
Limitations, 32, 62–63
  of conclusions, 62–63
  failure to include, 65
  measures as, 63
  practice implications of, 64
  of research reports, 32, 62–63
  of research studies, 32
  sample as, 62
  study design as, 63
Literature review, 39, 205–211. See also Journals
  as critique, 210
  current studies in, 206
  definition of, 205
  errors in, 212–213
  examples of, 212

Literature review *(continued)*
    peer-reviewed journals in, 207
    primary sources in, 206
    purposes of, 206, 206*b*
    research design and, 210–211
    research problem and, 202, 204–205
    in research process, 47, 47*f*
    secondary sources in, 206, 213
    as synthesis, 210
Logistic regression, 35
Longitudinal study, 187, 188

M
Manipulation, 189, 190
Mann–Whitney test, 97
MANOVA test, 96*t*, 100
Matched sample, 117
Maturation, internal validity and, 180, 180*b*
McNemar test, 97
Mean, 82, 91
    t distribution of, 92–93, 93*f*
Measurement effects, 181
Measures, 38. *See also* Instruments; Scale(s)
    of central tendency, 82–83, 83*f*
    as limitations, 63
    reliability of, 163–164
    repeated, 187, 190, 191*f*
    validity of, 164–167
Median, 82
    test, 97
Medical records, data collection from, 166
Member checks, 156
Member(s). *See also* Subject(s)
    five rights of, 136–140, 136*t*
    informed consent of, 135–143
    in qualitative studies, 114. *See also*
        Sample/sampling
Meta-analysis, 42–46, 43*t*
    introduction in, 42, 43*t*
    problem in, 42, 43*t*
    results sections of, 43*t*, 44
Metasynthesis, 37, 37*t*, 39, 42–46
Methods, 149
    as limitation, 63
    in meta-analysis, 42, 43*t*
    qualitative, 35–36, 36*f*
    quantitative, 35–36, 36*f*
    in research report, 30*t*, 35–39, 36*f*, 48
    in systematic review, 43*t*, 44
Mild traumatic brain injury (mTBI), predictors of PCS
        at 3 months in individuals with, 271–282
Minnesota Evidence-based Practice Center, 6
Mixed method designs, 193
Mode, 82
Model testing design, 189, 189*f*, 191*t*
Mood and self-esteem in individuals with clinical
        mental health diagnosis, effect of single bout
        of exercise on, 286–290
Mortality, internal validity and, 180, 180*b*
Multifactorial design, 190
Multiple analysis of variance (MANOVA)
        test, 96*t*, 100

Multivariate analysis, 34, 72
Multivariate statistical concepts, 34
Multivariate studies, 34
Multivariate tests, 95–102, 96*t*

N
National Institute of Nursing Research, 4
National Institutes of Health, 3, 4
New England Journal of Medicine, 4
Nondirectional hypothesis, 209
Nonequivalent control group pretest–posttest
        quasi-experimental design, 190
Nonparametric statistics, 94–95
Nonprobability sampling, 116–117, 123
Nonresearch-based evidence, 15*f*, 16
Normal curve, 80, 81*f*, 83*f*
Novelty effects, 181
Null hypothesis, 102, 209–210
Nurse, intuition of, 9
Nursing practice
    evidence-based. *See* Evidence-based
        practice (EBP)
    nursing research and, 200–202, 201*f*
    nursing theory and, 200–202, 201*f*
    research problems in, 200–202, 201*f*
    students' choices of field of, 339–343, 344–345
Nursing process *vs.* research process, 40–46, 41*t*
Nursing research. *See also* Research
    funding for, 229
    nursing practice and, 200–202, 201*f*
    nursing theory and, 200–202, 201*f*
    systematic, 42–46, 43*t*
Nursing Research, 4
Nursing theory
    nursing practice and, 200–202, 201*f*
    nursing research and, 200–202, 201*f*
    research problems in, 200–202, 201*f*
Nutrition Research, 4

O
Observation(s), 157, 158, 202
    documentation of, 223–224
    participant, 153
Occupational Therapy Journal of Research, 4
Office for Human Research Protections (OHRP),
        144, 145*f*
One-way analysis of variance test, 95, 96*t*, 100
Online journals, 21
Open-ended question, 153
Operational definition, of variable, 149
Ottawa model, of evidence-based practice, 6, 8*f*
Outcomes research, 5
Overweight or obese students' perceptions of caring
        in urban physical education programs, 242–252

P
Parametric statistics, 94–95
Participant(s). *See also* Subject(s)
    five rights of, 136–140, 136*t*
    informed consent of, 135–143
    observation, 153

in qualitative studies, 114. *See also* Sample/
  sampling
Patient care questions, 8–9
  sources of answers to, 8–22
PDCA model. *See* Deming Cycle
Pearson product–moment correlation, 99
Peer review, 20, 207
People living with HIV/acquired immunodeficiency
    syndrome (PLWH)
  reasons for, excluding individuals from their
    chosen families, 327–337
Phenomenologic method, 183–184, 183*t*, 191*t*
Physiologic measurements, 157
PICO/PICOT method, 13, 14*b*, 56*t*, 70*t*, 268
Pilot study, defined, 230
Populations. *See also* Sample/sampling; Subject(s)
  common characteristics of, 110–111
  criteria for participation, 112, 139
  definition of, 110
  identification of, 111–112
  sample *vs.*, 110–113
Postconcussion syndrome (PCS), 272
Power analysis, defined, 123
Practice, defined, 135
Practice implications
  of conclusions, 50–51, 64
  of limitations, 64
  of research discussions, 61–62
  of systematic reviews, 64
Predictive validity, 166
Predictor (independent) variables, 73*t*, 77, 149
Pretest–posttest experimental design, 190, 190*f*
Primary sources, 17, 18, 18*t*–19*t*
  in literature review, 206
Printed indexes, 18–19, 18*t*–19*t*
Privacy, of research subjects, 136, 136*t*,
    139–140, 143*t*
Probability, 92–94
  sampling, 118–120
Problem(s)
  in meta-analysis, 42, 43*t*
  in research report, 28, 30*t*, 39–40, 43*t*, 48, 202–205,
    212–213
  in systematic review, 43*t*, 44
  with tables, 85
Procedures, 37–39
  qualitative, 38
  quantitative, 38
  in research reports, 37–39
Process improvement, 45
Prospective designs, 186–187
Psychological morbidity three months after intensive
    care, investigating risk factors for, 297–313
Purposive samples/sampling, 114, 117, 120*t*, 121*t*, 184,
    188, 189
p value, 34, 93, 94, 94*t*, 97

Q

Qualitative research
  data analysis, 73–76, 75*f*
  data collection errors in, 152–156, 156*t*, 169
  descriptive results in, 73–76

ethnographic, 183*t*, 184
goals of, 35, 38, 60–61
grounded theory method in, 183*t*, 184–185
historical, 183*t*, 185–186
informants in, 114
members, 114
participants, 114
phenomenologic, 183–184, 183*t*
purpose of, 73
vs. quantitative research, 36, 36*f*
rigor in, 154–156, 156*t*
sample size in, 115
sampling in, 113–116, 120*t*, 121*t*–122*t*,
    123–124, 124*t*
strengths and weaknesses of, 115
studies, 35, 37
study design in, 182–186, 182*f*, 183*t*
terminology for, 73–76, 74*b*
variables in, 73, 149–151
volunteers in, 114
Quality improvement studies, 43*t*, 44, 46
Quantitative research
  data analysis, 76–83
  data collection errors in, 157–168, 167*t*
  descriptive results in, 76–83
  goals of, 60–61, 123–124
  inferential results in, 90–107
  methods in, 38
  purpose of, 73
  vs. qualitative research, 36, 36*f*
  sample size in, 122–123
  sampling in, 113, 116–123, 120*t*, 121*t*–122*t*,
    123–124, 124*t*
  strengths and weaknesses of, 120–122
  studies, 35, 37
  study design in, 186–191, 186*f*
  terminology for, 76–83
  variables in, 73, 149–151, 157–162
Quasi-experimental design, 189–191, 190–191,
    191*f*, 191*t*
Questionnaires, 159, 160*b*, 167–168
  Brunel Universal Mood States (BRUMS), 288
  in data collection, 48, 159, 160*b*, 167–168
  open-ended question, 153
Questions
  designing clinical questions, 14*b*
  open-ended, 153
  patient care, 8–9
  research, 8–22, 176–178, 176*b*, 208
  semistructured, 158, 160*b*
  structured, 158–159
Quota sample, 117, 120*t*, 122*t*

R

Random assignment, 121
  in experimental study, 190
Random number table, 118, 118*f*, 119*b*
Random sampling, 118, 120*t*
  simple, 118, 118*f*, 120*t*, 121*t*–122*t*
  stratified, 118, 120*t*, 121*t*–122*t*
Reactivity effects, 181
Records, as data source, 154, 166

Refereed journals, 207
Regression analysis, 101
Reliability, 163–164, 167t
  definition of, 163
  internal consistency, 164, 167t
  interrater, 163, 167t
  of scales, 163–164
  test–retest, 164, 167t
  validity and, 166
Repeated measures, 187, 190, 191f
Replication study, 58–59
Research. *See also* Healthcare research
  abstracts, 21–22
  vs. healthcare decision making processes,
    230–231, 231t
  exemption, 143–144
Research articles
  body satisfaction and psychological functioning
    and weight-related cognitions and behaviors
    in overweight adolescents, 237–240
  effect of single bout of exercise on mood and
    self-esteem in individuals with clinical
    mental health diagnosis, 286–290
  investigating risk factors for psychological
    morbidity three months after intensive care,
    297–313
  leg length discrepancy (LLD), in cementless total
    hip arthroplasty (THA), 255–259
  mild traumatic brain injury (mTBI), predictors of
    PCS at 3 months in individuals with, 271–282
  overweight students' perceptions of caring in PE,
    242–252
  people living with HIV/acquired
    immunodeficiency syndrome (PLWH)
    reasons for, excluding individuals from their
     chosen families, 327–337
  quality-of-life outcomes between mastectomy alone
    and breast reconstruction, 316–324
  teaching and reinforcing evidence-based medicine
    (EBM) literature searching skills, during
    clinical years, 261–269
  use of postoperative restraints in children with cleft
    lip/palate repair, 292–295
Research-based evidence, 11, 15f
Research design, 63, 174–196. *See also* Research
    studies
  control factors in, 177, 177f, 182f, 186f, 187–188
  correlational, 188–189, 189f, 191t, 192
  cross-sectional, 187
  definition of, 175
  descriptive, 183, 188–189, 191t
  errors in reporting of, 194
  ethnographic, 183t, 184, 191t
  examples of, 191t, 196
  experimental, 189–191, 189b, 191t
  fit of, 176–178, 192–194
  functions of, 176, 177f, 182, 182f, 186f, 188–191
  goals of, 175–182
  grounded theory, 183t, 184–185
  historical, 183t, 185–186
  literature review and, 210–211
  longitudinal, 187, 188

mixed method, 193
model testing, 189, 189f, 191t
multifactorial, 190
phenomenologic, 183–184, 183t, 191t
prospective, 186–187, 191t
qualitative, 182–186, 182f, 183t
quantitative, 186–191, 186f
quasi-experimental, 189–191, 190–191,
  191f, 191t
questions, 176–178
of research reports, 195
retrospective, 186, 191t
rigor and, 178–179
selection of, 194
systematic review, 16, 23–25, 41t, 42–46,
  64–65, 191t
time factors in, 177, 177f, 186–187, 186f
validity and, 178–182, 178f
Research findings. *See also* Conclusions; Results
  dissemination of, 49, 50, 225–227
  implementation of, 47f, 49–50, 223–224, 229–230
Research hypothesis, 102, 208, 209–210
Research in Nursing & Health, 4
Research literacy, 5
Research objective, 204
Research plan, development of, 46–49, 47f,
  221–223, 223b
Research problem
  conceptual framework for, 203–205
  context for, 202
  definition of, 201
  development of, 202
  example of, 201
  literature review and, 202, 204–205
  practice-based, 200–202, 201f
  refinement of, 203–205, 221–222
  sources of, 200–202
  statement of, 202–205
  theoretical framework for, 203–205
  theory-based, 200–202, 201f
Research process, 16, 217–233
  assumption identification in, 220–221
  characteristics of, 227b
  data analysis in, 47f, 49, 224–225
  disseminating findings in, 49, 50, 225–229
  documentation of, 224–225
  enjoyment of, 230–231
  factors affecting, 229–230
  vs. healthcare decision making process,
    230–231, 231t
  implementation stage of, 47f, 49–50, 223–224,
    229–230
  interpreting results in, 224–225
  knowledge foundation for, 220
  knowledge gap identification in, 47f, 48, 219–221
  literature review in, 47, 47f
  nursing process, 40–46, 41t
  planning stage of, 48–49, 221–223, 223b
  refining research problem in, 221–222
  research purpose identification in, 220–221
  research reports and, 46–51, 227–229, 227f
  steps in, 47–49, 47f

Research purpose, 204, 208. *See also* Research
  questions
  identification of, 220–221
Research questions, 8–22, 176–178, 176*b*, 208
  directional, 208
  nondirectional, 208
  study design and, 176–178
  types of, 176*b*
Research reports, 225–227. *See also* Journals
  abstracts, 21–22
  accessing, 18–21, 18*t*–19*t*
  background section in, 51*f*–52*f*, 202–205
  comparison in, 58–59, 58*t*
  components of, 30–40, 30*t*
  conclusions in, 30–32, 30*t*, 57, 58*t*, 62–65
  critical reading results sections of, 85–86, 85*b*
  data analysis, 39
  data collection section of, 169–170
  errors in
    background section, 212–213
    data collection section, 168–169
    literature review section, 212–213
  evaluation of, 232
  finding, 17–18
  introduction in, 28, 30*t*, 39, 43*t*, 48, 202–205,
    211–212
  language and style of, 30*t*, 50
  levels of development in, 208, 208*f*
  limitations in, 32, 61, 62–63. *See also* Limitations
  literature review in, 39, 205–211
  methods in, 30*t*, 35–39, 36*f*, 48, 63
  vs. nonresearch reports, 17
  overinterpretation in, 65
  problem in, 28, 30*t*, 39–40, 43*t*, 48, 202–205,
    212–213
  procedures in, 37–39
  research design section of, 195
  research process and, 46–51, 227–229, 227*f. See
    also* Research process
  results section, 30*t*, 32–35, 33*b*
  sample in, 36–37, 62, 128
  sources of, 18–21, 18*t*–19*t*
  systematic analysis, 42–46
Research studies
  comparison group in, 188
  control group in, 188, 189
  correlational, 188–189, 189*f*, 191*t*, 192
  cross-sectional, 187
  descriptive, 183, 188–189, 191*t*
  design of. *See* Research design
  ethnographic, 183*t*, 184, 191*t*
  grounded theory, 183*t*, 184–185
  historical, 183*t*, 185–186
  limitations in, 32, 62–63
  longitudinal, 187, 188
  multivariate, 34
  phenomenologic, 183–184, 183*t*, 191*t*
  prospective, 186–187, 191*t*
  qualitative, 35, 37. *See also* Qualitative research
  quality improvement, 43*t*, 44, 46
  quantitative, 35, 37. *See also* Quantitative research
  results of, 30*t*, 32–35, 33*b*

retrospective, 186, 191*t*
  synthesis, 195–196
Research summaries, 22–23
Research synthesis studies, 195–196
Research utilization, 3
Respiratory Research, 4
Response rate, in sampling, 127, 127*t*
Results
  conclusions and, 30–32, 30*t*, 33*b*, 84, 103–105.
    See also Conclusions
  credibility of, 156, 156*t*
  data collection and, 170–171
  descriptive, 33, 70–86. *See also* Descriptive results
  differing interpretations, 64
  discussions of, 57–62, 58*t*, 64
  generalizability of, 61, 122, 155
  inferential, 90–107. *See also* Inferential results
  interpretation of, 225
  in meta-analysis, 43*t*, 44
  overinterpretation in, 65
  in research reports, 30*t*, 32–35, 33*b*
  of research studies, 30*t*, 32–35, 33*b*
  sampling and, 128–129
  in systematic review, 43*t*, 44
  terminology of, 72–83
  transferability of, 155–156, 156*t*
Retrospective designs, 186, 191*t*
Rich samples, 113
Rigor, 154–156, 156*t*
  research design and, 178–179
Risk–benefit ratio, 138
Rosenberg Self Esteem scale, 288

S
Sample/sampling, 36–37, 110–131. *See also* Subject(s)
  bias, 116, 126, 127*t*, 180, 180*b*
  cluster, 119, 120*t*, 122*t*
  conclusions and, 128–129
  control in, 187–188
  convenience, 114, 120*t*, 121*t*
  data collection and, 170–171
  errors in reporting of, 128
  five rights and, 136–140, 136*t*
  goals of, 124*t*, 139
  informed consent of, 135–143
  language of, 113, 124*t*
  as limitation, 62
  matched, 117
  nonprobability, 116–117, 123
  vs. populations, 110–113
  probability, 118–120
  problems with, 124–127, 126*t*, 127*t*
  purposive, 114, 120*t*, 121*t*, 184, 188, 189
  in qualitative research, 113–116, 120*t*, 121*t*–122*t*,
    123–124, 124*t*
  in quantitative research, 113, 116–123, 120*t*,
    121*t*–122*t*, 123–124, 124*t*
  quota, 117, 120*t*, 122*t*
  in research reports, 36–37, 128
  response rate and, 127, 127*t*
  results and, 128–129
  sampling unit in, 122

Sample/sampling *(continued)*
  selectivity in, 126
  simple random, 118, 118*f*, 120*t*, 122*t*
  size of, 115, 122–123
  snowball, 114, 120*t*, 121*t*
  stratified random, 118, 120*t*, 122*t*
  systematic, 119, 120*t*, 122*t*
  terminology for, 113–114
Sampling frame, 116
Sampling unit, 122
Saturation, 115
Scale(s)
  external factors affecting, 168
  Likert-type response, 160*b*, 161, 161*f*
  reliability of, 163–164, 167*t*
  validity of, 164–167
  visual analog, 161, 162*f*
Scatter plot, 98*f*
SCID (Structured Clinical Interview for Axis I
    DSM-IV Disorders) scale, 150, 158
Search engines, 20
Secondary sources in literature review, 206, 213
Selection bias, 180, 180*b*
Selectivity, in sampling, 126
Self-determination, for research subjects,
    136*t*, 139, 143*t*
Semistructured questions, 158, 160*b*
Significance, 34, 92–94
Sign test, 97
Simple random sample, 118, 118*f*, 120*t*, 122*t*
Skewed curve, 81*f*, 82, 83*f*
Snowball sampling, 114, 120*t*, 121*t*
Software
    database, 18*t*–19*t*, 20–21
    data collection, 155, 225
Specific aim, 204, 208
Speculation, 59–61
Standard deviation, 79–80, 91
Statement of purpose, 204
Statistical concepts
    alpha coefficient, 164
    beta (β) value, 101
    central tendency, 77, 78*t*, 82–83
    correlation, 97–99, 98*f*
    covariance, 97–99, 98*f*
    distribution, 80
    factor, 102
    frequency distribution, 80, 81*f*
    logistic regression, 35
    mean, 82, 91
    median, 82
    mode, 82
    multivariate, 34
    normal curve, 80, 81*f*, 83*f*
    null hypothesis, 102
    p value, 34
    regression, 101
    significance, 34, 92–94
    skew, 81*f*, 82, 83*f*
    standard deviation, 79–80, 91
    variance, 77–79, 78*t*
Statistical significance, 34, 93, 94

conclusions, 103–105
Statistical tests. *See* Test(s)
Statistics, 33
    descriptive, 34, 70–86. *See also* Descriptive results
    inferential, 70–72, 90–107. *See also* Inferential
        results
    nonparametric, 94–95
    parametric, 94–95
    significant, 34, 92–94
Stratified random sample, 118, 120*t*, 122*t*
Structured Clinical Interview for Axis I DSM-IV
        Disorders (SCID) scale, 150, 158
Structured question, 158–159
Study design, 63
Study populations. *See* Populations
Subjective judgment, 9–10, 15
Subject(s). *See also* Sample/sampling
    anonymity rights of, 136, 136*t*, 138, 143*t*
    assent of, 143
    coercion of, 139
    confidentiality rights, 136, 136*t*, 138, 143*t*
    criteria for participation for, 112
    dignity rights of, 136*t*, 139–140, 143*t*
    fair treatment of, 136*t*, 138, 143*t*
    five rights of, 136–140, 136*t*
    informed consent of, 135–143
    privacy rights of, 136, 136*t*, 139–140, 143*t*
    protection from discomfort and harm for, 136*t*,
        140*b*–141*b*, 143*t*
    recruitment of, 138
    self-determination rights of, 136*t*, 139, 143*t*
    withdrawal of, 139
Synthesis research studies, 195–196
Systematic observation, 158
Systematic reviews, 16, 23–25, 64–65, 191*t*
    conclusions in, 42, 43*t*
    introduction in, 43*t*, 44
    methods in, 43*t*, 44
    problem in, 43*t*, 44
    results in, 43*t*, 44
Systematic sample, 119, 120*t*, 122*t*

T
Tables
    descriptive results in, 84–85
    problem with, 85
    random number, 118, 118*f*, 119*b*
t distribution, 92–93, 93*f*
Terminology
    examples of, 28
    for qualitative studies, 73–76, 74*b*
    for quantitative studies, 76–83. *See also* Statistical
        concepts
    of research reports, 29, 30*t*, 42
    of results, 72–83
    for sampling, 113, 114
Testing, internal validity and, 180, 180*b*
Test–retest reliability, 164, 167*t*
Test(s)
    ANOVA, 95, 96*t*, 99–100
    bivariate, 95–102, 96*t*
    multivariate, 95–102, 96*t*

for structure/components of, 101–102
    t, 92–93, 95, 96*t*, 99, 103
The Joint Commission (TJC), 45
Themes, 32–33, 75
Theoretical definition, of variable, 149, 152
Theoretical framework, for research problem, 203–205
Theory, 40
    definition of, 201
    Lazarus's theory of stress and coping, 40, 40*f*
    practice and, 200–202, 201*f*
Time factors, in research designs, 177, 177*f*,
        186–187, 186*f*
TJC (The Joint Commission), 45
Total Quality Management (TQM), 45
Transcription, of interview, 224–225
Transferability, 155–156, 156*t*
Translation, errors in, 168
Triangulation, 156
Trustworthiness, 154, 156*t*
t test, 92–93, 95, 96*t*, 99, 103

U

Univariate analysis, descriptive, 72–73, 83
Unstructured interview, 152

V

Validity, 164–167, 167*t*
    concurrent, 166, 167*t*
    construct, 166, 167*t*
    content, 165, 167*t*
    criterion-related, 165–166, 167*t*
    external, 178–179, 178*f*, 179*t*
        threats to, 179*t*, 180–182
    face, 165

internal, 178–180, 178*f*, 179*t*
    threats to, 179–180, 180*b*
predictive, 166
reliability and, 166
research design and, 178–182, 178*f*
Variables
    in bivariate analysis, 73
    definition, 72
        operational, 149
        theoretical, 149, 152
    dependent, 73*t*, 76–77
    error in, 150–151
    identification of, 149–151
    independent (predictor), 73*t*, 77, 149, 190
    positive and negative relationship,
        209–210, 209*f*
    in qualitative research, 73, 149–151
    in quantitative research, 73, 149–151, 157–162
    in research purpose, 204, 208
    in univariate analysis, 72–73
Variance, 77–79, 78*t*
Visual analog scales, 161, 162*f*
Volunteers. *See also* Subject(s)
    five rights of, 136–140, 136*t*
    informed consent of, 135–143
    in qualitative studies, 114. *See also* Sample/
        sampling
Vulnerable populations, 138

W

Web sites, 12, 18*t*–19*t*
Western Journal of Nursing Research, 4
Wilcoxon signed-ranks test, 97
Withdrawal from study, 139